Critical Di

D

A

Critical Diagnostic Thinking
IN
Respiratory Care

A CASE-BASED APPROACH

JAMES K. STOLLER, MD
Vice Chairman, Division of Medicine
Head, Section of Respiratory Therapy
Professor of Medicine
Department of Pulmonary and Critical Care Medicine
The Cleveland Clinic Foundation
Cleveland, Ohio

ERIC D. BAKOW, MA, MPM, RRT
Process Improvement Specialist
Institute for Performance Improvement
University of Pittsburgh Medical Center
Pittsburgh, Pennsylvania

DAVID L. LONGWORTH, MD
Chairman, Department of Infectious Diseases
The Cleveland Clinic Foundation
Cleveland, Ohio

W.B. SAUNDERS COMPANY
A Harcourt Health Sciences Company
Philadelphia   London   New York   Sydney   St. Louis   Toronto

W.B. SAUNDERS COMPANY
A Harcourt Health Sciences Company

The Curtis Center
Independence Square West
Philadelphia, Pennsylvania 19106

NOTICE

Pharmacology is an ever-changing field. Standard safety precautions must be followed, but as new research and clinical experience broaden our knowledge, changes in treatment and drug therapy may become necessary or appropriate. Readers are advised to check the most current product information provided by the manufacturer of each drug to be administered to verify the recommended dose, the method and duration of administration, and contraindications. It is the responsibility of the treating physician, relying on experience and knowledge of the patient, to determine dosages and the best treatment for each individual patient. Neither the publisher nor the editor assumes any liability for any injury and/or damage to persons or property arising from this publication.

Acquisitions Editor: Karen Fabiano
Developmental Editor: Mindy Copeland
Project Manager: Linda McKinley
Production Editor: Kristin Hebberd
Designer: Julia Ramirez

Last digit is print number: 9   8   7   6   5   4   3   2   1

CONTRIBUTORS

LOUTFI S. ABOUSSOUAN, MD
Assistant Professor of Medicine
Division of Pulmonary and Critical
   Care Medicine
Wayne State University School
   of Medicine
Detroit, Michigan

SANDRA G. ADAMS, MD
Division of Pulmonary Diseases/
   Critical Care Medicine
Department of Medicine
The University of Texas Health
   Science Center
San Antonio, Texas

ALEJANDRO C. ARROLIGA, MD, FCCP
Head, Section of Critical Care
Department of Pulmonary
   and Critical Care Medicine
The Cleveland Clinic Foundation
Cleveland, Ohio

RICHARD D. BRANSON, BA,
   RRT, FAARC
Associate Professor of Surgery
University of Cincinnati
University Hospital
Cincinnati, Ohio

HOWARD CHRISTIE, PA-C, RRT
Physician's Assistant, Department
   of Pulmonary and Critical Care
   Medicine
The Cleveland Clinic Foundation
Cleveland, Ohio

EDGAR DELGADO, BS, RRT
Education/Quality Improvement/
   Research Coordinator
Department of Respiratory Care
University of Pittsburgh Medical Center
Pittsburgh, Pennsylvania

MICHAEL A. DEVITA, MD, FACP
Assistant Professor of Anesthesiology/
   Critical Care Medicine and Internal
   Medicine
University of Pittsburgh Medical Center
Pittsburgh, Pennsylvania

RAED A. DWEIK, MD
Staff Physician
Department of Pulmonary and Critical
   Care Medicine
The Cleveland Clinic Foundation
Cleveland, Ohio

GARY W. FALK, MD
Staff Physician
Center for Swallowing and
   Esophageal Disorders
Department of Gastroenterology
The Cleveland Clinic Foundation
Cleveland, Ohio

ROBERT GERBER, MD
Senior Fellow, Department of
   Pulmonary and Critical Care
   Medicine
The Cleveland Clinic Foundation
Cleveland, Ohio

LAWRENCE GOLDSTEIN, MD
Eastern Ohio Pulmonary Consultations
Boardman, Ohio

JOHN E. HEFFNER, MD
Professor of Medicine
Vice Chair, Department of Medicine
Medical University of South Carolina
Charleston, South Carolina

EDWARD HOISINGTON, RRT
Supervisor, Section of
    Respiratory Therapy
Department of Pulmonary
    and Critical Care Medicine
The Cleveland Clinic Foundation
Cleveland, Ohio

TAREQ JAMIL, MD
Fellow, Division of Pulmonary
    and Critical Care Medicine,
Wayne State University School
    of Medicine,
Detroit, Michigan

MANI S. KAVURU, MD
Staff Physician
Director, Pulmonary Function
    Laboratory
Department of Pulmonary and Critical
    Care Medicine
The Cleveland Clinic Foundation
Cleveland, Ohio

LUCY KESTER, MBA, RRT, FAARC
Education Coordinator, Section
    of Respiratory Therapy
Department of Pulmonary
    and Critical Care Medicine
The Cleveland Clinic Foundation
Cleveland, Ohio

PAUL A. LANGE, MD, FCCP
Assistant Professor of Medicine
Division of Pulmonary and Critical
    Care Medicine
Case Western Reserve University
Director of Lung Transplantation
    Services
University Hospitals of Cleveland
Cleveland, Ohio

R. WAYNE LAWSON, MS, RRT
Assistant Professor
Department of Respiratory Care
University of Texas Health
    Science Center
San Antonio, Texas

BRIAN M. LEGERE, MD
Staff Physician
Coastal Pulmonary Medicine
Wilmington, North Carolina

NEIL R. MACINTYRE, MD, FAARC
Professor of Medicine
Respiratory Care Services
Duke University Medical Center
Durham, North Carolina

ATUL C. MEHTA, MD
Professor of Medicine
Vice Chairman, Department
    of Pulmonary and Critical Care
    Medicine
Head, Section of Bronchology
The Cleveland Clinic Foundation
Cleveland, Ohio

ALISON G. MORRIS, MD
Department of Critical Care Medicine
University of Pittsburgh Medical
    Center
Pittsburgh, Pennsylvania

DOUGLAS ORENS, RRT, MBA
Manager, Section of Respiratory Care
Department of Pulmonary and Critical
    Care Medicine
The Cleveland Clinic Foundation
Cleveland, Ohio

SANJAY A. PATEL, MD
Fellow, Division of Pulmonary,
    Allergy, and Critical Care Medicine
University of Pittsburgh Medical Center
Pittsburgh, Pennsylvania

JAY I. PETERS, MD
Professor
Division of Pulmonary Diseases/
    Critical Care Medicine
Department of Medicine
The University of Texas Health
    Science Center
San Antonio, Texas

ALBERT L. RAFANAN, MD
Senior Fellow, Department of
  Pulmonary and Critical Care
  Medicine
The Cleveland Clinic Foundation
Cleveland, Ohio

SUNDER SANDUR, MD
Attending Physician
Department of Pulmonary
  and Critical Care Medicine
Saint Mary's Hospital
Waterbury, Connecticut

BIPIN D. SARODIA, MD
Senior Clinical Fellow, Department
  of Pulmonary and Critical Care
  Medicine
The Cleveland Clinic Foundation
Cleveland, Ohio

FRANK C. SCIURBA, MD
Associate Professor of Medicine
Division of Pulmonary, Allergy, and
  Critical Care Medicine
Director, Emphysema Research Center
University of Pittsburgh Medical Center
Pittsburgh, Pennsylvania

DAVID SHELLEDY, PHD, RRT
Chairman, Department
  of Respiratory Care
The University of Texas
  Health Science Center
San Antonio, Texas

LAURENCE A. SMOLLEY, MD
Clinical Assistant Professor
  of Internal Medicine
The Cleveland Clinic Foundation
Cleveland, Ohio;
Chairman, Pulmonary Department
Cleveland Clinic Florida
Fort Lauderdale, Florida

PATRICK J. STROLLO, JR, MD
Director, Pulmonary Sleep Evaluation
  Laboratory
Associate Professor of Medicine
Division of Pulmonary, Allergy,
  and Critical Care Medicine
University of Pittsburgh Medical Center
Pittsburgh, Pennsylvania

IRAWAN SUSANTO, MD, FACP
Associate Clinical Professor
Director, Pulmonary Consultation
  and Procedures
Pulmonary and Critical Care Medicine
UCLA School of Medicine
Los Angeles, California

LYNN T. TANOUE, MD
Associate Professor of Medicine
Yale University School of Medicine
New Haven, Connecticut

FRAN WHALEN, MD
Montefiore University Hospital
University of Pittsburgh Medical Center
Pittsburgh, Pennsylvania

PREFACE

As all clinicians recognize, the challenge of clinical medicine is to integrate massive amounts of information into dichotomous decisions, such as whether to treat hypertension or operate for a clinical problem.

Collecting volumes of clinical information, critically synthesizing and evaluating it, and applying evidence-based judgment and experience to make clinical recommendations require advanced training, discipline, and practice. This book addresses the acquisition and critical synthesis of diagnostic information. Critical and diagnostic thinking is the process by which clinicians gather the data to construct a *differential diagnosis* (list of suspected causes of a patient's condition) and then frame the diagnostic question for additional laboratory testing.

What are the elements of critical diagnostic thinking? First, clinicians must ask hypothesis-driven questions and listen carefully to the patient's responses, registering not only what is said, but also how it is said (e.g., tone of voice and affect, body attitude and language). The clinician's ability to elicit hypothesis-driven information grows with experience; the patient's response to one question triggers a more refined set of diagnostic possibilities, which in turn prompts the clinician's next questions.

Understandably, questions from the first-year respiratory therapist and beginning medical student often resemble a rote list of queries that review one organ system at a time, whereas the seasoned clinician's inquiry becomes much more focused but perhaps less exhaustive. With experience, the questions resemble tighter and tighter circles around the *target*, the cause of the patient's symptom.

For example, a patient's report of expectorating blood (hemoptysis) elicits the experienced clinician's questions about the source of bleeding (e.g., nose, intestinal tract, lungs; and if lungs, which lung and segment) and the character of the bleeding (e.g., how much, when, with what pattern). The purpose of the questioning is to determine the cause of the bleeding in order to determine how to treat and ideally cure the problem. Each subsequent question seeks to gain a more refined understanding of the source of the bleeding to define a course of treatment.

With the task defined, how do clinicians learn the process of critical diagnostic thinking? Our long-standing interest in this process of learning clinical medicine has convinced us that clinicians learn in a case-based way. To this point, we as editors can remember specific aspects of what we know about hemoptysis from specific patients with hemoptysis we have seen over the years. This insight has led us to organize the book as a series of clinical vignettes. Each chapter poses an important respiratory problem presented as a case with an accompanying description of the history and physical examination. Because a hypothesis-driven approach to diagnostic thinking is driven by knowledge of the possible causes (differential diagnosis), the next section of each chapter reviews common and uncommon causes of the patient's symptom. The following part and tables discuss the ways in which specific features of the history and physical examination influence the likelihood of a specific cause of the symptom. For example, having massive hemoptysis makes tuberculosis, bronchiectasis, and lung abscess more likely than bronchitis, which would better explain non-massive hemoptysis. Finally, each chapter closes with a discussion of pitfalls in the diagnosis—those issues observed to be frequently confused or especially challenging.

The book begins with an introduction to the process of critical diagnostic thinking. Using a variety of examples of respiratory problems, Drs. Shelledy and Stoller explain and demonstrate how the astute clinician uses information from the history and physical examination to develop an ordered list of likeliest causes, or the differential diagnosis.

The second part of the book, written by respiratory care colleagues, presents cases that involve common outpatient respiratory issues, including symptoms (e.g., cough, wheezing, dyspnea, phlegm production, sleepiness) and signs (e.g., clubbing, hypercapnia, chest x-ray infiltrate, nodule, hilar adenopathy).

The third part addresses common respiratory problems in the non-ICU adult inpatient (e.g., post-operative hypoxia, nosocomial pneumonia, atelectasis, preoperative respiratory assessment).

The final part of the book addresses critical diagnostic thinking in the adult ICU patient. Unlike earlier discussions on symptoms, these chapters present common ICU problems that invite critical diagnostic reasoning.

This book's goal is to clarify the process of clinical reasoning so that respiratory care clinicians can progress from hearing the patient's symptoms and observing signs to understanding the next diagnostic step and ultimately providing treatment. The insights into the reasoning process will translate into more effective care for patients. The critical reader will find this a useful guide along the path of enhancing clinical acumen.

The book assembles contributions from many talented, experienced respiratory care clinicians to whom we, as editors, are deeply indebted. Also, we gratefully acknowledge the capable editorial staff at Harcourt Health Sciences, who supported and assisted ably in the production of the manuscript.

JAMES K. STOLLER
ERIC D. BAKOW
DAVID L. LONGWORTH

CONTENTS

PART I

BACKGROUND

CHAPTER 1

AN INTRODUCTION TO CRITICAL DIAGNOSTIC THINKING

David Shelledy
James K. Stoller

Key Terms

- Diaphoresis
- Dyspnea
- Angina pectoris
- Pneumoconiosis
- Hemoptysis
- Digital clubbing
- Ascites
- Pectus excavatum
- Pectus carinatum
- Kyphosis
- Kyphoscoliosis
- Anklylosing spondylitis
- Cheyne-Stokes breathing
- Biot's breathing
- Forced vital capacity (FVC)
- Forced expiratory volume in 1 second (FEV_1)
- Forced expiratory volume in 3 seconds (FEV_3)
- Peak expiratory flow rate (PEFR)
- Total lung capacity (TLC)

▼ THE IMPORTANCE OF CRITICAL THINKING AND PROBLEM SOLVING

Critical diagnostic thinking is an essential attribute of the capable respiratory care practitioner. Respiratory care clinicians are called on to care for patients with a variety of clinical problems. Skills to identify not only the source of the patient's problem (i.e., the diagnosis) but also the best available treatment are indispensable for everyday practice. Thus critical diagnostic thinking deserves a great deal of attention at the beginning of a book regarding diagnostic reasoning for respiratory care clinicians.

Clinical reasoning, critical thinking, diagnostic reasoning, decision analysis, and *problem solving* are all terms used to describe how clinicians make clinical decisions. Problem-based learning, evidence-based medicine, protocol-directed care, and critical pathways have been implemented in various settings to improve the quality of clinical decision-making.

Critical diagnostic thinking is first addressed by identification of the elements of critical diagnostic thinking. The discussion continues with ways in which basic data-gathering skills for respiratory care clinicians (e.g., taking a history, performing a physical examination) are directed at the elements of critical diagnostic reasoning. Next follows a discussion of the process used to formulate and evaluate hypotheses to include the use of laboratory evaluations. Finally, pitfalls and common mistakes in critical diagnostic reasoning are reviewed.

The Elements of Critical Diagnostic Reasoning

Box 1-1 presents core critical thinking skills needed for the respiratory care clinician to practice critical diagnostic reasoning. These skills include interpretation, analysis, and evaluation of data; making clinical inferences; and providing explanation. Self-regulation is a key part of maintaining and improving skills.

Core critical thinking skills needed by respiratory care clinicians may also include the ability to prioritize, anticipate, troubleshoot, communicate, negotiate, make decisions, and reflect on experiences. Finally, critical diagnostic reasoning requires the integration of many different pieces of information derived from a patient history, a careful and focused physical examination, and a broad knowledge of the causes of various diseases (i.e., the differential diagnosis).

As testimony to the importance of these skills, various instruments and surveys have been developed to assess respiratory care clinicians' critical thinking and problem-solving abilities. For example, the board examinations for advanced level respiratory therapists include clinical simulations that attempt to measure information-gathering and decision-making skills.

Still, the question remains: How does one do critical thinking? The approach to clinical diagnostic thinking should include certain key elements of problem solving that are integral to the scientific method and should form the foundation for problem solving. These key elements are (1) identifying the perceived problem; (2) gathering additional information to clarify the problem, i.e., by cataloging signs and symptoms; (3) formulating possible explanations or hypotheses by making a list of "likely suspects;" (4) testing explanations (hypotheses), i.e., by identifying signs and symptoms in common and verifying with appropriate diagnostic testing; (5) formulating and implementing solutions, i.e., by making a diagnosis; and (6) monitoring and reevaluating.

Box 1-1
Core Critical Thinking Skills for Respiratory Care Clinicians

Interpreting	**Evaluating**	**Explaining**
Categorizing	Assessing claims	Stating results
Decoding significance	Assessing arguments	Justifying procedures
Clarifying meaning		Presenting arguments
	Inferring	
Analyzing	Querying evidence	**Self-Regulating**
Examining ideas	Conjecturing alternatives	Self-examining
Identifying arguments	Drawing conclusions	Self-correcting
Analyzing arguments		

From Facione PA: *Critical thinking, a statement of expert consensus for purposes of educational assessment and instruction,* ERIC Document Reproduction Service No. ED 315 423, 1990.

The Impact of Evidence-Based Medicine on Critical Diagnostic Reasoning

Currently, evidence-based medicine (EBM), which is defined as the integration of the best research evidence with clinical expertise and patient values, is widely advocated to guide clinical practice. Besides defining practice according to the best available scientific support, EBM also can provide a structured approach to clinical problem solving and decision making. The move to EBM is driven, in part, by the need for valid, current information about the causes, diagnosis, treatment, prognosis, and prevention of specific conditions and the fact that textbooks may be out of date, inaccurate, or based on opinion rather than scientific evidence. EBM combines the need to ask relevant, answerable clinical questions with methods to find the current best evidence. Questions may relate to diagnosis and screening, prognosis, treatment, or prevention. Sources of answers to questions may include evidence-based textbooks, journals, and clinical practice guidelines, electronic databases (e.g., evidence-based medical reviews, the Cochrane Library, and MEDLINE), and evidence-based information services.

With respect to critical diagnostic thinking, EBM can help answer whether a diagnostic test is accurate, how well the test distinguishes between patients who do and do not have a specific disorder, and whether a test is appropriate to a specific patient. An EBM approach also may be useful in the assessment of data about patient prognosis. Where possible, an EBM approach may be preferred to select a treatment because treatment is based on the best scientific evidence available. Ideally, treatment decisions should be based on the results of multiple randomized, controlled trials (RCTs) in which the lower limit of the confidence interval for the treatment effect exceeds the minimally important clinical benefit. In the absence of multiple trials that agree, evidence from single RCTs may be used. Other types of evidence, from most to least preferable, include results from concurrent non-randomized cohort studies, historic cohort studies, and case studies. Guidelines used to assess evidence are outlined in Table 1-1.

**TABLE 1-1
Levels of Evidence and Grades of Recommendations
for Therapy**

Level of Evidence	Grades of Recommendation
Level 1	**Grade A**
Level 1	Results come from a single RCT in which the lower limit of the CI for the treatment effect exceeds the minimal clinically important benefit.
Level 1+	Results come from a meta-analysis of RCTs in which the treatment effects from individual studies are consistent, and the lower limit of the CI for the treatment effect exceeds the minimal clinically important benefit.
Level 1−	Results come from a meta-analysis of RCTs in which the treatment effects from individual studies are widely disparate, but the lower limit of the CI for the treatment effect still exceeds the minimal clinically important benefit.
Level 2	**Grade B**
Level 2	Results come from a single RCT in which the CI for the treatment effect overlaps the minimal clinically important benefit.
Level 2+	Results come from a meta-analysis of RCTs in which the treatment effects from individual studies are consistent, and the CI for the treatment effect overlaps the minimal clinically important benefit.
Level 2−	Results come from a meta-analysis of RCTs in which the treatment effects from individual studies are widely disparate, and the CI for the treatment effect overlaps the minimal clinically important benefit.
Level 3	**Grade C**
	Results come from non-randomized concurrent cohort studies.
Level 4	**Grade C**
	Results come from non-randomized historic cohort studies.
Level 5	**Grade C**
	Results come from case series.

RCT, Randomized, controlled trial; *CI,* confidence interval.
From Cook DJ, Guyatt GH, Laupacis A, et al: *Chest* 108:227S-230S, 1995.

An Approach to Critical Thinking and Problem Solving

Various techniques have been used to improve critical diagnostic thinking. These include the use of problem-oriented medical records, algorithms for diagnosis, and treatment and calculation of diagnostic probabilities. However, the most widely accepted and studied models of critical diagnostic thinking are based on the scientific method.

Critical diagnostic thinking begins with identifying of the problem and gathering information. This includes obtaining a patient history, performing a physical examination, and laboratory testing. The patient history includes the patient profile, chief complaint, history of the present illness, past medical history, social and oc-

Box 1-2
Common Clinical Problems Related to Respiratory Care

Allergy/Immunology
Wheezing patient
Patient with allergies
Immunosuppressed patient

Cardiovascular
Chest pain
Hypertensive patient
Edema
Murmur
Mitral valve prolapse
Palpitations
New-onset congestive heart
  failure
Chronic congestive heart
  failure
Acute ischemia
Chronic, stable angina
Abnormal stress test
Atrial arrhythmias
Asymptomatic ventricular
  arrhythmias
Congenital heart disease
Aortic valve disease
Syncope
Claudication
Abdominal aortic aneurysm
Hyperlipidemia

Critical Care
Acute pulmonary embolus
Severe airway obstruction
Massive gastrointestinal
  bleeding
Chest pain
Comatose or obtunded
  patient
Hyperthermic patient
Hypothermic patient
Pulseless and apneic patient
Acute respiratory failure
Shock
Sepsis syndrome
Anuria/oliguria/heart failure
Agitated patient
Dying patient

Infectious Disease
Upper respiratory infection
Sore throat
Active tuberculosis
Pneumonia/bronchitis
HIV infection
Febrile patient
Septic patient

Pulmonary
Cough
Dyspnea

Pulmonary—cont'd
Pulmonary infiltrate
Hemoptysis
Asthma
Chronic obstructive pul-
  monary disease
Solitary pulmonary nodule
Pulmonary embolism/deep
  vein thrombophlebitis
Pleural effusion
Broken rib
Pneumothorax

**Other Common
Problems**
Substance abuse (tobacco,
  alcohol, sedatives/narcotics,
  cocaine, drug overdose)
Cancer
Acute renal failure
Diabetes mellitus
Neurologic problems (stroke,
  seizures, headaches,
  dementia)
Accidents and trauma
  (multiple trauma, chest
  trauma, head trauma,
  gunshot wounds, etc.)

Modified from Bennett JC, Plum F (eds): *Cecil textbook of medicine*, ed 20, Philadelphia, 1996, WB Saunders.
HIV, Human immunodeficiency virus.

cupational history, family history, and a review of systems. The physical examination, in turn, includes inspection, palpation, auscultation, and percussion.

Common diagnostic tests for the respiratory care patient may include a chest
x-ray, oximetry, arterial blood gases, pulmonary function tests (e.g., spirometry,
lung volume measurements, and diffusing capacity), sputum examination (Gram's
stain, culture, sensitivity, cytology, stains for acid-fast bacilli [AFB], such as mycobacteria, and silver stain for fungi and *Pneumocystis carinii*), hematology (complete blood count, hemoglobin, hematocrit), and blood chemistry (serum electrolytes, enzymes, glucose). Other tests may include analysis of blood for tumor
markers or drug concentrations. History, physical examination, and laboratory testing provide the foundation for development and verification of a specific patient
diagnosis. Examples of common cardiovascular, pulmonary, and infectious disease
problems encountered by the respiratory care clinician are listed in Box 1-2. In the

sections that follow, the history, physical examination, and laboratory testing are reviewed as they relate to aspects of critical diagnostic reasoning.

▼ IDENTIFYING THE CLINICAL PROBLEM: PATIENT HISTORY AND PHYSICAL EXAMINATION

The first step in critical diagnostic thinking is to identify and clarify the problem by performing a patient history. The patient history begins with the patient profile and chief complaint.

Patient Profile

Before the process of critical thinking begins, some basic information about the patient, sometimes known as the *patient profile,* must be gathered. The patient profile provides a narrative description or "snapshot" of the patient (i.e., the "who, why, what, where, and when" of the patient's current condition). The patient's name, address, gender, ethnicity, admitting diagnosis (if available), and any other already identified problems (to include why the patient sought medical care) should be noted. Other helpful information used to describe the patient may include place of birth, home environment, education, socioeconomic status, marital status, and languages spoken. If a medical record or chart is available, any previous blood gas levels, chest x-rays, pulmonary function tests, and other reports, the results of diagnostic studies including sputum AFB stains, culture, sensitivity, cytology, and silver stain should be sought and reviewed. Previously performed history and physical examination reports and consultations found in the patient's medical record also can be extremely helpful because they may establish the patient's baseline from which current findings may differ in ways that provide important diagnostic clues.

Chief Complaint

The next step in critical diagnostic thinking is to identify the perceived problem or "chief complaint." The chief complaint is often provided by the patient or family when they are questioned as to why they are seeking medical care. The classic "Why are you here?" question is a fast way to identify the patient's perceived problem. However, it is important NOT to jump to conclusions based on information provided by any one source: the patient, the family, or other health care workers. For example, an important caution is not to label the patient's problems based on preliminary information, lest the subsequent testing and treatment be misdirected at the wrong problem. Rather, the practitioner should consider all the available information from the complete history, physical examination, and laboratory test results when determining a diagnosis to which treatment is directed.

For respiratory care patients, common chief complaints are shortness of breath (dyspnea), cough, sputum production, hemoptysis, and chest pain. Each will be discussed briefly here but are discussed in greater detail in later chapters.

Cough

Cough has been described as the "watchdog" of the lung. As discussed in Chapter 2, development of a cough or a change in a chronic cough may signal development of lung disease or a change in a chronic respiratory condition. Common causes of cough include post-nasal drip, acute or chronic bronchitis, asthma, and gastroesophageal reflux. Cough may be the only symptom of asthma and can result from gastroesophageal reflux, even in the absence of classic symptoms of heartburn. In this context, the challenge for the respiratory care clinician is to use information from the patient's history, physical examination, and laboratory testing to determine which of the possible causes or etiologies account for *this* patient's cough.

Sputum Production

As discussed in Chapter 3, sputum production is another common pulmonary symptom and may result from acute or chronic infection or inflammation. The diagnostic criterion for chronic bronchitis is the presence of a productive cough (often of a tablespoon or more of sputum) on most days for at least 3 months of the year in at least 2 consecutive years.

Hemoptysis

As reviewed in Chapter 8, hemoptysis can have many etiologies and is usually classified as either being massive (e.g., >600 mL of expectorated blood/day) or non-massive. Because it may be life threatening, massive hemoptysis represents a respiratory emergency. In contrast, non-massive hemoptysis less commonly poses an emergency from airway compromise, though its occurrence may signal a significant underlying problem for which definite and prompt diagnosis and treatment are needed (e.g., pulmonary embolism). To work through these issues, the respiratory care clinician must have knowledge of the causes of massive and non-massive hemoptysis (i.e., the differential diagnosis) and features of the history, physical examination, and relevant laboratory tests that suggest a specific cause of hemoptysis. In other words, the respiratory care clinician must integrate critical diagnostic reasoning with a rich fund of knowledge about causes and treatment of hemoptysis.

Dyspnea

As reviewed in Chapters 4 and 5, dyspnea is another common pulmonary symptom with many different etiologies. In assessing the specific cause of dyspnea in an individual patient, the respiratory care clinician is aided by understanding the pace with which the dyspnea began, the characteristics of the dyspnea (e.g., occurring only with activity, on lying down, or on simply standing upright), the presence of any accompanying symptoms (e.g., dyspnea in a patient who wheezes possibly suggesting asthma as a cause of both symptoms), triggers of the dyspnea, the usual duration and character of the dyspnea, and any maneuvers that help relieve the dyspnea (e.g., use of a family member's bronchodilator, rest, etc). This focus on understanding the character, pace, duration, triggers, and relievers of a symptom provides a useful guideline that helps clarify the specific etiology of a patient's symptom.

Chest Pain

The three main types of chest pain are substernal, pleuritic, and musculoskeletal. Substernal chest pain is associated with angina pectoris and myocardial infarction (MI). The patient may complain that it feels as if someone is sitting on his/her chest. The pain may radiate down the arms or up to the jaw. Unexplained severe central chest pain lasting 2 minutes or longer in at-risk patients may indicate an MI, even in patients without known cardiac disease, and action should be taken accordingly. Pleuritic chest pain is often a sharp, localized pain, often at the periphery of the chest. Musculoskeletal pain may be caused by rib fractures or chest trauma. Musculoskeletal pain often varies as the patient breathes and moves about. The onset and duration of chest pain and whether the pain is associated with trauma, coughing, movement, or a lower respiratory infection should be noted. Associated symptoms, such as shallow breathing, fever, uneven chest expansion, coughing, anxiety about getting air, or radiation of the pain to the neck or arms, also should be noted during the patient interview. Treatment or medications taken for pain should be reviewed. Chapter 15 describes the approach to the patient with pleuritic chest pain. Evaluation of the patient with non-pleuritic chest pain is described in Chapter 16.

Oxygenation, Ventilation, and Respiratory Failure

In addition to having a working knowledge of common pulmonary symptoms, the respiratory care clinician also must be knowledgeable about causes of impaired oxygenation, ventilation, and respiratory failure.

Early signs and symptoms of acute hypoxia include tachycardia, increased blood pressure, tachypnea, hyperventilation, restlessness, disorientation, dizziness, excitement, headache, blurred vision, and confusion. Severe hypoxia is associated with slowed, irregular respirations, bradycardia, hypotension, loss of consciousness, somnolence, convulsions, and coma. Also, severe hypoxia may lead to cardiac or respiratory arrest.

Acute ventilatory failure is defined as a sudden rise in arterial P_{CO_2} with a concomitant fall in pH. The clinical manifestations of acute ventilatory failure are similar to those of hypoxia. Marked increases in P_{CO_2} (hypercarbia) may also cause vasodilatation, sweating, redness of the skin, hallucinations, seizures, and coma.

The Additional Elements of the History

Identifying the perceived problem is only the starting point in critical diagnostic thinking. For a systematic approach, the respiratory care clinician needs to gather more information, which includes obtaining a patient history and performing a physical examination. The history should include the history of the present illness, the past medical history, the family history, current medications, allergies, and occupational and smoking history. Box 1-3 summarizes items that should be included in the pulmonary history.

Box 1-3
Items to be Included in a Pulmonary History

Cough
Onset: sudden, gradual; duration
Nature: dry, moist, wet, hacking, hoarse, barking, whooping, bubbling, productive, non-productive
Pattern: occasional, regular, paroxysmal; related to time of day, weather, activities, talking, deep breaths; change over time
Severity: tiring, sleep disruption, chest pain
Associated symptoms: dyspnea, chest pain, headache, choking
Efforts to treat: medications, other

Sputum Production
Amount: milliliters, tablespoons, teaspoons
Frequency: daily, mornings, Mondays
Color: green, yellow, brown, colorless, "red brick," frothy pink
Consistency: purulent, viscous, tenacious, watery, saliva
Odor: foul-smelling, sweet-smelling
Other: blood-tinged, bloody, mucous plugs

Hemoptysis
Color: bright red, brown
Amount: slight, blood-tinged sputum versus frank hemoptysis

Wheezing, Whistling, Chest Tightness
Onset, duration, frequency, associated events

Chest Pain
Nature, location, duration, associated activities or events

Breathlessness (Dyspnea)
Onset, position, exercise, associated symptoms, level of activity associated with dyspnea (severe exertion, stairs, walking, at rest)

Smoking History
Cigarettes, cigars, pipes, other
Frequency and amount (pack-years for cigarettes)
Attempts to quit

Current Medications
Respiratory (bronchodilators, anti-inflammatory agents, other)
Antibiotics
Cardiac drugs
Other

Current Respiratory Care
Oxygen
Ventilatory support
Bronchial hygiene and airway care (chest physiotherapy, PEP therapy, flutter, artificial airways, humidifiers, nebulizers, etc.)

The History of Present Illness

As summarized in Box 1-3, the patient should be asked to describe his or her principal symptoms in terms of onset (date, time, character [e.g., sudden, gradual]), nature of the complaint (quality and quantity), and location (Where is the pain, discomfort or other symptom? Does it spread? If so, to what destination?). Progression over time (the course of the complaint) should be noted. The patient should be asked about features that cause the symptom to worsen or to improve (triggers, relievers). Previous treatment and its effect on the symptom also should be noted (What has been done about this symptom in the past?).

In addition to clarifying the principal symptoms, the history should include questions regarding the presence or absence of cough, sputum production, hemoptysis, wheezing, whistling or chest tightness, chest pain, and breathlessness.

The patient's smoking history, current medications, and any current respiratory care (including home care) also should be assessed. More specifically, the patient should be questioned about current and past tobacco use and the type of tobacco product used (cigarettes, pipes, cigars). The number of years smoked and the number of packs smoked per day are often multiplied to create a measure called "pack-years." Also, any previous attempts to quit smoking should be noted and the method used (e.g., nicotine patches, gum, smoking-cessation programs, etc.). Because of embarrassment or the desire to please their health care provider, patients may underreport current tobacco use; the physical examination should include an inspection of the fingers for nicotine stains, which will help identify continuing smokers. Measurement of carboxyhemoglobin levels via cooximetry or measurements of urinary cotinine (a longer-lasting metabolite of nicotine) may also help identify "closet smokers." In addition to tobacco use, other inhaled drugs associated with lung injury include crack cocaine and marijuana. Alcohol use also should be noted. For example, alcoholics are prone to the development of an aspiration pneumonia.

Current Medications

All current medications and vaccination status should be recorded as part of a complete history. In particular, the clinician should inquire specifically about current use of bronchodilators (including over-the-counter drugs like Primatene Mist), anti-inflammatory agents (inhaled corticosteroids), antiasthmatic agents (e.g., cromolyn, nedocromil, zafirlukast, zileuton), mucolytics (e.g., acetylcysteine, dornase alpha, guainefesin) or aerosolized antiinfective agents (e.g., pentamidine, ribavirin, antibiotics). Nicotine replacement therapy (transdermal patch, gum, or nasal spray) as a part of a smoking cessation program also should be noted. An underrecognized genetic protein deficiency, alpha$_1$-antitrypsin deficiency, can lead to severe panacinar emphysema. In these patients, the use of alpha$_1$-proteinase inhibitors* should be noted. Use of nasal decongestants, antihistamines, expectorants, and cough and cold medications is important to record. Antibiotics, cardiac drugs (especially beta-blockers [which can exacerbate bronchospasm] and angiotension-converting enzyme inhibitors [which can cause cough]), antihypertensive medications, and diuretic use should be identified, as should medications for pain, anxiety, sleep, or psychotherapeutic agents.

The Past Medical History

A complete past medical history should include the patient's general state of health, childhood illnesses, adult illnesses, psychiatric illnesses, accidents and injuries, operations, hospitalizations, thoracic trauma or surgery, respiratory care received (oxygen, aerosol medications, etc.), pulmonary disease, cardiac problems, cancer (lung, other), and exposure to respiratory infections (tuberculosis [TB], influenza). Previous hospitalizations, including intensive care unit admissions, should be noted, as well as any history of intubation or mechanical ventilation.

Ancillary information regarding the patient's occupation, hobbies, and leisure activities may be helpful in pointing to a specific pulmonary problem. The patient also should be asked about the frequency of chest colds, bronchitis, or pneumonia,

---

*Prolastin, Bayer, West Haven, Conn.

and about whether he or she has ever been diagnosed as having any type of lung disease.

Occupational and Environmental History

Occupational exposure to aluminum, asbestosis, beryllium, sugar cane, cotton brac, barium, coal dust, moldy hay, clay, iron, silica dust, talc, and other substances can be associated with the development of lung disease. The development of occupational asthma has been associated with exposure to many substances, including animal-derived materials, plants and vegetable products, enzymes, chemicals (such as isocyanates used in plastic manufacture), drugs, wood dust, and metals.

A travel history may also be important in critical diagnostic reasoning. For example, the fungus coccidioidomycosis is prevalent in the San Joaquin Valley and parts of New Mexico, California, Texas, and Utah. Histoplasmosis is endemic to the Ohio and Mississippi River Valleys. Hanta virus is especially prevalent in the Four Corners region of New Mexico.

In the specific context of asthma, questions regarding exposure to dust mites, cockroaches, and animal danders may help to identify specific triggers. Hobby and leisure exposure to dusts, fumes, and pets also may help to identify specific contributors.

Timing of Signs and Symptoms as a Diagnostic Feature

Symptom modifiers (such as what brings on the symptom, what improves the symptom, and how the symptom is characterized by the patient) and temporal aspects of a symptom or sign are important characteristics that allow the astute clinician to narrow down the "list of suspects" and identify the specific cause in an individual patient. The following are among the time-related questions that might be posed when assessing the patient's symptom:

1. At what time of day (week, season, or year) does the symptom occur?
2. How does the symptom change over time? Does it steadily worsen, as in a crescendo pattern? Does it come and go with some "good days" and some "bad days?"

There are many examples of respiratory symptoms that have characteristic (though not uniform) timing characteristics. With regard to onset, occupational asthma or hypersensitivity pneumonitis may first become noticeable at the beginning of the work week, steadily worsen over the course of the week, and then remit during time off work (e.g., weekends and non-working holidays). Asthma may worsen at night and cause nighttime awakening in up to 15% of asthmatics, though it must be understood that nighttime onset also may be characteristic of other conditions that may mimic some features of the asthmatic patient. For example, postnasal drip may cause worsened cough in the supine position and therefore be confused with asthma. Also, like asthma, gastroesophageal reflux may worsen at night when the supine posture encourages headward movement of stomach acid. As another example of seasonal factors that may help to identify the cause of a symptom, one might imagine an accountant with asthma whose stress-induced symptoms worsen as the tax season approaches. In this instance, realizing that the patient is an accountant and that asthma is a condition that may be worsened by stress may allow the astute clinician to suspect asthma as the cause of the accountant's early spring cough.

In addition to the timing of onset, another very important diagnostic feature of illness is how the associated signs and symptoms change over time. This temporal pattern might be referred to as the "slope" of the disease, or, borrowing from aeronautic terminology, as the "glidepath" of the illness. Both the terms *slope* and *glidepath* are meant to elicit the image that the rate of change over time of the signs and symptoms can help the clinician identify the etiology. Again, many useful examples can be cited. In infectious disease, "tertan fever" or fever that occurs every 48 hours is a characteristic but not consistent feature of malarial infection due to either *Plasmodium vivax* or *Plasmodium ovale*. These causative organisms can sometimes be distinguished from another malarial species, *Plasmodium malariae*, which causes "quartan fever," or fever that occurs every 72 hours.

In respiratory disease, the timing of occurrence and the rate of change of signs and symptoms over time also can be very helpful diagnostic features. For example, chronic bronchitis is actually defined by the timing and chronicity of associated symptoms. Specifically, chronic bronchitis is defined as the occurrence of phlegm production, which occurs daily for at least 3 months of the year in at least 2 consecutive years. The dyspnea associated with intermittent asthma often can be characterized as occurring sporadically, with the patient having some "good days" and some "bad days." In contrast, dyspnea that occurs in an unrelentingly worsening pattern, especially if occurring progressively over the course of several months to years, would be more characteristic of a parenchymal lung illness, such as idiopathic pulmonary fibrosis, or a vascular process, such as pulmonary hypertension, rather than asthma. As a final example of the value of timing and rate of onset of a sign or symptom as a diagnostic criterion, digital clubbing is recognized as being caused by many conditions, including chronic suppurative lung illnesses (e.g., bronchiectasis), interstitial lung diseases (e.g., sarcoidosis), congenital cyanotic heart disease, chronic liver disease (e.g., cirrhosis), inflammatory bowel disease, hypothyroidism (in which it may be called *thyroid acropachy*), as a familial trait, or finally, as a complication of many malignancies, including lung cancer. However, among the common cell types of lung cancer (e.g., adenocarcinoma, squamous cell cancer, large cell cancer, and small cell cancer), clubbing is said to rarely accompany small cell cancer. The presumed reason is that the early predisposition to spread distantly (i.e., metastasize) with small cell lung carcinoma would more commonly cause the illness to present as a symptom or sign attributed to the metastatic focus. Put differently, the generally aggressive, rapid time course of small cell carcinoma would not allow digital clubbing (which presumably develops insidiously and slowly) to develop over the short time frame during which other constitutional or metastatic signs and symptoms would become pronounced.

Review of Symptoms

The next step of diagnostic critical thinking is the review of symptoms. To begin, the respiratory care clinician should write a complete problem list for the patient based on the symptoms noted during the patient history. The list may be organized by system as described in Box 1-4.

Box 1-4
Review of Symptoms–Typical Problems Related to Pulmonary Disorders

General symptoms: Fever, chills, malaise, fatigue, lethargy, night sweats, weight loss, restlessness, dizziness
Skin: Pale, cold and clammy, redness, cyanosis, rash, sweating
Skeletal: Pain, swelling, fractures, trauma
Head: Headache, dizziness, head injury
Eyes: Blurred vision, diplopia, conjunctivitis
Ears: Pain, hearing loss, vertigo
Nose: Sinus pain, colds, nasal obstruction or runny nose, sneezing, nasal flaring, post-nasal drip
Throat: Hoarse, voice change, sore throat, tooth pain or abscess, ulcers
Endocrine: Thyroid enlargement, diabetes, pregnancy
Respiratory: Cough, sputum production, hemoptysis, dyspnea, orthopnea, wheezing, whistling or chest tightness, chest pain, exposure to TB, etc
Cardiac: Chest pain or discomfort, palpitations, edema
Hematologic: Anemia, bruising, bleeding, blood loss
Lymph nodes: Tender, enlargement
Gastrointestinal: Diet, appetite, digestion, food problems, heartburn, nausea, vomiting, diarrhea
Genitourinary: Urine output
Neurologic and mental status: Fainting, seizures, convulsions, coma, paralysis or weakness, tremors, headache, depression, anxiety, sleep disturbances, disorientation, excitement, confusion, somnolence

▼ FORMULATION AND EVALUATION OF HYPOTHESES

As mentioned, commonly identified respiratory problems may include shortness of breath, cough, sputum production, and hemoptysis. Other possible problems might include chest pain, restlessness, nervousness, excitement, tremors, headache, palpitations, disorientation, dizziness, headache, blurred vision, daytime sleepiness, fatigue, or confusion. Each problem should be described in some detail as to its nature, onset, location, and progression over time. After the problem list is written, the clinician creates another list of diseases or conditions that produce these symptoms. This is the respiratory care clinician's list of "likely suspects." The initial hypotheses can be generated from this list, which can then guide the subsequent physical examination and laboratory studies. For example, shortness of breath, cough, sputum production, and fever may generate the hypothesis that these problems are caused by a respiratory tract infection. While performing the physical examination, the respiratory care clinician should specifically look for signs that can help evaluate this hypothesis, such as increased respiratory rate, other signs of hypoxemia, abnormal findings on chest examination, etc.

The Physical Examination

As reviewed in Table 1-2, the physical examination should include an assessment of the patient's general appearance (e.g., Does the patient appear acutely ill, chronically

TABLE 1-2
Elements of the Physical Examination and Key Findings Associated with Pulmonary Disorders

Elements	Key Findings
Ancillary Equipment in Use	Intravenous catheters, cardiac monitors, chest tubes, respiratory care equipment
General Appearance	Distress, malnourishment, position
Vital signs	Tachycardia, bradycardia, hypertension, hypotension, tachypnea, bradypnea, fever
Level of consciousness	Awake and alert versus restlessness, anxiety, excitement, confusion, sleepiness, lethargy, somnolence, coma
Extremities	Cyanosis, pale, cold, clammy extremities, edema, digital clubbing, nicotine-stained fingers
Respiratory rate and pattern	Tachypnea, increased or decreased depth, irregular breathing patterns
Skin (color, temperature, condition)	Cyanosis, rash, warmth, cold and clammy, cherry-red color (carbon monoxide), sweating, surgical scars, wounds, radiation markers
Head, eyes, ears, nose, and throat	Cyanosis (lips, gingiva), pursed-lip breathing, nasal flaring, pupils dilated or contracted
Neck	Jugular vein distension, accessory muscle use, subcutaneous emphysema
Chest (inspection, palpation, percussion, auscultation)	Increased AP diameter, deformities, scars, trauma, flail, asymmetric motion, retractions Tactile fremitus, symmetry of chest wall expansion, tracheal shift Resonance versus hyperresonance or dullness Absent or diminished breath sounds, crackles, rhonchi, wheezing, rubs, "E to A" egophony, bronchovesicular breath sounds over periphery
Cardiovascular	Abnormal rate and/or rhythm
Abdomen	Obesity, ascites, pregnancy, scars, trauma

AP, Anteroposterior.

ill, older than his/her stated age?), vital signs, and then a systematic analysis of the various organ systems, especially as they relate to respiratory problems. Highlights should include assessment of the patient's level of consciousness, oxygenation, perfusion, skin color and characteristics, nail beds, mucosa, and capillary refill. The chest examination is also essential and should include inspection, palpation, auscultation, and percussion. The respiratory care clinician should evaluate for tactile and vocal fremitus, abnormal chest excursion, tracheal position, dullness, hyperresonance, and so-called adventitious sounds (e.g., crackles, wheezes).

Inspection

Careful observation is an essential step in clarifying the problem and identifying possible causes. Inspection should include an assessment of the patient's general appearance, level of consciousness, extremities, respiratory rate and pattern, retractions, color, presence of diaphoresis, and position. Dyspnea that occurs when the patient lies down for the examination (which is called *orthopnea*) may be associated with congestive heart failure and diaphragmatic dysfunction. As a matter of the history, the degree of orthopnea often is measured by the number of pillows that the patient requires to lie down.

Another important aspect of inspection is to notice the patient's use of any ancillary equipment or devices. For example, cardiac monitors, chest tubes, suction apparatus, intravenous catheters, or other equipment at the bedside can provide the clinician with important clues regarding the patient's condition.

Other aspects of inspection, including assessment of skin color, temperature, and condition, may help evaluate a respiratory condition. Cyanosis is associated with severe hypoxemia, but the presence or absence of cyanosis must be interpreted cautiously. Patients with anemia may be severely hypoxemic without having cyanosis (because they have insufficient hemoglobin to generate the blue color of desoxyhemoglobin), whereas patients with polycythemia (as may occur with chronic hypoxemic lung disease) may turn blue after only small decreases in arterial oxygen saturation.

A pale, cold, clammy appearance may be associated with hypotension and shock. Elevated carbon dioxide levels may cause the patient to appear flushed. Skin rash may be associated with allergic or drug reactions, whereas elevated carbon monoxide levels result in a bright, cherry-red skin color. Sweating (diaphoresis) is often associated with acute distress.

The patient's level of consciousness and response to verbal questions should be observed. Hypoxemia may cause changes in central nervous system (CNS) function, with mental status and level of consciousness ranging from restlessness and dizziness to frank coma and seizures. In assessing the patient's mental status, the clinician should ask the following questions: Is the patient alert, oriented, and aware of person, place, and time? Is the patient obtunded, stuporous, or comatose?

Extremities

The fingers should be assessed for capillary refill, digital clubbing, and nicotine stains (as evidence of active smoking). Assessing capillary refill can be helpful in the assessment of circulation. For example, cold, clammy extremities with poor capillary refill may indicate poor perfusion and circulation. Edema, especially in the ankles and feet, may be associated with fluid overload (as in renal failure) or congestive heart failure.

The differential diagnosis of digital clubbing of the fingers is broad and includes congenital cyanotic heart disease, chronic pulmonary infection (e.g., bronchiectasis, lung abscess), interstitial lung disease, chronic liver disease, inflammatory bowel disease, various cancers, thyroid disease, and familial clubbing. As another example of critical diagnostic reasoning, assessing the specific cause of an individual patient's clubbing requires the integration of information from other aspects of the physical examination (e.g., Is there other evidence of cancer, of chronic liver disease, etc?) and from the history (e.g., Do other family members have clubbing? Is there a history of hemoptysis, weight loss, chronic alcohol ingestion, etc?). A common pitfall regarding clubbing is to think that clubbing can result from chronic obstructive pulmonary disease (COPD) with hypoxemia. This is not the case; alternate causes should be sought in patients with COPD who also have clubbing.

Inspection of the head and neck may reveal cyanosis of the lips and gums, pursed-lip breathing, nasal flaring, and/or jugular vein distension. Pursed-lip breathing is sometimes seen in patients with COPD as an adaptation to reduce air-trapping. Nasal flaring is a sign of respiratory distress, especially in children. Jugular vein distension is associated with congestive heart failure and fluid overload. Use of the accessory muscles of the neck on inspiration is a sign of increased work of breathing—a common finding in acute exacerbations of COPD.

Inspection of the Chest

Inspection of the chest should include assessment of the anteroposterior (AP) diameter of the chest, presence of chest wall or spinal deformity, and observation for the presence of unilateral apparent hyperexpansion. Right-to-left symmetry of respirations and intercostal retractions should be noted, as well as the presence of chest trauma, multiple rib fractures, or flail chest (a part of the chest wall that moves paradoxically, i.e., inward when the patient inspires and the rest of the chest is expanding). Abdominal disorders (obesity, ascites), pregnancy, scars (trauma, surgery), and radiation markers (radiation therapy) also should be noted during the chest inspection.

An increased AP diameter ("barrel chest") may be associated with air-trapping or pulmonary overinflation. Barrel chest is a common finding in COPD and is sometimes seen in cystic fibrosis and in acute asthma. The appearance of unilateral hyperexpansion may be due to a decrease in compliance on one side, pneumothorax, or bronchial intubation.

Chest wall or spinal deformities include pectus excavatum, pectus carinatum, kyphosis, kyphoscoliosis, and ankylosing spondylitis. These disorders may decrease thoracic compliance and impair ventilation, resulting in a restrictive ventilatory defect. Obesity, pregnancy, or ascites may indirectly reduce thoracic compliance, as well as limiting a patient's inspiratory capacity. Obesity also may predispose the patient to obstructive sleep apnea and disorders of ventilatory control.

The patient's respiratory rate, respiratory pattern, and the presence of tachypnea, bradypnea, and periodic breathing should be noted. Cheyne-Stokes or Biot's breathing, as well as abnormally deep breathing, should be noted. The thorax and abdomen should rise and fall together as the patient breathes. Ventilatory muscle fatigue leading to ventilatory failure is sometimes associated with asynchronous or spasmodic contractions of the diaphragm. In the circumstance of bilateral diaphragm dysfunction (as may accompany ventilatory failure, bilateral phrenic nerve dysfunction, or neuromuscular disease), the diaphragm moves inward when the patient inspires. This movement may be especially prominent when the patient is supine. Sedatives, narcotics, severe hypoxia, or CNS problems may lead to bradypnea followed by respiratory arrest.

Traumatic multiple rib fractures of adjacent ribs (also known as *flail chest*) may cause chest wall instability and paradoxical chest wall movement. A flail chest is caused by two to three consecutive rib fractures, with each rib broken in two or more places. Chest wall instability may cause paradoxic chest wall movement in which the chest wall sinks in on inspiration on the affected side. A severe flail may lead to hypoxemia and acute ventilatory failure requiring mechanical ventilatory support. Pneumothorax and lung contusions are common in patients with flail chest.

Marked increases in inspiratory effort may cause intercostal, supraclavicular, or substernal retractions. Causes of retractions include upper airway obstruction, decreased lung compliance, or inadequate inspiratory gas flow during mechanical ventilation. Hyperinflation also may cause dimpling, or inward contraction of the chest wall, at the site of diaphragm insertion in patients with COPD. This is known as *Hoover's sign.*

Asymmetric movement of the chest may be caused by bronchial intubation, unilateral pneumonia, major atelectasis, pneumothorax, pneumonectomy, other unilateral disorders of lung, or chest wall expansion. Right-to-left symmetry of respiration can be assessed by placement of both hands parallel to one another on the chest wall (right and left) while observing chest expansion. If one side "lags" behind the other, right-left chest wall movement is asymmetric.

Finally, the presence of surgical scars resulting from pneumonectomy, lobectomy, or thoracotomy is of obvious interest, as is sternal scarring from prior open heart surgery. Radiation markers or small, pointlike tattoos on the chest wall for focusing radiation therapy also should be noted.

Palpation

Palpation of the chest wall may be used to determine chest expansion and to assess for the presence of tactile fremitus, tactile rhonchi, or tracheal deviation. The degree and symmetry of chest expansion are evaluated by positioning the tips of each thumb at approximately the eighth thoracic vertebra along the posterior chest wall as the patient takes a deep breath. Bilateral limitation to chest expansion may be noted with COPD and neuromuscular disease, whereas unilateral limitation may occur with lobar pneumonia or atelectasis on one side.

The clinician assesses tactile fremitus by placing the ulnar surface of the hand on the chest wall as the patient repeatedly speaks the number "99." The vibrations created are referred to as *tactile fremitus.* Air is a poor transmitter of sound, whereas fluid enhances transmission. Conditions that increase the air in the lung (e.g., pneumothorax, emphysema) decrease fremitus, whereas conditions that increase tissue density (e.g., consolidation, atelectasis) increase fremitus.

Subcutaneous emphysema is air under the skin, usually present in the neck and face. On palpation, the skin feels "crackly," similar to the feeling when one balls up a sheet of waxed paper. Because subcutaneous emphysema represents air that has escaped the lung and dissected into the tissues, the presence of subcutaneous emphysema also should suggest the possibility of pneumothorax (especially tension pneumothorax) or pneumomediastinum.

Tracheal deviation is movement or shift of the trachea away from the midline. The clinician can feel the position of the trachea by placing the index finger in the suprasternal notch. Tracheal deviation toward the affected side may be caused by massive atelectasis or severe pneumonia. Tension pneumothorax or bronchial intubation may shift the trachea away from the affected site.

Percussion

Percussion is performed by striking the patient's chest wall with the fingertip. There are two methods of percussion—mediate and intermediate. With mediate percussion, the clinician taps directly on the chest wall. With intermediate percussion, the clinician places the first and second finger of one hand between the chest wall and the hand used for percussion. Chest percussion allows for assessment of the density of the underlying lung tissue. Percussion over normal air-filled lung tissue has been compared to the sound heard by tapping on a watermelon, referred to as a *resonant percussion note*. Increased resonance can be compared to the sound heard when striking a hollow log, often referred to as *hyperresonance* or *tympany*. Conditions that increase the air in the lung increase resonance. Hyperresonant (tympanic) percussion notes are associated with hyperinflation (asthma, emphysema) or pneumothorax. Decreased air-to-lung tissue ratios decrease resonance— often referred to as dullness. Decreased resonance can be compared to the sound associated with striking a solid log. A dull percussion note may be due to pleural effusion, empyema, atelectasis, consolidation, or percussion over the liver, heart, or kidneys.

Auscultation

Auscultation used to assesss breath sounds is an essential part of the chest examination. The clinician should auscultate from side to side over both anterior and posterior aspects of the chest in a systematic fashion.

The character of normal breath sounds varies by position on the chest. For example, tracheal and bronchial breath sounds (which are coarse, harsh, loud sounds) are normally heard over the trachea and right and left mainstem bronchi. Bronchovesicular breath sounds are normally heard posteriorly over the area between the scapulae and anteriorly over the sternum. These sounds are not as loud or high-pitched as tracheal breath sounds. Vesicular breath sounds are heard over normal lung tissue throughout the rest of the thorax (i.e., in most places on the chest except over the large airways). Vesicular sounds are softer in intensity and lower in pitch. Adventitious breath sounds may indicate the presence of an abnormality affecting the lung parenchyma and/or the airways. Regarding adventitious parenchymal lung sounds, bronchial breath sounds may develop over areas of consolidated lung. Diminished breath sounds are associated with hypopnea, as noted with neuromuscular disease and sedative overdose or with an increase in the air-to-tissue ratio in the lung as occurs with emphysema and pneumothorax.

Abnormal airway sounds, such as wheezes, may be classified as continuous or discontinuous. Continuous sounds maintain a uniform pattern for at least one tenth of a second, whereas discontinuous sounds are shorter in duration. Wheezing and stridor are continuous sounds associated with airway narrowing. Stridor is a loud, high-pitched sound that can sometimes be heard without the use of a stethoscope. Stridor is a sign of upper airway obstruction and is a classic finding in laryngotracheobronchitis or croup and in conditions causing glottic narrowing (e.g., fixed narrowing at the level of the vocal cords).

Wheezes are generated by the vibration of the wall of a narrowed or compressed airway as air passes through at high velocity. During an asthma attack, the diameter of the airway can be reduced due to mucosal edema, secretions, and bronchospasm. When listening to breath sounds, the clinician should note the pitch, intensity, and portion of the respiratory cycle occupied by the wheeze. Wheezes vary in pitch by the site of origin and degree of narrowing. Wheezing due to severe bronchospasm during an acute asthma exacerbation is high in pitch. Obstruction of the bronchi that develops with chronic bronchitis as large amounts of tenacious sputum narrow the airways leads to a wheeze that is low in pitch. During an asthma attack, wheezing is usually heard on auscultation unless the airflow obstruction is so severe that airflow is markedly diminished (i.e., the "silent chest" of very severe asthma). Improvement in the patient's airway caliber can affect the pitch and intensity of the wheeze and the portion of the respiratory cycle occupied by the wheeze. High-pitched wheezes at end-expiration indicate less airflow obstruction than a lower-pitched wheeze throughout inspiration and expiration.

Crackles are discontinuous sounds associated with the sudden opening of small airways upon inspiration or the flow of gas through airway secretions. Crackles associated with sudden opening of small airways are described as "Velcro" crackles and are noted with pulmonary edema or pulmonary fibrosis. Crackles due to secretions may clear or improve after an effective cough.

Diminished or absent breath sounds are associated with decreased ventilation of that portion of the lung. Causes of diminished or absent breath sounds include severe COPD, pneumothorax, pleural effusion, atelectasis, or bronchial intubation. Rhonchi, which may clear following a cough, are coarse inspiratory sounds often associated with secretions in larger airways. "E-A" egophony is an audible "A" sound when the patient says "E." This sign is associated with consolidation. A pleural friction rub is a loud, dry, creaky, coarse, and leathery sound associated with pleural irritation.

Although the breath sound classification system described is widely used, clinicians often disagree about auscultatory findings and use these terms in various ways. As a crude classification scheme, these authors divide breath sounds into inspiratory and expiratory sounds. Inspiratory sounds include stridor, crackles (rales), rubs, and rhonchi. Wheezes are expiratory sounds.

Differential Diagnosis of the Clinical Problem

Critical diagnostic thinking requires the clinician to identify the problem, gather additional information, formulate possible explanations or hypotheses, test explanations, and make a diagnosis. The first step is identification and clarification of the problem. As noted, the patient history is used to identify specific patient problems or complaints. After identification of specific problems, the clinician performs the physical examination. The physical examination also may provide evidence that may be used to support, reject, or revise specific hypotheses as to the causes of the patient's problems. Finally, the physical examination may identify additional problems in the form of specific signs. For example, physical examination of the respiratory care patient may identify alterations in vital signs (tachypnea, tachycardia, fever); signs related to increased work of breathing (e.g., accessory muscle use); abnormal breath sounds (wheezing, crackles, rhonchi, and absent, diminished, or bronchial breath sounds); or alterations in mental status (e.g., anxiety, confusion, lethargy, somnolence, etc). Taken together, the signs and symptoms identified on history and physical examination make up the patient's problem list.

The next step in critical diagnostic thinking is to formulate possible solutions or generate a hypothesis. Each sign and symptom previously identified is listed, along with more common and less common causes of this sign or symptom. Table 1-3 lists common problems seen in the respiratory care patient, along with common causes

Text continued on p. 25.

TABLE 1-3
Differential Diagnoses of Cough, Sputum Production, Dyspnea, Hemoptysis, and Chest Pain

Problem	Common Causes	Less Common Causes
Acute cough	Viral upper respiratory infection (pharyngitis, rhinitis, tracheo-bronchitis, serous otitis) Bacterial infection (tracheo-bronchitis, acute bronchitis, mycoplasma, pneumonia, ear infection, sinusitis, abscess) Asthma Sinusitis Gastroesophageal reflux CHF, pulmonary edema Inhalation of irritants (smog, smoke fumes, dusts, cold air) Bronchiolitis (RSV)	Tumor, neoplasm Pulmonary emboli Aspiration (foreign body, liquid) Laryngitis ACE inhibitor medication Pleural disease Diaphragm irritation Mediastinal disease Extrabronchial lesions Fungal lung disease Ornithosis
Chronic cough	Post-nasal drip (sinusitis, allergic rhinitis) Smoking Asthma Chronic bronchitis Gastroesophageal reflux CHF Type I ACE inhibitor HIV Bronchiectasis Neoplasms, bronchogenic carcinoma Lung abscess Recurrent aspiration Aspiration (foreign body, liquid) Mycoplasma pneumonia Pulmonary tuberculosis Pulmonary fibrosis Cystic fibrosis	Chronic pulmonary edema Mitral stenosis Laryngeal inflammation or tumor Fungal pneumonia External or middle ear disease Bronchogenic cyst Mediastinal mass Zenker's diverticulum Aortic aneurysm Vagal irritation Pacemaker wires Pleural disease Pericardial, mediastinal, or diaphragm irritation Psychogenic cough
Acute dyspnea	Acute asthma (intermittent dyspnea) COPD exacerbation (chronic bronchitis, emphysema) Tracheobronchitis Pneumonia or other parenchymal inflammation Left-sided CHF Pulmonary edema (acute) Acute pulmonary emboli Myocardial ischemia (coronary artery disease, acute or chronic) Pneumothorax Hyperventilation (anxiety, metabolic acidosis)	Pulmonary hypertension Fever Anemia Pericardial tamponade Lung cancer Diaphragmatic paralysis Inhalation of noxious fumes or gases Space occupying lesions of the thorax Anaphylaxis Botulism Increased intracranial pressure

RSV, Respiratory syncytial virus; *ACE,* angiotensin-converting enzyme; *HIV,* human immmunodeficiency virus; *COPD,* chronic obstructive pulmonary disease; *CHF,* congestive heart failure.

TABLE 1-3

Differential Diagnoses of Cough, Sputum Production, Dyspnea, Hemoptysis, and Chest Pain—cont'd

Problem	Common Causes	Less Common Causes
Acute dyspnea —cont'd	Hypoxemia Large pleural effusion Upper airway obstruction (stridor, croup, epiglottis, laryngitis, laryngeal edema, foreign body aspiration) Non-cardiogenic pulmonary edema Aspiration (gastric liquid, foreign body) Atelectasis Chest trauma (pulmonary contusions, rib fractures, flail chest) Acutely increased work of breathing (decreased compliance and/or increased resistance) Shock Neuromuscular disease	
Chronic dyspnea (intermittent or persistent)	COPD (chronic bronchitis, emphysema, cystic fibrosis) CHF Asthma Interstitial fibrosis Hypoxemia Pulmonary hypertension Neuromuscular disease Poor physical conditioning with obesity Anemia Ascites Metabolic acidosis Aortic or mitral valve stenosis Arterial hypertension Chronically increased work of breathing (decreased compliance and/or increased resistance) Neuromuscular disease Bronchiectasis	Pulmonary alveolar proteinosis Alveolar microlithiasis Lipoid pneumonia Lung resection Recurrent pulmonary emboli Lung cancer Persistent large pleural effusion Kyphoscoliosis Tracheal stenosis Mitral stenosis Abdominal mass Pregnancy Congenital heart disease Abnormal hemoglobin Thyroid disease Idiopathic pulmonary hemosiderosis Aortic or mitral valve stenosis or regurgitation
Acute sputum production	Viral infection (tracheobronchitis, bronchiolitis, pneumonia) Bacterial infection (tracheobronchitis, pneumonia) Mycoplasma pneumonia Lung abscess Asthma Inhalation of irritants (smoke, smog, dusts, fumes)	Tuberculosis Lung abscess Neoplasms–lung tumor Foreign body aspiration

Continued

TABLE 1-3
Differential Diagnoses of Cough, Sputum Production, Dyspnea, Hemoptysis, and Chest Pain—cont'd

Problem	Common Causes	Less Common Causes
Chronic sputum production	COPD (chronic bronchitis, cystic fibrosis) Cigarette smoking Asthma Chronic sinusitis with drainage	Bronchiectasis Tuberculosis Lung abscess Bronchopleural fistula with empyema Recurrent aspiration
Hemoptysis	Bronchitis (acute and chronic) Bronchiectasis Lung abscess Tuberculosis Pneumonia (includes necrotizing pneumonias) Neoplasms–bronchogenic carcinoma Pulmonary embolism–pulmonary infarction Cystic fibrosis	Trauma Fungal lung disease (includes allergic bronchopulmonary aspergillosis) Empyema Aspiration (foreign body) Inhalation of toxic gases Arteriovenous fistula Broncholithiasis Goodpasture's syndrome Idiopathic pulmonary hemosiderosis Mycetoma Parasitic infection Wegener's granulomatosis Bronchogenic cyst Pulmonary endometriosis (catamenial hemoptysis)
Pleuritic or chest wall pain	Pleuritis Pneumonia Pulmonary embolism Empyema Tuberculosis Trauma Rib fracture Pneumothorax Hemothorax	Pulmonary infarction Irritation of intercostal nerves (herpes zoster, spinal nerve root disease) Costochondritis Irritation of the diaphragm
Visceral chest pain	Tumor, neoplasm of major bronchi, mediastinum Abnormalities of the heart, aorta, pericardium Esophageal pain (reflux, tumor) Acute bronchitis	Peptic ulcer Cocaine use Cholecystitis
Substernal pain	Myocardial ischemia, angina pectoris Myocardial infarction Esophagitis, esophageal pain Arrhythmias Myocarditis Pericarditis	Dissecting aortic aneurysm Congenital cardiovascular anomalies Aortic stenosis Mitral regurgitation Mitral valve prolapse Psychogenic chest pain

RSV, Respiratory syncytial virus; *ACE,* angiotensin-converting enzyme; *HIV,* human immmunodeficiency virus; *COPD,* chronic obstructive pulmonary disease; *CHF,* congestive heart failure.

and less common causes of these problems. This list of possible causes makes up the "likely suspects," explanations, or hypotheses to be evaluated in determining the appropriate diagnosis. After generation of explanations as to possible causes of the problems listed, the clinician reviews possible causes for each sign and symptom to determine which explanations are common to multiple signs and symptoms.

For example, a patient may present with chronic cough, sputum production, and progressive, persistent exertional dyspnea. Physical examination may reveal tachypnea, tachycardia, and accessory muscle use. Wheezing, crackles, and bronchial breath sounds may be noted on auscultation. The differential diagnosis as to the most common possible causes for the patient's problems would include chronic bronchitis, asthmatic bronchitis, acute exacerbation of COPD, and bronchiectasis. Additional possible explanations may include respiratory infection, which in turn may be viral, bacterial, fungal, or mycoplasmal in origin.

Clinical Features that Suggest a Specific Cause

After developing a list of the patient's problems (signs and symptoms), as well as the most common and less common causes, the respiratory care clinician must then relate specific aspects of the history and physical examination to generate a leading diagnosis. The process of development of a leading diagnosis must take into account the prevalence of specific diseases and typical presentation and should coincide with possible causes (hypotheses) generated on review of the patient's signs and symptoms. Development of a leading diagnosis depends on the patient's symptoms (history) and physical examination (signs). Confirmation or rejection of the leading diagnosis then depends on the results of additional diagnostic tests and laboratory studies. Typical presentations for common pulmonary disorders are described in Table 1-4.

▼ Laboratory Evaluation

Laboratory studies that are often helpful in evaluating the patient with pulmonary symptoms include arterial blood gas analysis, chest x-ray, pulmonary function testing, complete blood count, blood chemistry, and sputum analysis. A brief discussion of each type of laboratory test follows, with specific attention paid to ways in which the results of laboratory tests must be interpreted in the context of the history and physical examination. The chapters that follow discuss these tests more extensively in the specific context of pulmonary symptoms (what the patient experiences) and signs (what the clinician observes). The excellent clinician orders laboratory tests sparsely and only to help refine the diagnosis and/or to optimize the patient's management. Because laboratory tests may confer risks to the patient and incur expense, tests should be ordered only when their results will affect management in a reasoned way.

Arterial Blood Gases

Arterial blood gas (ABG) analysis remains the gold standard for the assessment of oxygenation, ventilation, and acid-base balance. A normal arterial oxygen tension

TABLE 1-4
Typical Presentations of Common Respiratory Disorders

	History	Physical Examination	Laboratory Tests
Viral upper respiratory infection	Nasal congestion, runny nose, scratchy sore throat, laryngitis, cough, sputum production	Mucopurulent nasal discharge, fever, pale, boggy, swollen pharynx Breath sounds may show gurgles or coarse rhonchi	Chest radiograph may be clear, throat culture to rule out streptococcal infection
Sinusitis	Post-nasal drip, cough, sneezing, nasal congestion, facial pain, pressure or fullness	Headache pain worsened by touch	Sinus CT scan
Mycoplasma bronchitis or pneumonia	Dry hacking cough progressing to cough with purulent sputum	Fever, crackles, signs of pneumonia	Chest radiograph–signs of pneumonia, Gram's stain negative except for neutrophils, bedside cold agglutinins positive, ESR elevated
Pneumonia	Cough, purulent or rusty sputum, fever, chills, dyspnea, pleuritic chest pain	Sudden onset, spiking fever with rigors, mental status changes associated with hypoxemia, tachycardia, tachypnea, cyanosis, crackles, bronchial breath sounds, egophony, vocal fremitus, diminished breath sounds, dull percussion note	New or progressive infiltrate on chest radiograph, sputum analysis (color, amount, consistency, odor, Gram's stain, direct fluorescent antibody stain, fungal stains, acid-fast stains, culture and sensitivity), WBC with differential
Atelectasis	History of recent abdominal or thoracic surgery, immobilization, chest wall pain, muscular weakness, thoracic or abdominal limitation to diaphragmatic excursion (ascites, obesity, peritonitis, thoracic deformity,	Decreased chest wall movement over affected side, absent or diminished breath sounds, dull percussion node, crackles	Findings associated with atelectasis on chest radiograph, decreased inspiratory capacity, vital capacity

etc.), weakness, neuromuscular disease, pneumonia or other acute restrictive disease, other chronic restrictive pulmonary disease, sedatives or narcotics

COPD exacerbation (chronic bronchitis, emphysema)	Chronic cough with sputum production (chronic bronchitis), increased dyspnea, orthopnea, decreased mobility	Diffuse wheezing, cyanosis (chronic bronchitis), dependent edema, clinical manifestations of hypoxemia, increased AP diameter, accessory muscle use, pursed lip breathing, diminished breath sounds, prolonged expiration, wheezing, crackles, rhonchi	Decreased FEV_1/FVC; hyperinflation on chest radiograph, possible new infiltrates
Pleural effusion	Dyspnea, pleuritic chest pain, cough	Chest wall movement reduced over affected side, dull percussion note, absent or diminished breath sounds over effusion, egophony and/or bronchial breath sounds above effusion, pleural rub may be present	Chest x-ray consistent with pleural effusion, thoracentesis, pleural fluid analysis (appearance, WBC and differential, Gram's stain, culture, glucose, amylase)
Pneumothorax	Chest pain, dyspnea	Tachycardia, tachypnea, respiratory distress, tracheal deviation to opposite side with tension, decreased chest wall movement on affected side, resonant or hyperresonant percussion note, absent or decreased breath sounds	Chest x-ray consistent with pneumothorax, arterial blood gases, oximetry may show hypoxemia with or without hypercapnea

CT, Computed tomography; ESR, erythyrocytic sedimentation rate; WBC, white blood cells; FEV₁, forced expiratory volume in 1 second; FVC, forced vital capacity; AP, anteroposterior.

(PaO$_2$) is 80 to 100 torr (or mm Hg), which should result in an arterial oxygen saturation (SaO$_2$) of about 95% to 97%. Mild, moderate, and severe hypoxemia can be defined as an arterial PaO$_2$ of <80 torr, <60 torr, and <50 torr, respectively. However, in the acute care setting, a minimal PaO$_2$ of at least 60 torr is often satisfactory, resulting in an SaO$_2$ ≥90%. As a rough guideline, a PaO$_2$ of 50 torr corresponds to an SaO$_2$ of about 85% and a PaO$_2$ of 40 torr corresponds to an SaO$_2$ of about 75%. Measurement of SpO$_2$ via pulse oximetry is often relied on as a substitute for ABG analysis and actual measurement of SaO$_2$ and PaO$_2$. However, the correlation between SpO$_2$ and measured SaO$_2$ is much weaker than is often assumed. In addition, SpO$_2$ should not be relied on in the presence of increased levels of carboxyhemoglobin or methemoglobin. Pulse oximetry also can be inaccurate in the presence of low blood pressure, poor perfusion, and very low oxygen levels. The SpO$_2$ also is less reliable in the presence of artificial or painted fingernails, vascular dyes, jaundice, and darkly pigmented skin.

It also should be noted that arterial oxygen content (CaO$_2$) depends on PaO$_2$, SaO$_2$, and hemoglobin levels. Oxygen delivery (DO$_2$) is determined by CaO$_2$ and cardiac output (Q$_T$) where DO$_2$ = CaO$_2$ × Q$_T$. A normal CaO$_2$ is about 20 mL O$_2$/100 mL of blood, with a normal DO$_2$ being about 1000 mL of O$_2$/minute. Decreased hemoglobin levels or reductions in cardiac output can result in profound decreases in DO$_2$, even in the face of an otherwise adequate PaO$_2$ and SaO$_2$. Evaluation of the patient with hypoxia is described in Chapter 23, and refractory hypoxemia is discussed in Chapter 34.

Measurement of arterial pH establishes the patient's overall acid-base balance. Acidemia is defined as a pH of less than 7.35, normal as a pH of 7.35 to 7.45, and alkalemia as a pH of greater than 7.45. The terms *acidemia* and *alkalemia* refer to the net effect of changes in respiration and metabolic status on pH, whereas the terms *acidosis* and *alkalosis* refer to trends in the carbon dioxide tension and bicarbonate concentration that contribute to the net effect. For example, the patient with a profound metabolic acidosis (decreased serum bicarbonate) may have a net alkalemia if an accompanying respiratory alkalosis (decreased PCO$_2$) of sufficient degree is present.

Arterial blood pH is determined primarily by the ratio of base (HCO$_3$⁻) to acid (PaCO$_2$). The kidneys control the level of bicarbonate (HCO$_3$⁻), the major base in the blood, whereas the level of ventilation determines the arterial carbon dioxide level (PaCO$_2$). Increased PaCO$_2$ or decreased HCO$_3$⁻ can lead to acidosis, whereas a decreased PaCO$_2$ or increased HCO$_3$⁻ may cause an overall alkalosis. Common causes of a metabolic acidosis (decreased HCO$_3$⁻) include lactic acidosis, ketoacidosis, renal failure, and severe diarrhea. Ingestion of acids, such as aspirin, antifreeze (ethylene glycol), methanol, and hydrochloric acid, also may cause a metabolic acidosis. Common causes of metabolic alkalosis (increased HCO$_3$⁻) include vomiting, nasogastric suction, diuretics, hypochloremia, hypokalemia, hypovolemia, and NaHCO$_3$⁻ ingestion or infusion.

Normal ventilation maintains arterial PaCO$_2$ values between 35 and 45 mm Hg. Hyperventilation (respiratory alkalosis) can be defined as a PaCO$_2$ <35 mm Hg and hypoventilation (respiratory acidosis) as a PaCO$_2$ >45 mm Hg. Acute ventilatory failure is a sudden rise in PaCO$_2$ (>45 to 50 mm Hg) with a corresponding drop in pH. Chronic ventilatory failure is suggested when an elevated PaCO$_2$ is accompanied by an elevated serum HCO$_3$⁻ and a resulting normal or near-normal pH.

Common causes of acute ventilatory failure include severe pneumonia, acute pulmonary edema, sedative or narcotic drug overdose, and trauma to the head, chest, or high spinal cord. Chronic ventilatory failure is often associated with stable, severe COPD. Common causes of a respiratory alkalosis (hyperventilation) include hypoxemia, anxiety, pain, fever, pulmonary emboli, liver disease, and sepsis. Patients with acute asthma, pneumonia, pulmonary edema, or pulmonary emboli also may present with hypoxemia and respiratory alkalosis, which may then progress to acute ventilatory failure as the patient's condition worsens.

Chest Radiography and Medical Imaging

Because the chest radiograph is an indispensable tool in the evaluation of patients with lung disease, the well-prepared respiratory care clinician should have an excellent working knowledge of the chest x-ray. Careful interpretation of the film enhances critical diagnostic thinking by enhancing diagnostic skills and by improving the appreciation of response to therapy.

With regard to diagnosis, the plain chest x-ray can help detect and diagnose a variety of conditions, including atelectasis, pneumonia, acute lung injury and acute respiratory distress syndrome (ARDS), pulmonary edema, pleural effusion, tumor, cavitary lung disease and lung abscess, interstitial pulmonary fibrosis, pneumothorax, and lung hyperinflation. The most common disturbances on chest x-ray relate to changes in air or fluid volume. Air is less dense than fluid on x-ray and appears radiolucent or dark. Fluid, bone, and soft tissue are more dense and appear radiopaque, with bone appearing densest and frankly white.

Atelectasis is the loss of lung volume due to collapse of alveoli. The manifestation on the chest x-ray may be as subtle as small white streaks due to alveolar collapse or a large density when an entire lobe or lung develops atelectasis. Atelectasis of a lung segment or lobe may cause narrowing of the rib spaces and movement of lung fissure lines and hilar structures toward the affected area. A rise in the hemidiaphragm on the affected side also may be observed as an indirect sign of atelectasis.

Hyperinflation is another important finding on the chest x-ray and may be due to air trapping as in asthma, chronic bronchitis, emphysema, or cystic fibrosis. Hyperinflation causes the lung fields to appear darker or more radiolucent. Other radiographic changes associated with hyperinflation include widening of the rib spaces, low, flat diaphragms, and a narrow heart shadow.

Pneumothorax is defined as air in the pleural space. As the pleural space fills with air, the lung collapses toward the hilum on the affected side. The chest x-ray shows a radiolucent or dark area without vascular markings on the affected side. Pneumothorax may be spontaneous or traumatic. The application of positive pressure breathing by manual resuscitator bag or mechanical ventilator can cause a tension pneumothorax, a life-threatening event if unrecognized and untreated. In tension pneumothorax, tracheal and mediastinal shift occurs away from the affected side on the chest x-ray.

Increased fluid in the lung increases the opacity or whiteness on the chest film. Pleural fluid often appears "hazy" with obliteration of the costophrenic angle on the affected side. Interstitial fluid is sometimes described as "dots and lines" or as branching, linear, streaky infiltrates. Alveolar filling may be described as soft, fluffy, and poorly demarcated or as having a "ground glass" appearance. With alveolar filling, air bronchograms may be present. Air bronchograms are caused by parenchymal consolidation that is adjacent to an air-filled bronchus.

The silhouette sign is another important finding on a chest x-ray and refers to the loss of the normal radiographic edge of a structure (e.g., the heart or aorta) when the adjacent tissue has the same density. For example, normally, the heart shadow is clearly distinguished from the lung because the air in the lung is less dense than the fluid density in the heart and the contrast allows the edge of the heart to be seen. However, when the lung adjacent to the heart is consolidated (e.g., filled with a fluid density like water or pus), the edge of the heart no longer can be seen but blends into or is hidden by the adjacent lung that has the same density. In this case, a "silhouette sign" is present, or the heart border is said to be "silhouetted" by the fluid-filled lung. The presence and position of a silhouette sign can help identify the location of a pulmonary infiltrate. For example, an infiltrate that obscures the right heart border is probably in the right middle lobe, whereas a nearby infiltrate that obscures the right hemidiaphragm but not the heart border is more likely to be in the right lower lobe.

The plain chest x-ray can be very helpful in the diagnosis and management of pulmonary edema, which occurs when a transudative (plasma-like) fluid fills the interstitial and then the alveolar spaces. The chest x-ray findings may include pulmonary edema, enlargement of the heart shadow (e.g., cardiomegaly), pleural effusions (often bilateral), and so-called cephalization of blood flow, meaning that the vessels feeding the apices of the lung appear fuller than normal. Acute lung injury and ARDS may also produce a picture of pulmonary edema, though due in this case to a "non-cardiogenic" cause; specifically, capillary damage in the lung allows fluid to leak from pulmonary capillaries into the interstitial tissues nearby or into the alveoli themselves. Unlike the pulmonary edema due to congestive heart failure, non-cardiogenic pulmonary edema typically demonstrates diffuse, bilateral infiltrates on chest x-ray, a normal heart size, and lower (<18 mm Hg) pulmonary artery occlusion pressure.

Pneumonia may be diagnosed based on the development of a new or progressive infiltrate on chest x-ray in conjunction with two or more of the following: fever, increased white blood cell count, and/or purulent sputum. Clinical signs and symptoms might appear before the development of radiologic changes. Lobar consolidation may suggest a bacterial pneumonia, whereas an interstitial infiltrate may suggest a non-bacterial cause (e.g., *P. carinii*, viral, fungal, or so-called atypical pneumonia of which *Mycoplasma pneumoniae* is one cause). Bacterial pneumonia may cause a purulent exudate to fill the affected lung tissue with fluid, causing lobar consolidation, as is sometimes seen with streptococcal and klebsiella pneumonias. As an important clue on the chest x-ray, the location of the infiltrate may be helpful in establishing a cause of the infiltrate. For example, an apical infiltrate should suggest the possibility of tuberculosis, whereas an infiltrate in the dependent lung segments (lower lung zones) could be due to aspiration, with gravity causing the consolidation in lower lung areas.

A pleural effusion is fluid in the pleural space and typically causes a hazy border of the lung and blunting or obscuring of the costophrenic angle on chest film. The differential diagnosis of pleural effusion is very extensive (e.g., includes congestive heart failure, abdominal problems [ascites, pancreatitis, surgery], infection [bacterial pneumonia, TB], trauma, malignancy, pulmonary embolism, pulmonary infarction, collagen vascular disease, and hypoalbuminemia [e.g., due to cirrhosis, starvation, or kidney disease]). Determining the specific cause of a pleural effusion may require sampling and analyzing the fluid but also may depend on careful integration of the features of the history and physical examination. In this way, information from the chest x-ray is useful to the respiratory clinician in critical diagnostic reasoning.

Other important findings on the plain chest x-ray for the respiratory care clinician include the position of the endotracheal tube in intubated patients and the position and course of other tubes and catheters, such as chest tubes, central venous lines, and pulmonary artery catheters. The tip of the endotracheal tube in intubated patients should lie in the middle third of the trachea at least 3 cm above the carina.

Finally, although the plain chest x-ray is an immensely helpful tool, other imaging techniques may be needed to best evaluate lung conditions. A working knowledge of other imaging studies, such as computed tomography, ventilation-perfusion scanning, and pulmonary angiography, enhances the respiratory care clinician's critical diagnostic skills.

Hematology

Assessment of the patient's red and white blood cell counts and characteristics is another important element of diagnostic reasoning. The complete blood count (CBC) includes an analysis of red blood cells (RBCs) and white blood cells (WBCs). RBC analysis includes the RBC count, hemoglobin level (Hgb), hematocrit, and erythrocyte indices. The normal RBC count is 4.6 to 6.2 × 106/mm^3 for men and 4.2 to 5.4 × 106/mm^3 for women. Hemoglobin is the molecule packaged within the RBC that carries oxygen. Normal adult Hgb values are about 15 g/dL, with a range of about 12 to 16 g/dL. Hematocrit (Hct) is the percentage of RBC volume to total blood volume. Adult values should be about three times the Hgb level or about 38% to 54%. Polycythemia refers to an increase in RBC mass and is commonly caused by chronic hypoxemia, which triggers the release of erythropoietin and stimulates the bone marrow to produce more RBCs. The resultant increase in RBCs increases Hgb and total oxygen-carrying capacity of the blood. Anemia or blood loss causes a decrease in RBC count and Hgb and thus reduces the oxygen-carrying capacity of the blood. The CaO_2 may be calculated as: $CaO_2 = (1.34 \times Hgb \times SaO_2) + 0.003 (PaO_2)$. Given a normal PaO_2 of 100 mm Hg, an (SaO_2) of 97% (0.97) and an Hgb of 15g/dL, the resultant CaO_2 would have a normal value of 19.8 ml O_2/100 mL of blood (19.8 volumes %). In the face of anemia or blood loss causing an Hgb of only 5g/dL, CaO_2 would drop to 6.8 mL O_2/100 mL blood even if the PaO_2 and SaO_2 remained normal. Thus, although anemia does not generally affect the PaO_2, anemia can compromise the oxygen-carrying capacity of the blood and must be considered in patients with evidence of perfusion impairment.

Analysis of the WBCs (leukocytes) includes measurement of the total number, as well as the percent distribution of the various types of WBC (e.g., polymorphonuclear leukocyte, eosinophil, basophil, lymphocyte, etc). A normal WBC count is 4500 to 11,500/mm^3. An elevated WBC count, called *leukocytosis*, may be associated with infection. A decrease in the WBC count, *leukopenia*, may be sometimes caused by a viral infection, although other causes, such as chemotherapy, radiation therapy, or certain drugs that suppress the bone marrow production, also must be considered.

The WBC differential count measures the types of WBCs by number and percentage per 100 WBCs. Neutrophils (segmented and band forms) make up 40% to 75% of the WBC count. Neutrophils provide the major defense against bacterial infections. Neutrophilia (increased neutrophils) is commonly associated with inflammation and infection, such as a bacteria pneumonia. Bands are immature neutrophils. Bands normally comprise up to 6% of the WBC count. A so-called left shift refers to an increase in the number of immature neutrophils, usually bands, due to stress, infection, or inflammation. Neutropenia (decreased neutrophils) may occur with overwhelming infection but may occur from all the causes cited for leukopenia.

Lymphocytes normally comprise 20% to 45% of the total WBCs. As a generalization, T lymphocytes are involved in cellular immunity and B lymphocytes are concerned with production of antibodies. Although many other causes exist, a common cause of lymphocytosis (increased lymphocytes) is viral infection, including viral pneumonia and mononucleosis. Lymphocytopenia (decreased lymphocytes) can occur as a result of trauma, various infections, or progression of human immunodeficiency virus (HIV) infection.

Monocytes normally represent 2% to 10% of the differential count. Monocytosis may be seen with malignancies and chronic infections such as tuberculosis, syphilis, and some fungal lung diseases.

Eosinophils normally comprise up 6% of the WBCs. Common causes of eosinophilia include allergic reactions, asthma, and parasitic infections. Basophils comprise up to 1% of the WBC count and do not generally play a role in pulmonary disorders.

Platelets are the blood component responsible for clot formation; a decrease in the platelet count can cause bleeding or hemorrhage. Causes of a decreased platelet count include bone marrow suppression (e.g., by drugs) or replacement (e.g., by invading cancer), excess breakdown of platelets (e.g., caused by reactions to drugs or autoimmune disorders), or consumption of platelets (e.g., by an enlarged spleen). Coagulation studies include platelet count, bleeding time, activated partial thromboplastin time (APTT), and the prothrombin time (PT) or international normalized ratio (INR). The APTT and INR also are used to monitor anticoagulant therapy (heparin and warfarin, respectively), which often is used to treat or prevent pulmonary emboli.

Clinical Chemistry

Basic blood chemistry values include measurement of electrolytes, serum enzymes, and glucose. Serum electrolytes include sodium (Na^+), potassium (K^-), chloride (CL^-), and bicarbonate (HCO_3^-). Of special interest to the respiratory care clinician is the effect of electrolyte disturbances on acid-base balance. Hypokalemia, hypochloremia, and HCO_3^- infusion may cause a metabolic alkalosis, whereas loss of HCO_3^-, hyperkalemia, and hyperchloremia may contribute to a metabolic acidosis. Calculation of the patient's so-called anion gap (where the anion gap = $[Na^+]$ − ($[Cl^-]$ + (HCO_3^-)) is helpful in the evaluation of the cause of metabolic acidosis. A normal anion gap is 9 to 14 mEq/L.

A metabolic acidosis with an increased anion gap (a so-called gap or delta acidosis) may be due to the accumulation of lactic acid or ketoacids, renal failure, or ingestion of ethylene glycol, methanol (wood alcohol), or aspirin overdose. Metabolic acidosis with a normal anion gap (so-called non-gap acidosis) can be caused by diarrhea, pancreatic fistula, renal tubular acidosis, drugs called *carbonic anhydrase inhibitors* (such as acetazolamide, sometimes used to treat glaucoma), the ingestion of ammonium chloride, or intravenous hyperalimentation.

Kidney function can be assessed by analysis of serum creatinine and blood urea nitrogen (BUN). Kidney disease, shock, heart failure, and hypotension may increase the BUN. Elevated creatinine levels often are associated with a decrease in glomerular function or in diseases associated with muscle breakdown (which spills creatinine precursors into the circulation).

Finally, glucose levels are important in the diagnosis of diabetes mellitus (i.e., when the blood sugar is abnormally elevated) and in monitoring the effect of drug therapy for diabetes. Low glucose levels can occur when the dose of drugs for diabetes are too high or in other conditions (e.g., sepsis, adrenal insufficiency, hypothyroidism).

Microbiologic Evaluation

The diagnosis of infections depends on the ability to stain and or culture the responsible organisms that are causing disease. Various tissues and body fluids can be sampled for staining and culture, including urine, blood, cerebrospinal fluid (CSF, the fluid around the spinal cord), and sputum. In the assessment of pneumonia, sputum examination, Gram's stain (a standard staining technique that distinguishes organisms that take up the stain [gram positive] from those that do not take up the stain [gram negative]), culture, and sensitivity can help identify the specific cause of pneumonias that are caused by bacteria, fungi, protozoa, or viruses.

Other stains (e.g., silver, acid-fast stain, Giemsa, etc.) can be used to demonstrate other organisms (e.g., *P. carinii*, fungus, mycobacteria). For example, the Kinyoun stain for AFB is useful when examining sputum specimens for the presence of mycobacteria. India ink preparation may identify cryptococci present in the CSF, whereas Giemsa-stained blood smears may identify patients with blood parasitic infections. Methenamine silver staining of the sputum may help to identify *P. carinii* as the causative agent of pneumonia.

Other tests that enhance the diagnosis of infection include antibody titers (i.e., measuring the levels of antibodies produced to infectious agents) and serum concentrations of infectious agents (e.g., viral amounts or titers in HIV infection).

Pulmonary Function Studies

Pulmonary function testing may include simple spirometry (forced expiratory volume in 1 second [FEV_1], forced vital capacity [FVC], and peak expiratory flow rate [PEFR]), measurement of lung volumes (functional residual capacity [FRC], residual volume [RV], and total lung capacity [TLC]), flow-volume studies, tests for diffusion capacity (DLCO), airway resistance, response to a bronchodilator, methacholine challenge, and cardiopulmonary exercise testing.

Simple spirometry can be quickly accomplished with a variety of compact devices that meet American Thoracic Society standards. Restrictive pulmonary disorders are characterized by a decrease in the TLC, often with decreased FVC, whereas obstructive disorders are associated with decreased expiratory flow rates (FEV_1, FEV in 3 seconds [FEV_3], and PEFR). Measurement of FVC and FEV_1 are the most commonly used measures for assessing restrictive and obstructive pulmonary disease. Restrictive pulmonary diseases typically exhibit FVC values below 80% of those predicted, with a normal FEV_1/FVC ratio ($FEV_1/FVC \geq 0.75$). Chronic restrictive disorders include interstitial lung disease such as pulmonary fibrosis, sarcoidosis, or pneumoconiosis. Acute restrictive parenchymal disorders include pneumonia, acute lung injury, ARDS, and pulmonary edema. Pleural disease (effusion, pneumothorax) also may acutely reduce lung volumes. Extrapulmonary restrictive disorders include chest wall deformities (such as kyphoscoliosis, pectus excavatum), neuromuscular disease, obesity, ascites, and diaphragmatic paralysis. Pregnancy and congestive heart failure also may cause a reduction in lung volumes measured by pulmonary function testing. As a rough guideline, the degree of impairment with restrictive disease in patients who also do not have an obstructive defect ($FEV_1/FVC \geq 0.75$) can be classified as follows:

FVC <80% predicted—mild restriction
FVC <60% predicted—moderate restriction
FVC <50% predicted—severe restriction

In the presence of obstruction, measurement of TLC should be used to assess the degree of restriction. A TLC <80% predicted can be classified as mild, <70% predicted as moderate, and <60% of predicted as severe restriction.

Obstructive lung disease typically causes a decrease in FEV_1/FVC ratio to less than 0.75. Obstructive disorders include asthma, emphysema, chronic bronchitis, bronchiectasis, and cystic fibrosis. As a decreased D_{LCO} often reflects the loss of alveolocapillary units, patients with emphysema who experience loss of alveolar walls characteristically have decreased values of D_{LCO}. In contrast, with "pure" chronic bronchitis and asthma, where alveoli are preserved, the D_{LCO} is classically normal. As a general guideline, the degree of obstruction can be classified as follows:

FEV_1/FVC <0.75—mild obstruction
FEV_1/FVC <0.60—moderate obstruction
FEV_1/FVC <0.40—severe obstruction

Obstructive and restrictive defects may coexist, such as in a patient with COPD (obstructive disease) who also has pulmonary fibrosis or congestive heart failure. In such patients, a decreased TLC may be accompanied by a decreased FEV_1/FVC.

Response to a bronchodilator can help evaluate whether the patient has a component of reversible airway obstruction. Criteria for a significant response to a bronchodilator include a rise in the FEV_1 and/or FVC by at least 12% (from pre- to post-bronchodilator) and 200 mL. Notably, although the presence of a bronchodilator response establishes the presence of reversible airflow obstruction, the absence of a bronchodilator response does not rule out reversibility.

A methacholine challenge test, in which the cholinergic agent, methacholine, is given in increasing concentrations while expiratory flow rates and airway resistance are serially measured, can help evaluate patients in whom airway hyperreactivity is suspected. In patients with hyperactive airways, the FEV_1 will fall by at least 20% at a concentration of methacholine below 25 mg/mL. Such an abnormal result may permit a trial of asthma therapy for the presenting symptom, e.g., cough.

Finally, cardiopulmonary exercise testing may help determine if the patient's exercise limitation is due to pulmonary disease, cardiac disease, or deconditioning.

▼ ASSESSMENT OF THE EFFECT OF THERAPY

For some signs and symptoms, an important aspect of clinical assessment is evaluation of the response to treatment. For example, the effect of the administration of a bronchodilator to a wheezing patient provides important diagnostic information. A reduction in wheezing and an improvement in PEFR and/or FEV_1 after bronchodilator therapy provide good evidence for the presence of reversible bronchospasm consistent with a diagnosis of asthma. On the other hand, absence of a response to a bronchodilator may point to other causes of the wheezing, such as partial airway obstruction due to a tumor. Response to oxygen therapy also can help determine the differential diagnosis of hypoxemia. For example, hypoxemia due to diseases that cause low ventilation-to-perfusion (low $\dot{V}/\dot{Q}$) ratio often respond well to the administration of low-to-moderate concentrations of oxygen. Examples include asthma, chronic bronchitis, emphysema, bronchiectasis, and cystic fibrosis. On the other hand, hypoxemia due to anatomic shunt generally does not respond well to low-to-moderate concentrations of oxygen. Moderate-to-high concentrations of oxygen with the application of positive end-expiratory pressure (PEEP) may be required to reverse hypoxemia in conditions associated with significant, diffuse alveolar collapse such as ARDS.

▼ PITFALLS AND COMMON MISTAKES

Common mistakes made in critical diagnostic thinking include faulty hypothesis generation, faulty context formulation, faulty information gathering and processing, faulty estimation of disease prevalence when evaluating a specific hypothesis, anchoring, vertical line failure, and faulty hypothesis verification.

Faulty hypothesis generation refers to the failure to consider possible causes that should be considered. Faulty hypothesis generation is more likely to occur in the presence of atypical or unusual presentations of common diseases and also may occur when the clinician is faced with uncommon or unfamiliar disease states or conditions.

Faulty context formulation occurs when the clinician only considers a narrow range of specific diagnoses based on the close resemblance to a typical disease presentation. In this case, the clinician may consider only obvious causes to the exclusion of alternative possible causes. A similar error can occur when the clinician considers only an exotic possible diagnosis. Uncommon diseases are often over-represented in the literature, which may cause the clinician to favor a more exotic but incorrect diagnosis.

Faulty information gathering and processing includes failure to obtain relevant information, failure to effectively link key features of a patient's presentation, and failure to consider possible errors in laboratory and diagnostic testing. For example, appropriate laboratory tests relevant to a specific diagnosis may not be ordered. Alternatively, the clinician may fail to recognize the possibility of false-positive or false-negative laboratory test results. The probability of a positive test in a patient who has the disease in question is referred to as the *sensitivity* of the test. The probability of a negative test in a patient who does not have the disease in question is referred to as the *specificity* of the test. As the specificity of a test increases, the sensitivity decreases, and vice versa.

Faulty estimation of disease prevalence also may result in errors in critical diagnostic thinking, including failure to consider common problems and failure to consider uncommon problems. The novice respiratory care clinician may be inappropriately drawn to an exotic diagnosis at the expense of carefully considering more common causes of a patient's specific signs and symptoms. Alternatively, a more exotic, but possible cause may not be considered, and appropriate testing may not be ordered after the more common causes of specific signs and symptoms have been ruled out.

Anchoring refers to the common error of accepting a label previously assigned to a patient without adequately considering alternative hypotheses. A diagnosis that has been assigned to a patient before the clinician's careful assessment and evaluation always must be considered as provisional. For example, a COPD patient admitted to the emergency department may be in the hospital for reasons that have nothing to do with the COPD diagnosis. Furthermore, the label of COPD may be inappropriately given. Imagine the consequences of assuming that the patient's current problem is COPD, when the patient may have really suffered a stroke or MI. As a rule, the clinician should confirm the evidence supporting the patient's diagnosis.

Vertical line failure refers to erroneous conclusions based on an assumed progression for the patient's condition. For example, the COPD patient who arrives in the emergency department is assumed to be suffering from an acute exacerbation. This assumption is based on knowledge of the typical progression of COPD; however, this assumption may be in error. Lateral or non-vertical line thinking is required to consider alternative hypotheses as to causes of the patient's condition, such as stroke or MI.

Finally, faulty hypothesis verification involves failure to perform a final check before a specific diagnosis is accepted. For example, a less likely diagnosis may be rejected in favor of a more common diagnosis simply because the clinician has failed to pursue the less common hypothesis, which can occur because of fatigue, difficulty in assessment, cost, or unfamiliarity with a less common diagnostic path.

▼ SUMMARY

The use of critical diagnostic thinking skills by the respiratory care clinician is essential to provide patients with appropriate care and monitoring while minimizing misallocation of resources. The most commonly used approach to critical diagnostic thinking involves the application of the scientific method to clinical problem solving. The first step in critical diagnostic thinking is identification of the perceived problem. Initially, the patient's problems are identified and clarified and a patient history and physical examination are obtained. Hypotheses as to possible causes of the problem then are generated and a list of "likely suspects" identified. Next, additional diagnostic tests are identified and performed to evaluate each hypothesis, moving from most common to less common causes. Based on test results and related observations, hypotheses are revised, accepted, or rejected. The differential diagnosis takes into consideration the prevalence, as well as clinical features and typical presentations of specific disease states and conditions.

Common pitfalls in critical diagnostic thinking include failure to consider possible causes (hypotheses) that should be considered, pursuit of an exotic diagnosis in favor of a more common cause of the observed signs and symptoms, failure to recognize false-positive and false-negative test results, acceptance of an early diagnosis without adequate verification, drawing of erroneous conclusions by assuming a natural progression to a disease state or condition that is incorrect, and failure to consider a less likely cause after the more prevalent causes of the patient's signs and symptoms have been ruled out.

The process of diagnosis involves integration of the patient's symptoms and signs with a comprehensive list of "suspect" conditions, which could plausibly explain them. Because the comprehensive list of suspect conditions is often large (except in the rare instances in which the patient's symptoms are characteristic of only a few underlying causes), the process of critical diagnostic reasoning involves two simultaneous activities: (1) considering a separate "list of suspects" for each of the patient's relevant symptoms and searching for "suspects" common to all these lists, and (2) considering which underlying conditions best explain the characteristics of the patient's symptoms. An important aspect of this second activity is fully characterizing the patient's symptoms according to what elicits the symptom, what alleviates the symptom, when it occurs, how long it lasts, whether it waxes and wanes or progressively worsens, and whether there is a pattern to its occurrence. By integrating the information obtained from a careful history, physical examination, and carefully selected laboratory tests with full knowledge of the suspect conditions, the clinician is capable of establishing a diagnosis. This process of data gathering and integration represents critical diagnostic thinking that is the subject of the chapters that follow.

▼ BIBLIOGRAPHY

Adler SN, Gasbarra DB, Adler-Klein D: *A pocket manual of differential diagnosis*, ed 4, Philadelphia, 2000, Lippincott, Williams & Wilkins.

Andreoli TE, Bennett JC, Carpenter CCS, et al: *Cecil essentials of medicine*, Philadelphia, 1997, WB Saunders Co.

Bates B: *Guide to clinical thinking*, Philadelphia, 1995, JB Lippincott Co.

Bennett JC, Plum F, (eds): *Cecil textbook of medicine*, Philadelphia, 1996, WB Saunders Co.

Dains JE, Baumann LC, Scheibel P: *Advanced health assessment and clinical diagnosis in primary care*, St. Louis, 1998, Mosby.

Friedman, HH: *Problem-oriented medical diagnosis*, ed 6, Boston, 1996, Little, Brown & Co.

George RB, Matthay MA, Light RW, et al: *Chest medicine: essentials of pulmonary and critical care medicine*, ed 3, Baltimore, 1995, Williams & Wilkins.

Goodfellow LT, Valentine T, Holt ME: Construction of an instrument to assess critical thinking in respiratory care: an empirical process, *Resp Care Educ Ann* 8:13-25, 1999.

Healey PM, Jacobson ES: *Common medical diagnoses: an algorithmic approach*, ed 3, Philadelphia, 2000, WB Saunders Co.

Kovaes G, Croskerry P: Clinical decision making: an emergency medicine perspective, *Acad Emerg Med* 6(9):947-952, 1999.

Mishoe SC, MacIntyre, NR: Expanding roles for respiratory care practitioners, *Respir Care* 40(1):71-86, 1997.

Sackett DL, Straus SE, Richardson WS, et al: *Evidence-based medicine*, ed 2, Edinburgh, 2000, Churchill Livingston.

Seller RH: *Differential diagnosis of common complaints*, ed 4, Philadelphia, 2000, WB Saunders Co.

Smith DS: *Field guide to bedside diagnosis*, Philadelphia, 1999, Lippincott, Williams & Wilkins.

PART II

COMMON PRESENTATIONS IN THE OUTPATIENT SETTING

CHAPTER 2

CHRONIC COUGH

James K. Stoller

▼ Key Terms

▼ Cough
▼ Post-nasal drip
▼ Gastroesophageal reflux
▼ Endobronchial lesion

▼ Bronchitis
▼ Angiotensin-converting
enzyme (ACE) inhibitor
(type I)

▼ Bronchiectasis
▼ Methacholine
challenge test
▼ Lung cancer

▼ THE CLINICAL PROBLEM

A 50-year-old man presents with a 5-month history of daily non-productive cough. He reports that the cough is somewhat worse at night and is accompanied by some voice raspiness, but he denies breathlessness or wheezing. There is no hemoptysis. He denies a history of heartburn or known gastroesophageal reflux.

He has never smoked and has had no prior lung problems. His past medical history is notable for hypertension, and he is currently being treated with a beta-blocker but not with an angiotensin-converting enzyme (ACE) inhibitor.

On physical examination, his blood pressure is 155/88 in his right arm sitting. Examination of the head, eyes, ears, nose, and throat shows some clear nasal discharge but no sinus tenderness. His chest is clear to percussion and auscultation. Cardiac examination is unremarkable, as is the remainder of the physical examination.

Box 2-1
Differential Diagnosis of Cough

Common Causes	Less Common Causes
Asthma (hyperreactive airways)	ACE inhibitor drugs (type I) (e.g., captopril, lisinopril)
Bronchitis	Endobronchial lesions (both benign and malignant)
Post-nasal drip	Bronchiectasis
Gastroesophageal reflux	Interstitial lung disease (e.g., usually interstitial pneumonitis)
	CHF
	Hair irritating the tympanic membrane

CHF, Congestive heart failure.

Laboratory tests available at this initial visit include a chest x-ray, which shows a normal-sized heart and clear lung fields with no pleural effusions.

What is the differential diagnosis for this patient's cough, and what is the most likely cause?

Differential Diagnosis of Cough

Four common causes of cough explain the majority of presentations. Specifically, these include post-nasal drip, gastroesophageal reflux, bronchitis, and asthma (or hyperreactive airways). Other less common causes of cough include complications of medications such as ACE inhibitors (type 1), endobronchial lesions, psychogenic or functional causes, and a variety of miscellaneous causes (e.g., bronchiectasis, interstitial lung disease, hair impinging on the tympanic membrane, etc.). See Box 2-1 for common and less common causes of cough.

The mechanism by which post-nasal drip causes cough is believed to be the irritation of receptors in the hypopharynx, which triggers the cough reflex (Table 2-1). As a result, post-nasal drip, similar to gastroesophageal reflux and asthma, can be made worse when the patient assumes the supine posture, as occurs when the patient retires to go to sleep. Gastroesophageal reflux–related cough may be induced by the direct irritation of airway receptors, but evidence also suggests the cough may be precipitated when upper esophageal vagal reflex receptors are triggered.

Cough can be one of the cardinal manifestations of asthma, earning the designation "cough-variant asthma," even in the absence of a history of demonstrated wheezing or of demonstrable airflow obstruction on spirometry. The mechanism of cough in patients taking type I ACE inhibitors is believed to be due to the accumulation of proinflammatory or inflammatory mediators, such as bradykinin, prostaglandins, or substance P, all of which can raise the sensitivity of the cough reflex. Finally, airway lesions may induce cough by direct physical irritation, which triggers the cough reflex.

TABLE 2-1
Interpreting Signs and Symptoms in the Patient with Cough

Possible Causes	Mechanisms	Suggestive Clinical Features
Post-nasal drip syndrome (due to rhinitis or sinusitis)	Mechanical stimulation of afferent limb of the cough reflex in the upper airway	Presence of a dripping sensation, hoarseness, or throat-clearing; worsening with supine posture; presence of a "cobblestone" appearance of oropharyngeal mucosa
Asthma	Unknown	Presence of non-specific airway hyperresponsiveness (e.g., to methacholine, etc.), family history of asthma, response to a trial of corticosteroids
GERD	Direct irritation of the airway (e.g., microscopic or gross aspiration), triggering a distal esophageal vagal reflex	May cause cough in the absence of other symptoms; at times may have heartburn, regurgitation, sour taste, possibly worsening when supine
Bronchitis	Irritation of airway cough receptors	Phlegm production, acute or chronic (i.e., on most days >3 months/year over >2 consecutive years)
Bronchogenic cancer	Irritation of cough receptors by an endobronchial process	Endobronchial signs and symptoms (e.g., hemoptysis, localized wheeze, atelectasis) in central tumors, especially squamous and small cell carcinoma; adenocarcinoma and large cell cancers more commonly peripheral, thus present based on an abnormal chest x-ray or metastatic signs or symptoms
ACE inhibitor (type I)	Increased sensitivity of the cough reflex due to the accumulation of mediators like bradykinin, prostaglandins, etc.	Non-productive cough characterized by a tickling or irritating sensation in the throat; onset as soon as hours after first dose or as late as months later
Interstitial lung disease	Unknown; possibly stimulation of cough receptors in small airways or increased airway tension due to decreased lung compliance	Non-productive and usually associated with dyspnea; chest x-ray shows interstitial changes, chest examination may show rales, digits may show clubbing

GERD, Gastroesophageal reflux disease.

Clinical Features that Suggest a Specific Cause of Cough

In this case, clinical features suggest that post-nasal drip is an important contributor to this patient's cough. Specifically, the cough worsens when the patient is supine because of the increased hypopharyngeal irritation that occurs with post-nasal drip. Also, the clear nasal discharge is suggestive, as is the absence of other causes, such as a history of asthma, known gastroesophageal reflux, and so on.

At the same time, it is well known that more full-blown suggestive features of gastroesophageal reflux (e.g., heartburn, waterbrash) can be absent even in the presence of gastroesophageal reflux that causes cough. Similarly, patients with asthma may have cough as the sole manifestation of asthma and yet lack wheezing or breathlessness. Since the patient is not taking a type I ACE inhibitor drug, cough caused by an ACE inhibitor can be confidently excluded in this patient. A clear chest x-ray, although reassuring, does not absolutely exclude an endobronchial lesion.

Available data suggest that cough can frequently have multiple causes in a single patient. Thus the clinician who is suspicious of a particular etiology should not exclude the possibility of other contributing factors.

Diagnostic Testing in the Evaluation of the Patient with Cough

Various diagnostic tests have proven useful in the evaluation of the patient with cough; these tests include spirometry, methacholine challenge or other tests of non-specific airway hyperreactivity (e.g., histamine, cold air, or exercise challenge), the plain chest x-ray, and tests directed at demonstrating gastroesophageal reflux, such as barium swallow or a 24-hour pH probe monitoring. Because features of underlying causes of cough may be clinically occult, some investigators advocate an algorithmic approach to the assessment of patients with cough, starting with aggressive management of post-nasal drip, proceeding to spirometry and/or methacholine challenge testing if the cough persists, and ending with consideration of gastroesophageal reflux or possibly bronchoscopy. Figure 2-1 contains the American College of Chest Physicians' guidelines for evaluating chronic cough in the immunocompetent patient.

This algorithm calls for an initial chest x-ray, which leads to further appropriate assessment if abnormal. A normal chest x-ray prompts the clinician to ask about the use of an ACE inhibitor, which, if the patient is taking one, is stopped for several weeks in the hope that the cough remits. Persistent cough at this point leads to an evaluation of the common causes, starting with post-nasal drip (e.g., by initiating specific therapy), followed by asthma (e.g., with spirometry and post-bronchodilator testing or assessing non-specific bronchial hyperresponsiveness with methacholine or histamine challenge), and then gastroesophageal reflux, which is assessed most accurately with 24-hour pH monitoring. Persistence of cough after a thorough pursuit of the common causes should prompt consideration of uncommon causes, including subclinical congestive heart failure or an unsuspected endobronchial lesion.

In evaluating the current patient's cough, suspicion of post-nasal drip as the primary cause reasonably would lead to recommending treatment for post-nasal drip at the outset. Specifically, the patient might be offered both a nasal corticosteroid and a non-sedating antihistamine to dry up secretions and eliminate any

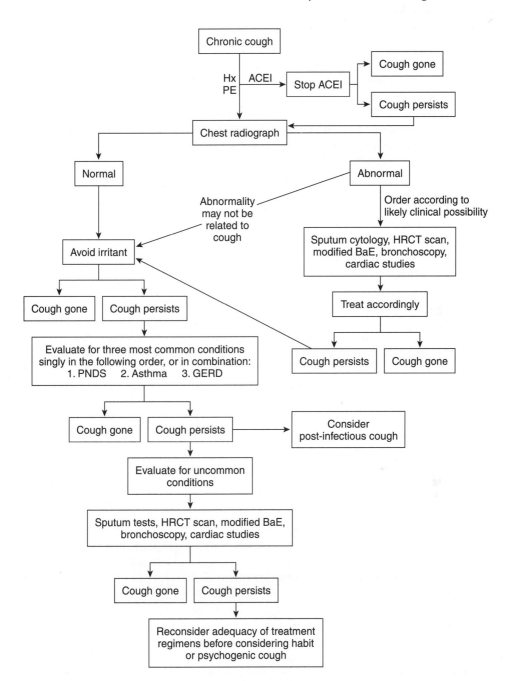

▼ **Figure 2-1**   Guidelines for evaluating chronic cough in immunocompetent adults. *ACEI,* Angiotensin-converting enzyme inhibitor; *BaE,* barium esophagography; *GERD,* gastroesophageal reflux disease; *HRCT,* high-resolution computed tomography; *Hx,* history; *PE,* physical examination; *PNDS,* post-nasal drip syndrome. From Irwin RS: *Chest* 114(suppl):166S, 1998.

inflammatory components of the coryza. If a 10- to 14-day trial of such therapy proves ineffective, further testing might then involve spirometry with a bronchodilator, looking for evidence of reversible airflow obstruction. If an obstruction is present, it may justify treatment for asthma, possibly with an aggressive bronchodilator regimen (and either systemic or inhaled corticosteroids).

Incomplete resolution of the cough after a trial of bronchodilator therapy can justify consideration of gastroesophageal reflux. Diagnostic options here include performing a 24-hour pH probe test (looking for evidence of acid reflux to a significant degree and temporal correlation with cough). Alternatively, some clinicians advocate treating gastroesophageal reflux with antacid therapy, possibly including a histamine$_2$ blocker (e.g., ranitidine) or a proton-pump inhibitor medication (e.g., omeprazole). Experience suggests that a 2- to 5-month trial of such medications may be necessary to ablate any cough that is a result of gastroesophageal reflux.

A recommendation to perform bronchoscopy would be driven by the suspicion of an endobronchial lesion, although it must be recognized that bronchoscopy rarely elucidates the cause of cough for which the cause is not otherwise suspected. In the current case, the patient's chest x-ray was clear, and there was no history of smoking to suggest an increased risk of bronchogenic cancer. However, if the patient volunteers a history of hemoptysis or if the chest x-ray is abnormal in a way that suggests an endobronchial lesion (e.g., atelectasis, lung mass, and so on), then the diagnostic threshold for performing bronchoscopy to evaluate cough would be lower, and bronchoscopy would be recommended earlier in the evaluation. In the current case, in which suspicion of an endobronchial lesion is low, bronchoscopy might be deferred as a late test, only to exclude causes for which the index of suspicion is quite low.

Pitfalls and Common Mistakes in Assessment and Treatment of Cough

Common pitfalls in the assessment of the patient with cough include inadequate attention to historical features that might suggest a specific underlying cause such as the features of post-nasal drip, asthma, bronchitis, or gastroesophageal reflux. By the same token, failure to entertain an underlying cause when a classic symptom is missing is a mistake because the absence of suggestive features does not exclude any specific cause. Several of these underlying causes may cause similar symptoms. For example, both asthma and gastroesophageal reflux may worsen at night; the latter is due to increased acid exposure to the esophagus and/or tracheobronchial tree when the patient is in the supine posture. Similarly, post-nasal drip may worsen at night because increased drainage occurs with supine posture. Thus the clinician must look for ways to discriminate between these common causes that are based both on historical features and results of diagnostic tests. Although some clinicians undertake empiric therapy for patients with cough, the opportunity to identify a specific cause by judicious laboratory testing leads many to favor a systematic approach that attempts to make a secure diagnosis.

Another common pitfall in the assessment of cough is failure to recognize type I ACE inhibitors as a potential cause of cough and then failure to discontinue the medication when it is implicated. Also, remembering that cough may have multiple causes in a single patient is important, lest effective therapy be abandoned as new therapy is sought. Finally, clinicians must remember that cough that results from gastroesophageal reflux may be slow to resolve after treatment is begun, which avoids stopping promising therapy too soon.

▼ BIBLIOGRAPHY

Irwin RS, Boulet L-P, Cloutier ZMM, et al: Managing cough as a defense mechanism: a consensus panel report of the American College of Chest Physicians, *Chest* 114(suppl):133S-181S, 1998.

Irwin RS, Curley FJ, French Cl: Chronic cough: the spectrum and frequency of causes, key components of the diagnostic evaluation and outcomes of specific therapy, *Am Rev Respir Dis* 141:640-647, 1990.

Poe RH, Harder RV, Israel RH et al: Chronic persistent cough: experience in diagnosis and outcome using an anatomic diagnostic protocol, *Chest* 95: 723-738, 1989.

Pratter MR, Bartter T, Akers S, et al: An algorithmic approach to chronic cough, *Ann Intern Med* 119: 977-983, 1993.

CHAPTER 3

RECURRENT EPISODES OF PURULENT PHLEGM

Raed A. Dweik

Key Terms

▼ Phlegm
▼ Bronchiectasis
▼ Cystic fibrosis (CF)

▼ Hemoptysis
▼ Chronic bronchitis

▼ Infection
▼ Smoking

▼ THE CLINICAL PROBLEM

A 65-year-old man presents with a several-year history of daily productive cough. He produces 1 to 1½ cups of sputum a day. The sputum is usually tan or yellow in color. Occasionally it becomes green and is associated on rare occasions with streaks of blood. The patient denies any shortness of breath or wheezing. He is an active smoker of 1 pack/day for the past 40 years. The patient recalls that he had an episode of severe pneumonia 5 years ago that required mechanical ventilation; he was hospitalized for 2 weeks. He has no other known pulmonary problems. He takes no medications.

On physical examination, his blood pressure is 130/80. Examination of the head, eyes, ears, nose, and throat is normal. He has clubbing but no cyanosis or peripheral edema. His chest examination is clear to percussion and auscultation, and the rest of the physical examination is unremarkable. A chest x-ray reveals increased linear pulmonary markings in the right lower lung zone. There were no infiltrates or effusions.

What is your differential diagnosis for this patient's productive cough, and what is the most likely cause?

Mechanism of Sputum Production

Healthy airways produce mucus on a daily basis that lines the lumen of the bronchial tree and serves an important role in host defense against the environment. Mucus is produced by glands in the airway walls of the central bronchial tree and by specialized mucus-secreting epithelial cells (goblet cells) that are present throughout the bronchial tree. Normally the quantity of this mucus is minimal and is not enough to stimulate the cough receptors. Mucus is gradually moved to the hypopharynx by the mucociliary function, where it is either swallowed or expectorated.

Both mucus-secreting elements may become enlarged in disease states. Diseases of the airways may cause the mucous glands, which line the airways, to produce an abnormally increased amount of mucus. This excess mucus stimulates the cough receptors and causes the patient to produce a loose, productive cough. This phenomenon occurs in a variety of airway diseases like acute bronchitis, chronic bronchitis, and bronchiectasis, when the volume of bronchial mucous glands may increase by 50% to 100%. The population of epithelial goblet cells also may expand, particularly in the more distal airways where few goblet cells are normally seen. The hypertrophy and hyperplasia of the mucus-secreting elements (including bronchial mucous glands and the epithelial goblet cells) are prominent features in chronic bronchitis.

Differential Diagnosis of Productive Cough

The quantity and quality of expectorated sputum are important features in trying to determine the etiology of productive cough. Box 3-1 lists common and less common causes of productive cough, and Table 3-1 outlines some features that may be helpful in determining the etiology of productive cough. Sputum production should be recorded in terms of onset and duration, quantity, and color. The volume is best expressed in familiar household terms like teaspoons, tablespoons, or cups. The color could be described as clear, white, yellow, or green. Sputum that is clear and thick is described as mucoid and is commonly seen in patients with airway disease. Mucoid sputum usually indicates uninfected secretions. The characteristics of the respiratory secretions are modified by the addition of products from the bronchial walls or from the alveoli (e.g., pus cells, plasma proteins, sloughed cells, blood, etc.). Sputum that contains pus cells is described as purulent, suggesting a bacterial infection. Purulent sputum appears thick, colored, and sticky.

Bronchial casts and mucous plugs can be coughed by patients with asthma. Blood gives a distinctive red color to the sputum and is easily recognized and reported by patients. A fetid odor suggests anaerobic infection, as in lung abscess. A large amount of mucoid sputum, up to 1 L/day, is called *bronchorrhea* and can be seen in bronchoalveolar cell lung cancer. For patients with chronic productive cough, changes from baseline in either quality or quantity or both are important clues that suggest an acute infection.

Box 3-1
Differential Diagnosis of Productive Cough

Common Causes	Less Common Causes
Acute bronchitis	Bronchoalveolar cell carcinoma
Chronic bronchitis	Asthma
Pneumonia	Lung abscess
Bronchiectasis (including CF and ciliary dyskinesia)	Pulmonary edema

CF, Cystic fibrosis.

TABLE 3-1
Features of Expectorated Sputum and Selected Etiologies

Feature	Selected Etiologies
Duration	Acute: Acute bronchitis, pneumonia
	Chronic: Chronic bronchitis, bronchiectasis
Color	Clear: Asthma, chronic bronchitis
	Yellow green: Pneumonia, acute bronchitis, exacerbation of chronic bronchitis
Hemoptysis	Bronchiectasis, lung cancer, tuberculosis, acute and chronic bronchitis
Quantity	Small (spoonful): Chronic bronchitis, others
	Large (cupful): Bronchiectasis, bronchoalveolar cell carcinoma
Odor	Foul: Lung abscess
Mucous plugs	Asthma

Clinical Features that Suggest a Specific Cause of Productive Cough

The most common causes of short-term productive cough are acute bronchitis and pneumonia. Chronic productive cough lasting for months or years, however, is more likely due to chronic bronchitis, bronchiectasis, or, less commonly, cystic fibrosis. Table 3-2 lists the causes of productive cough with suggestive clinical features of each category.

Chronic bronchitis is a clinical disorder characterized by excessive mucous secretion in the bronchial tree manifested by chronic or recurrent productive cough. It occurs in up to 30% of smokers. Chronic bronchitis is defined in clinical terms as a condition in which chronic productive cough is present for at least 3 months per year for at least 2 consecutive years. The definition specifies further that other causes of chronic cough (e.g., gastroesophageal reflux, asthma, and post-nasal drip) have been excluded. Other common symptoms of chronic bronchitis include wheezing and shortness of breath, typically on exertion. Dyspnea often is slow but progressive in onset and occurs later in the course of the disease, characteristically in the late sixth or seventh decade of life. Physical examination of the chest in a

TABLE 3-2
Interpreting Signs and Symptoms in the Patient with Productive Cough

Possible Causes	Mechanisms	Suggestive Clinical Features
Chronic bronchitis	Inflammation and enlargement of mucus-secreting elements	History of smoking, dyspnea on exertion, wheezing
Bronchiectasis	Bronchial inflammation with destruction of normal structural components of the bronchial wall, impaired ciliary function, and ineffective mucus clearance	History of aspiration, severe pneumonia, hemoptysis; cough may be brought on by change in posture
Lung abscess	Anaerobic bacterial infection, parenchymal lung destruction, pus drainage from the abscess cavity	History of alcohol use, loss of consciousness, aspiration, fever, foul-smelling sputum, poor dentition
CF	Frequent bronchial infection, accumulation of viscid mucus, ciliary dysfunction with stasis and obstruction	Age, gastrointestinal symptoms, infection with resistant organisms (e.g., mucoid *Pseudomonas aeruginosa, Pseudomonas cepacia*)
Ciliary dyskinesia	Similar to CF	Similar to CF
Asthma	Airway inflammation, mucous plugs	Recurrent wheezing, intermittent shortness of breath, allergies; usually cough is non-productive, but patients may cough up clear sputum or mucous plugs
Lung cancer (bronchoalveolar cell carcinoma)	Tumor of mucin (mucus-producing) glands	Anorexia, weight loss, copious amounts of clear sputum, persistent radiographic infiltrates
Pulmonary edema	Fluid congestion in the lungs due to increased hydrostatic pressure in the left side of the heart	Orthopnea, lower extremity edema, jugular venous distension, frothy pink sputum
Acute bronchitis	Infection or inflammation of the airways	Time limited (usually less than 3 weeks but can be up to 6 to 8 weeks)
Pneumonia	Infection and pus production	Time limited (usually less than 3 weeks but can be up to 6 to 8 weeks); acute presentation is high fever, shortness of breath, chest pain

CF, Cystic fibrosis.

patient with chronic bronchitis may show wheezing or diminished breath sounds early. Later, signs of hyperinflation may be evident (i.e., increased anteroposterior diameter and diaphragm flattening). Other late signs of chronic bronchitis may include use of accessory muscles of respiration, edema due to cor pulmonale, or mental status changes due to hypercapnia (especially if acute, as in acute exacerbations of chronic, severe disease). However, clubbing is not a feature of chronic bronchitis, and if present (as in this patient), should prompt the search for another cause of clubbing.

Cystic fibrosis (CF) is an inherited disease that primarily affects the gastrointestinal and respiratory systems and is characterized by a triad of airflow obstruction, exocrine pancreatic insufficiency (resulting in malabsorption), and abnormally high sweat electrolytes. The hallmark of CF is the accumulation of viscid mucus, which is followed by stasis, obstruction, and bronchiectasis. Patients with CF develop airway obstruction and frequent bronchial infections with resistant strains of bacteria, particularly *Staphylococcus aureus* and various *Pseudomonas* species. Patients with CF present with recurrent cough productive of thick, tenacious sputum. Other respiratory features may include hemoptysis, pneumothorax, and respiratory failure with progressive disease. The clinical course of respiratory disease in cystic fibrosis is variable, but the average life span for those with CF has risen steadily, so that the current median survival is 29 years. The age of the patient presented here excludes CF as the etiology of his chronic cough.

In the current case, clinical features suggest the patient has bronchiectasis. These features include the large volume of sputum production, the history of severe pneumonia in the past, the presence of clubbing on physical examination, and linear pulmonary markings on the chest x-ray.

Bronchiectasis refers to abnormal, irreversible dilation of the bronchi caused by destructive and inflammatory changes of the airway walls. Bronchiectasis has the following three major anatomic patterns:

1. Cylindrical bronchiectasis: Airway wall is regularly and uniformly dilated.
2. Varicose bronchiectasis: An irregular pattern with alternating areas of constriction and dilation.
3. Cystic bronchiectasis: Progressive distal enlargement of the airways resulting in sac-like dilations.

Bronchiectasis is thought to result from damage to the bronchial wall by chronic inflammation. Predisposing conditions are listed in Box 3-2. The hallmark of bronchiectasis is the chronic production of large quantities of purulent sputum. Dyspnea is variable and depends on the extent of involvement and underlying disease. Hemoptysis occurs frequently and is usually mild, but severe hemoptysis can be seen. Radiographic studies confirm the diagnosis by demonstrating airway dilation. A chest x-ray may show cystic spaces and tram tracks (thin parallel lines representing the airway walls). High-resolution computed tomography (CT) scanning has replaced bronchography as the definitive diagnostic test for bronchiectasis. Because reversible airway changes consistent with bronchiectasis can follow pneumonia, evaluation for bronchiectasis should be deferred for 6 to 8 weeks after pneumonia resolves before a diagnosis of bronchiectasis can be made.

> **Box 3-2**
> **Selected Causes of Bronchiectasis**
>
> **Local Bronchiectasis**
> Foreign body
> Benign airway tumor (e.g., adenoma)
> Bronchial compression by surrounding lymph nodes (e.g.,
>   middle lobe syndrome)
>
> **Diffuse Bronchiectasis**
> CF
> Ciliary dyskinesia (including Kartagener's syndrome)
> Hypogammaglobulinemia
> Alpha$_1$-antitrypsin deficiency
> Allergic bronchopulmonary aspergillosis
> Rheumatoid arthritis
> Serious lung infection (e.g., whooping cough, measles,
>   or influenza)

CF, Cystic fibrosis.

Diagnostic Testing in the Evaluation of Patients with Chronic Productive Cough and Suspected Bronchiectasis

The chest x-ray is abnormal in the majority of patients with bronchiectasis. Abnormalities on the chest x-ray include increased parallel linear pulmonary markings (described as tram tracks and representing thickened bronchial walls), nodular densities, and tubular densities representing mucus-filled sacs and bronchi. Bronchography has generally been considered the most sensitive imaging modality for the diagnosis of bronchiectasis. The popularity of this procedure, however, has diminished significantly over the past 20 to 30 years, primarily due to the advent of high-resolution CT scanning. CT can diagnose bronchiectasis noninvasively and assess disease location and the extent of involvement. The main feature of bronchiectasis on a CT scan of the chest is bronchi with thickened walls that extend out to the lung periphery where they are not usually seen. Similar to what is observed on the chest x-ray, these bronchi are oriented horizontally within the CT section, and they have the appearance of parallel tram tracks. On cross-section, the bronchi will classically have a "signet ring" appearance in combination with the accompanying artery. Normally, the bronchus and its accompanying artery are of equal size. An airway diameter that is more than 1.5 times that of the adjacent vessel indicates bronchiectasis.

Pulmonary function tests are less helpful in distinguishing bronchiectasis from other common causes of chronic productive cough (like chronic bronchitis and cystic fibrosis) since all of them present with airway obstruction. Pulmonary function testing, however, provides functional assessment of the degree of pulmonary impairment. Most patients with bronchiectasis will have airway obstruction as evidenced by reduced FEV_1 and FEV_1/FVC ratio. A restrictive pattern also may be seen in patients with advanced disease.

In evaluating the current patient's cough, several issues need to be considered. Chronic bronchitis is definitely a possibility due to his past history of smoking. He should be strongly encouraged to quit smoking. The history of a severe pneumonia, the presence of clubbing, and the described "tram track" abnormalities on the chest x-ray are features suggestive of bronchiectasis. CT of the chest with thin slices (high-resolution CT) may be helpful in determining the location and extent of the disease and excluding any proximal airway obstruction as an etiology. A flexible bronchoscopy may be considered if hemoptysis becomes a major feature; the bronchoscopy should localize the source of bleeding, which may be helpful in planning therapy, if needed.

Antibiotics and bronchopulmonary hygiene are the mainstays of bronchiectasis management. Antibiotics can be given as needed or following a regularly scheduled regimen. Sputum cultures may be helpful in guiding antibiotic choice. Secretions can be cleared by chest physiotherapy with postural drainage, cough maneuvers, and humidification. Inhaled bronchodilators may be helpful in some patients because of accompanying airflow obstruction. In cases that are complicated by massive hemoptysis, embolization of the bleeding bronchial artery may be helpful. Surgical resection should be reserved for patients with localized disease who develop massive hemoptysis or who are severely symptomatic despite appropriate medical therapy.

▼ BIBLIOGRAPHY

Barker AF: Bronchiectasis, *Semin Thorac Cardiovasc Surg*, 7:112-118, 1995.

Barker AF, Bardana EJ Jr: Bronchiectasis: update of an orphan disease, *Am Rev Respir Dis* 137:969-978, 1988.

Davis PB, Drumm M, Konstan MW. Cystic fibrosis, *Am J Respir Crit Care Med* 154:1229, 1996.

Dweik RA, Stoller JK: Obstructive lung disease: COPD, asthma, and related diseases. In Scanlan CL, Wilkins RL, Stoller JK, eds: *Egan's fundamentals of respiratory care*, ed 7, Chicago, 1999, Mosby, pp. 441-462.

CHAPTER 4

PROGRESSIVE EXERTIONAL DYSPNEA

Loutfi S. Aboussouan

Key Terms

▼ Asthma
▼ Dyspnea
▼ Emphysema

▼ Bronchial hyperreactivity
▼ Wheezing
▼ Congestive heart failure (CHF)

▼ Cardiac asthma
▼ Blockpnea

▼ THE CLINICAL PROBLEM

A 45-year-old white man presents with a 10-month history of progressive exertional dyspnea. He has no associated fever, cough, or wheezing. There is no variability in the severity of his symptoms, and he is unable to identify specific triggers. His current activity is limited to climbing one flight of stairs with significant dyspnea.

His past medical history is negative. He is not taking any medication and has no known drug allergies. He had a 1 pack/day smoking history over the preceding 25 years but quit 4 months ago because of worsening dyspnea. His family history is significant for emphysema in his father.

On physical examination, he appears barrel-chested, and the lung examination reveals a hyperresonant percussion note with diminished air entry bilaterally. There is full excursion of the diaphragms with inspiration. On cardiovascular examination, heart sounds are distant with no murmurs, gallops, or rubs appreciated; there is no neck vein distension. The abdomen is soft with no hepatosplenomegaly and no abdominal paradox on supine examination. A neurologic examination reveals good motor strength and no fasciculations. There is no pedal or sacral edema. The rest of the physical examination is unremarkable.

Database includes a chest x-ray, which reveals hyperinflated lungs, flattening of both diaphragms, and bullous changes at both bases.

What is the differential diagnosis for this patient's dyspnea, and what is the most likely cause?

Differential Diagnosis of Dyspnea

Although about two thirds of patients with dyspnea are ultimately shown to have pulmonary or cardiac disorders, other possibilities need to be considered, depending on the clinical presentation and findings on physical examination (Box 4-1).

Pulmonary etiologies account for about 60% of cases of chronic dyspnea and for over 36% of cases of chronic dyspnea that remain unexplained after a thorough history, physical examination, chest x-ray, and spirometry. Fifty percent of pulmonary causes of chronic dyspnea are ultimately established as caused by asthma after either diagnostic testing with a methacholine challenge test or after clinical response to an empiric trial of bronchodilator therapy. Other pulmonary disorders include emphysema, interstitial lung disease, upper airway obstruction by tumor or vocal cord problems, or pulmonary vascular disorders such as embolism or pulmonary hypertension.

Cardiac conditions account for 10% to 14% of cases of chronic dyspnea and include congestive heart failure (CHF) (due to cardiomyopathy or valvular heart disease), intracardiac shunting, pericardial disease, and angina. Dyspnea has been reported to be the earliest presentation of coronary artery disease in about 3% of

---

Box 4-1
Differential Diagnosis of Dyspnea

Common Causes	Less Common Causes
Pulmonary Causes	**Pulmonary Causes**
Asthma	Upper airway obstruction
Emphysema	Pulmonary embolism
Interstitial lung disease	Pulmonary hypertension
Cardiac Causes	**Cardiac Causes**
CHF	Pericardial disease
Angina equivalent	Intracardiac shunt
Other Common Conditions	**Neuromuscular Causes**
Anemia	Amyotrophic lateral sclerosis
Deconditioning	Myasthenia gravis
Hyperventilation syndrome	
Gastroesophageal reflux	**Other Conditions**
Post-nasal drip	Liver dysfunction
	Thyroid dysfunction

patients (a condition sometimes referred to as *blockpnea*). Also, dyspnea was found to be associated with angina and to be an early marker for the subsequent development of coronary artery disease.

Neuromuscular diseases rarely present with primary pulmonary symptoms. However, about 5% of patients with amyotrophic lateral sclerosis present with an initial complaint of dyspnea.

Dyspnea can also be the presenting symptom in about 18% of patients with liver dysfunction, which often is associated with hypoxemia due to intraparenchymal shunting of blood. An important clinical clue is the presence of platypnea and orthodeoxia, representing shortness of breath and oxygen desaturation, respectively, when the patient assumes the upright position.

Other common disorders presenting with dyspnea as a primary complaint include anemia, thyroid dysfunction (with either hyperthyroidism or hypothyroidism), gastroesophageal reflux, post-nasal drip, metabolic acidosis, and deconditioning.

Dyspnea is also reported in 50% to 90% of patients with hyperventilation syndrome. This condition is a distinct form of dyspnea associated with either organic or psychogenic causes. Organic conditions that may lead to hyperventilation include liver disease, sepsis, pulmonary vascular and embolic disease, interstitial lung disease, and salicylate intoxication. Although psychogenic hyperventilation is usually attributed to anxiety, less than half of cases have an identified psychiatric disorder.

Finally, it is important to remember that a thorough evaluation may fail to elicit a definitive diagnosis for chronic dyspnea in about 20% of patients.

Pathophysiologic Basis for Dyspnea

Given the subjective nature of dyspnea and the complexity of its genesis, a single pathophysiologic mechanism is unlikely to provide an adequate explanation for most cases. Numerous receptors may contribute to the sensation of dyspnea, including vagal afferent mechanoreceptors, chemoreceptors, and vascular and central nervous system (CNS) receptors. The four major pathophysiologic mechanisms for the development of dyspnea that have been proposed are likely to operate in concert.

The first mechanism is sensation of chemoreceptor stimulation. Some studies report that elevation of end-tidal CO_2 in high-level quadriplegic patients supported with mechanical ventilation is associated with a sensation of air hunger. Since that sensation could not be associated with respiratory muscle contractions, a possible mechanism is direct projection from chemoreceptors to the sensory cortex.

A second mechanism is stimulation of pulmonary receptors. Interruption of vagal transmission in patients with interstitial lung disease or emphysema has been associated with improvement of dyspnea in some. Since the vagus nerves ferry impulses from airway and intrapulmonary receptors, stimulation of those receptors may play a role in the sensation of dyspnea.

A third mechanism involves the respiratory muscle receptors. The sensation of dyspnea associated with breath-holding can be alleviated by bilateral phrenic nerve block or by curare in healthy volunteers, along with an increase in breath-holding time. Since these interventions are expected to preserve the pulmonary afferent traffic, the sensation of dyspnea with breath-holding appears to be mediated by transmission of afferent discharges from muscle receptors (particularly the diaphragm) to the cerebral cortex.

Finally, sensation of respiratory motor command may play a role. This mechanism associates different levels of dyspnea sensation for separate tasks, even if those tasks result in an equivalent level of ventilation and thus a presumably similar degree of afferent information from chest and lungs. For instance, studies in healthy volunteers and patients with chronic obstructive pulmonary disease (COPD) show that the sensation of dyspnea is lessened when ventilation is achieved by voluntary effort, as opposed to a similar degree of ventilation achieved through either exercise stimulus or CO_2 inhalation.

In addition to these basic pathophysiologic mechanisms, a combination of factors may be at play (Table 4-1). For instance, some studies document an increase in bronchial hyperresponsiveness in patients with CHF (cardiac asthma). Also, the mechanism of dyspnea in hyperventilation requires both initiation and maintenance of the process with proposed mechanisms, including an exaggerated response to stress and a hypocapnic set-point.

Clinical Features that Suggest a Specific Cause of Dyspnea

More than two thirds of patients presenting with a progressive or chronic dyspnea are ultimately diagnosed as having a cardiac or pulmonary problem. The cardiopulmonary system should therefore be the focus of attention (Table 4-1).

In the current case, the history and physical examination, as well as the available chest x-ray data, strongly suggest emphysema. Features in the history that support emphysema include the progressive nature of the disorder, the predominant symptom of dyspnea, and the history of smoking. The lack of variability in the severity of his symptoms, the absence of identifiable triggers, and the lack of wheezing on physical examination reduce the likelihood of asthma but do not definitely exclude that diagnosis. The physical examination reveals hyperresonant lungs and decreased air entry, which are consistent with features of emphysema. The chest x-ray, with findings of hyperinflation, is a good clinical correlate for the diagnosis of emphysema.

Several other features of this patient's presentation should prompt further consideration of a diagnosis of alpha₁-antitrypsin deficiency as the cause of emphysema. This disorder is significantly underrecognized as a cause of emphysema and should be considered in patients with early-onset emphysema, and with a family history of emphysema, particularly when the smoking history is absent or modest. In the current patient, the relatively young age and a family history of emphysema in his father should prompt testing for alpha₁-antitrypsin deficiency. The chest x-ray, in addition to showing features typical of emphysema with hyperinflation and flat diaphragm, shows bilateral basilar bullous changes. These changes are in contrast to the regular apical distribution of bullous changes in patients with classical emphysema and is an additional clue to suggest alpha₁-antitrypsin deficiency. Other features not present in this patient that should suggest a diagnosis of alpha₁-antitrypsin deficiency are abnormal liver function tests and possible panniculitis.

Cardiac and neuromuscular causes of dyspnea have been considered in the history and examination and appear excluded from consideration.

TABLE 4-1
Interpreting Signs and Symptoms in the Patient with Dyspnea

Possible Causes	Mechanisms	Suggestive Clinical Features
Asthma	Bronchial hyperreactivity, chemoreceptor or pulmonary receptor stimulation	Wheezing, reversible airway obstruction, hyperresponsiveness on a methacholine challenge, family history
Emphysema	Loss of alveolar bed, chemoreceptor or pulmonary receptor stimulation	Smoking, family history of emphysema, hyperinflation on chest x-ray, barrel-shaped chest, diminished air entry
Pulmonary fibrosis	Pulmonary receptor stimulation, hypoxemia	Digital clubbing, "Velcro-like" crackles, chest x-ray with reduced lung volume and bilateral peripheral infiltrates
Pulmonary hypertension	Decreased pulmonary vascular bed, hypoxemia	Loud P_2, pruning, and prominent pulmonary arteries on chest x-rays
Pulmonary embolism	Dead space ventilation, chest pain	Prolonged travel, immobility, oral contraceptives, malignancy
Tracheal obstruction	Flow limitation	Stridor, localized wheeze
Heart failure: Valvular disease, cardiomyopathy	Interstitial receptor stimulation, bronchial hyperreactivity, hypoxemia	Gallop, displaced point of maximal impulse, cardiac murmur, crackles, peripheral edema, chest x-ray showing cardiomegaly and infiltrates
Arrhythmias	Decreased cardiac output	Irregular or slow heart rhythm
Intracardiac shunting	Hypoxemia	Platypnea, orthodeoxia
Ischemic heart disease	Angina equivalent	Cardiovascular risk factors: Hypertension, diabetes, smoking
Pericardial disease	Constrictive pericarditis	Prominent "x" and "y" jugular vein waves, pericardial knock
Anemia	Decreased oxygen delivery	Pallor
Neuromuscular disease	Respiratory muscle weakness	Paradox, limited diaphragmatic excursion, fasciculations
Liver cirrhosis	Hypoxemia due to shunting	Angiomas, jaundice, clubbing, cyanosis, platypnea, orthodeoxia
Gastroesophageal reflux	Vagally mediated, asthma trigger	History of heartburn
Post-nasal drip	Upper airway obstruction	Vasomotor rhinitis, sinusitis, cobblestoned oropharynx
Metabolic acidosis	Compensatory hyperventilation	Review medications (i.e., acetazolamide)
Deconditioning	Reduced maximal oxygen uptake	Sedentary lifestyle
Hyperventilation	Hypocapnic set-point	Anxiety, pain, liver disease, pulmonary embolism

Diagnostic Testing in the Evaluation of the Patient with Dyspnea

Laboratory investigations may include complete blood counts and evaluation of thyroid function, since anemia and both hypothyroid and hyperthyroid states have been associated with a sensation of dyspnea.

A complete pulmonary function test can be extremely helpful in the identification of pulmonary causes of dyspnea. Typical features of asthma on a pulmonary function test include airway obstruction (i.e., reduced FEV_1/FVC ratio) with a bronchodilator response. Since one cardinal feature of asthma is its reversibility, a normal test does not exclude the diagnosis. Further testing may include a methacholine bronchoprovocation challenge or an empiric trial of bronchodilators. Features of emphysema on pulmonary function tests include airway obstruction, evidence of hyperinflation (increased total lung capacity), or air trapping (increased residual volume), with a reduction in the diffusion capacity. Interstitial lung disease is associated with a reduction in total lung capacity and diffusion capacity.

The flow-volume loop identifies airway obstruction by the scooped appearance of the expiratory portion of the flow-volume curve. The loop also may identify the presence of intra-thoracic obstruction (with a truncation of the expiratory flow portion) or extra-thoracic obstruction (with a truncation of the inspiratory flow portion of the curve) (Figure 4-1). Usually a truncated appearance to the flow-volume curves is seen with a significant degree of airway narrowing (diameter of 8 to 10 mm).

A diffusion capacity that appears to be reduced out of proportion to the abnormalities noted on spirometry or lung volumes should raise the possibility of pulmonary vascular disease (e.g., pulmonary hypertension or pulmonary embolic disease).

More specialized pulmonary tests may be necessary to reach a diagnosis. Specialized tests may include a methacholine bronchoprovocation challenge test for the diagnosis of atypical asthma. In addition, tests of maximal inspiratory and expiratory respiratory pressures may support a diagnosis of neuromuscular disease.

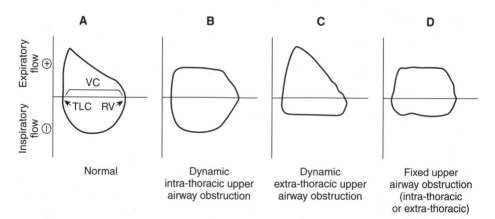

▼ **Figure 4-1** Patterns of normal (**A**) and abnormal (**B** to **D**) flow-volume loops. *VC*, Vital capacity; *TLC*, total lung capacity; *RV*, residual volume.

A simple chest x-ray provides a substantial degree of information. For example, pulmonary vascular congestion, increased interstitial markings, Kerley B lines, and cardiomegaly are consistent with CHF. Pulmonary vascular diseases may result in pruning of the vascular structures, prominent central pulmonary arteries, and possible right heart enlargement. The presence of bilateral hilar adenopathy with or without interstitial lung markings suggests a diagnosis of sarcoidosis in a young patient. A predominantly peripheral distribution of interstitial markings should raise the suspicion of interstitial lung disease. However, a chest x-ray may appear normal in 10% of cases of interstitial lung disease; therefore a high-resolution computed tomography (CT) scan of the chest may be necessary to pursue that diagnosis given the appropriate clinical presentation.

An evaluation of cardiac function is often best performed with an echocardiogram, which can evaluate left ventricular systolic function and valvular competence. The technicians performing the echocardiogram and the physicians interpreting it should be alerted to the suspected diagnoses. For example, the clinical suspicion of pulmonary hypertension should prompt close attention to right ventricular function and the possibility of tricuspid regurgitation, which allows the identification and quantification of possible pulmonary hypertension. Moreover, echocardiography may identify both intrapulmonary and intracardiac shunting. Intracardiac shunting may be determined by Doppler echocardiogram, whereas intrapulmonary shunting may require injection of agitated saline for a bubble echocardiography procedure.

If the etiology of dyspnea remains obscure, evaluation for possible embolic disease includes ventilation-perfusion lung scanning, pulmonary angiography, or Doppler venous studies of the legs. Specialized cardiopulmonary exercise testing often is the last resort for unexplained dyspnea but can identify cardiac versus pulmonary causes of dyspnea, deconditioning, or even psychogenic causes.

Assessment of the Effect of Therapy for Dyspnea

Clinical response to empiric therapy can be used as a diagnostic tool for dyspnea. For example, bronchodilators, decongestants, and proton pump inhibitors can be given for suspected asthma, post-nasal drip, or gastroesophageal reflux disease, respectively. In assessing this empiric response, several points need to be considered. For instance, even in cases where a definitive diagnosis is believed to have been reached, specific therapy relieves symptoms in only about 76% of subjects. Typically, conditions associated with a high success rate of empiric therapy include asthma, post-nasal drip, psychogenic causes, deconditioning, and gastroesophageal reflux. On the other hand, conditions such as COPD or interstitial lung disease (particularly idiopathic pulmonary fibrosis) may have a lesser success rate.

Pitfalls and Common Mistakes in Assessment and Treatment of Dyspnea

Common pitfalls include the lack of an appropriate history or physical examination. A patient presenting with the chief complaint of dyspnea may not volunteer a history of iron deficiency anemia, sickle cell anemia, or thalassemia. Also, a thorough medication history can offer important clues. Salicylates or ophthalmic medications containing beta-blocking agents may contribute to reactive airway disease but may not be readily reported by patients when listing their medications.

Also, many conditions are not initially suspected as causes of dyspnea, either because the condition is poorly recognized or because of an unusual initial presentation. Alpha$_1$-antitrypsin deficiency, for example, is a condition that can be treated by intravenous supplementation therapy, yet it remains significantly underrecognized, with delays of several years between onset of symptoms and a final diagnosis. Also, a neuromuscular cause of dyspnea, although rare, is often missed because the presenting symptom of dyspnea diverts the evaluation from the neuromuscular system to the pulmonary system. In addition, thyroid dysfunction, anemia, and deconditioning are often missed as causes of dyspnea.

Another pitfall is interpretation of diagnostic tests without consideration of the total clinical evaluation, which can lead to erroneous diagnoses. Both COPD and asthma are associated with evidence of airway obstruction, and both emphysema and interstitial lung disease reduce the diffusion capacity. Similarly, when performing a cardiopulmonary exercise test, it often is difficult to separate deconditioning from mild cardiac disease.

Finally, since many causes of dyspnea are common, several coexisting conditions may be encountered that potentially contributing to the symptoms.

▼ BIBLIOGRAPHY

Aboussouan LS, Stoller JK: New developments in alpha$_1$-antitrypsin deficiency, *Semin Respir Crit Care Med* 20:301-310, 1999.

Cook DG, Shaper AG: Breathlessness, angina pectoris and coronary artery disease, *Am J Cardiol* 63: 921-924, 1989.

Depaso WJ, Winterbauer RH, Lusk JA, et al: Chronic dyspnea unexplained by history, physical examination, chest roentgenogram, and spirometry, *Chest* 100:1293-1299, 1991.

Gillespie DJ, Staats BA: Unexplained dyspnea, *Mayo Clin Proc* 69:657-663, 1994.

Pratter MR, Curley FJ, Dubois J, et al: Cause and evaluation of chronic dyspnea in a pulmonary disease clinic, *Arch Intern Med* 149:2277-2282, 1989.

Short D, Stowers M: Earliest symptoms of coronary heart disease and their recognition, *Br Med J* 2:387-391, 1972.

Tobin MJ: Dyspnea. Pathophysiologic basis, clinical presentation, and management, *Arch Intern Med* 150:1604-1613, 1990.

CHAPTER 5

CHRONIC EXERTIONAL DYSPNEA

Sanjay A. Patel
Frank C. Sciurba

Key Terms

▼ Dyspnea
▼ Chronic obstructive pulmonary disease (COPD)

▼ Pulmonary hypertension
▼ Cardiopulmonary exercise test

▼ Airflow obstruction
▼ Emphysema

▼ THE CLINICAL PROBLEM

A 65-year-old white man presents with complaints of progressive shortness of breath for about 1 year. He describes dyspnea on exertion without any specific exacerbating factors. He has an intermittent dry cough but denies associated sputum production, hemoptysis, chest pain, fevers, chills, sweats, weight loss, or anorexia. Review of systems otherwise is unremarkable.

The past medical history is remarkable for hypertension and non-insulin-dependent diabetes mellitus. He smoked 1½ packs/day for 25 years. Medications include lisinopril, glyburide, and a daily aspirin. Family history is remarkable for a father with coronary artery disease. The patient worked as a radiology technician.

Physical examination reveals a moderately obese man breathing comfortably at rest. Vital signs are blood pressure 138/86, pulse 80, respiratory rate 16, temperature 98.8° F. Pulse oximetry on room air is 90%. Jugular venous distension measures 8 cm. Cardiac examination reveals a non-displaced point of maximal impulse, a normal S_1 and prominent S_2, particularly at the base, with a II/VI systolic murmur at the left lower sternal border. Lung fields are clear to auscultation and percussion. Extremities reveal 1+ pitting edema bilaterally and brawny skin changes of chronic venous stasis. The remainder of the examination is unremarkable.

Complete blood count, electrolytes, and renal and hepatic function tests are normal. Pulmonary function test results are as follows: forced expiratory volume in 1 second (FEV_1) 3.45 L (90% predicted), forced expiratory volume (FVC) 3.75 L (80% predicted), FEV_1/FVC 92%, total lung capacity (TLC) 6.13 L (88% predicted), residual volume (RV) 2.18 L (85% predicted), diffusing capacity of lung for carbon monoxide corrected ($DLCO_{corrected}$) 14.4 mm CO/min/mm Hg (55% predicted), room air arterial blood gas pH 7.43, PCO_2 38 mm Hg, PO_2 56 mm Hg, HCO_3^- 22 mg/dL, oxygen saturation 88%.

Chest x-ray shows normal lung fields with a mild cardiac enlargement. Electrocardiogram reveals normal sinus rhythm, right axis deviation, and right atrial abnormality. High resolution computed tomography (CT) scan reveals normal lung parenchyma with slightly enlarged pulmonary arteries.

What is the differential diagnosis for this patient's dyspnea, what is the most likely cause?

Definition of Dyspnea

Dyspnea is one of the most common presenting complaints in the outpatient and inpatient settings. It is a manifestation of a variety of disorders and probably encompasses a variety of different sensations. Thus a commonly accepted definition does not exist. A consensus statement of the American Thoracic Society defined dyspnea as ". . . a subjective experience of breathing discomfort . . . comprised of qualitatively distinct sensations . . . from interactions among multiple physiological, psychological, social, and environmental factors . . . ."

Differential Diagnosis of Chronic Dyspnea

The respiratory care clinician must understand the normal physiologic responses to exertion and the pathophysiologic mechanisms of dyspnea when evaluating a patient with chronic dyspnea. Only with this background can the respiratory clinician develop a logical and efficient diagnostic approach to chronic dyspnea.

Physiology of Exercise

The pulmonary, cardiac, vascular, hematologic, and musculoskeletal systems interact during exercise. These systems act to couple cellular respiration to pulmonary respiration. They deliver oxygen to the cellular organelles and eliminate carbon dioxide (CO_2), which is the by-product of cellular respiration. This interactive system preserves homeostasis during varying levels of external work.

During exercise, physiologic adaptations accommodate these increased gas exchange requirements. The adaptations involve all systems (Figure 5-1). The cardiac

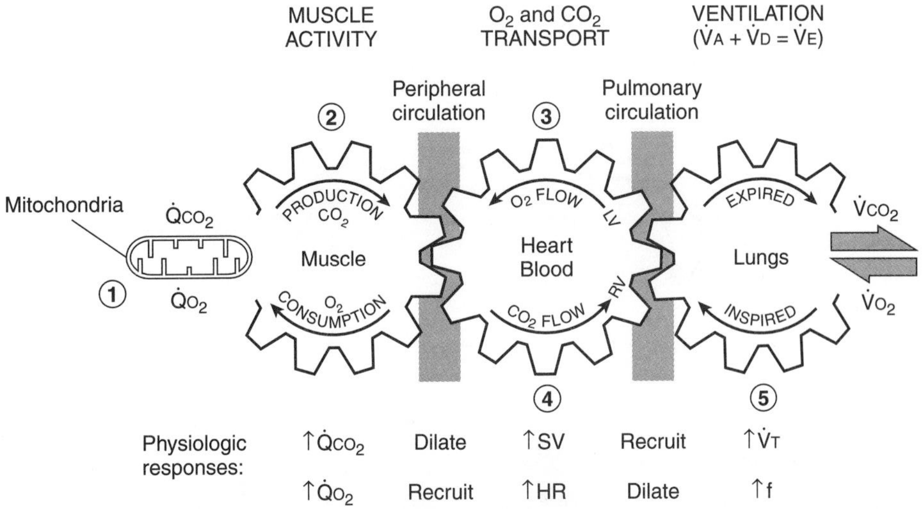

MUSCLE   O$_2$ and CO$_2$ VENTILATION
ACTIVITY   TRANSPORT   ($\dot{V}$A + $\dot{V}$D = $\dot{V}$E)

▼ **Figure 5-1**   Physiologic responses to exercise. Mechanisms by which cellular respiration is coupled to pulmonary respiration. The gears represent functional interdependence of the components of the system. The increase in oxygen utilization by the muscles during exercise is achieved by five major mechanisms: (1) increased oxygen extraction by the muscles ($\dot{Q}o_2$), (2) dilation of selected peripheral vascular beds, (3) increased cardiac output via increase in stroke volume (*SV*) and heart rate (*HR*), (4) increased pulmonary blood flow by recruitment and dilation of pulmonary vasculature, and (5) increased ventilation via increased tidal volume (*V$_T$*) and respiratory rate (*f*). The increase in CO$_2$ expiration is accomplished by mechanisms 2 to 5. *LV*, Left ventricle; *RV*, right ventricle; $\dot{V}$A, alveolar ventilation; $\dot{V}$D, dead space ventilation; $\dot{V}$E, minute ventilation. From Wasserman K: *Principles of exercise testing and interpretation*, Baltimore, 1999, Lippincott, Williams & Wilkins.

output increases via an increase in heart rate and stroke volume, and the pulmonary circulation is recruited and vasodilates. The peripheral circulation also is recruited and vasodilates, improving blood flow to active muscles. The skeletal muscles extract a higher fraction of the delivered oxygen, and the lungs increase minute ventilation by increasing tidal volume and respiratory rate.

Derangements in this integrated system commonly manifest as exercise intolerance and dyspnea. However, they may also manifest in non-specific ways such as fatigue, weakness, or chest pain. Mild abnormalities, which may not manifest as symptoms at rest, commonly become apparent with exertion.

Mechanisms of Dyspnea

Although the neurophysiologic mechanisms involved in producing the sensation of dyspnea are still incompletely understood, many clinically useful models have been postulated. A simplified, clinically useful model is illustrated in Figure 5-2. Dyspnea is perceived when there is an increase in ventilatory drive because of abnormally increased ventilation requirements or deranged mechanics. Ventilation requirements may change as a result of increased dead space ("inefficient" ventilation as in severe parenchymal lung disease or pulmonary vascular disease) or metabolic acidosis (as occurs in states of inadequate oxygen delivery or deconditioning). Deranged mechanics can be due to any obstructive or restrictive lung disease.

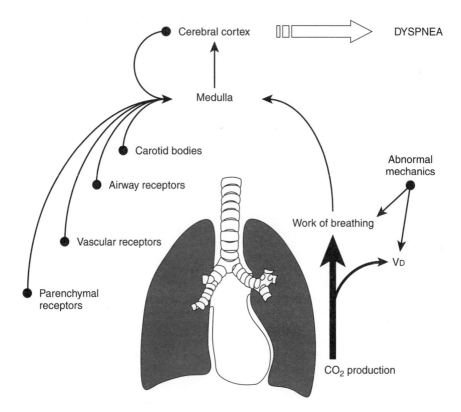

▼ **Figure 5-2**   Mechanisms of dyspnea. Abnormal lung mechanics commonly cause dyspnea by increasing the work of breathing by (1) increased direct mechanical workload and (2) increasing dead space ventilation, which increases the total minute ventilation required for a given level of CO_2 production. Hypoxemia of any etiology is sensed at the carotid bodies and also can independently elicit dyspnea. In addition, pulmonary airway, parenchymal, and vascular receptors, as well as higher centers in the CNS, can modulate and independently elicit dyspnea. V_D, Dead space ventilation.

Hypoxemia sensed at the carotid bodies is another important mechanism that produces dyspnea. Other afferent neural inputs to the respiratory centers may independently increase ventilatory drive and elicit dyspnea. These include pulmonary parenchymal receptors (J-receptors), pulmonary vascular "stretch" receptors, and upper airway receptors. In addition, higher centers of the central nervous system (CNS) can modulate respiratory drive and dyspnea (e.g., anxiety states).

Determining the Differential Diagnosis

With this background of exercise physiology and the model of dyspnea perception, the differential diagnoses of chronic dyspnea are organized (Box 5-1), which helps develop a clinically useful approach to the problem. The differential diagnoses are divided by common and uncommon causes, as well as by pathophysiologic mechanism. It should be remembered that these differential diagnoses are quite different than those of acute dyspnea.

Box 5-1
Differential Diagnosis of Chronic Dyspnea

Common Causes	Less Common Causes
Primary Lung Abnormalities	
Ventilatory-Obstructive Defect	
COPD (emphysema and chronic bronchitis)	Bronchiectasis (e.g., CF)
Asthma	Upper airway obstruction
Ventilatory-Restrictive Defect	
Parenchymal (interstitial lung processes)	
Pleural	*Pleural*
Pleural effusion	Pleural fibrosis
Chest wall abnormalities	*Chest wall abnormalities*
Kyphoscoliosis	Congenital abnormalities
Diaphragm dysfunction	*Diaphragm dysfunction*
Large ascites	Phrenic neuropathies
Obesity	Neuromuscular junction abnormalities
	Diaphragm myopathies
Oxygenation Defect	
Capillary destruction	*Pulmonary vascular diseases*
Emphysema	Primary pulmonary HTN
Diffusion block	Secondary pulmonary HTN
Interstitial lung processes	Chronic thromboembolic disease
Idiopathic pulmonary fibrosis	Arteriovenous malformations
Sarcoidosis	*Intra-cardiac shunts*
Occupational diseases	Congenital heart disease
Autoimmune diseases	Patent foramen ovale
Lymphangitic carcinomatosis	*Chronic alveolar filling diseases*
Interstitial edema	
Inadequate Oxygen Delivery	
Impaired Oxygen-Carrying Capacity	
Anemia	Hemoglobinopathies
Impaired Cardiac Output	
Systolic dysfunction	*Systolic dysfunction*
Cardiac ischemia	Non-ischemic cardiomyopathy
Ischemic cardiomyopathy	*Valvular heart disease*
Diastolic dysfunction (hypertensive heart)	
Skeletal Muscle Abnormalities	
Deconditioning	Skeletal myopathies

COPD, Chronic obstructive pulmonary disease; *CF*, cystic fibrosis, *HTN*, hypertension.

Patients with lung diseases commonly have dyspnea that results from abnormal lung mechanics (obstructive or restrictive), as well as increased dead space fraction, and both increase the work of breathing and the ventilatory drive and elicit dyspnea. In addition, these patients commonly have hypoxemia, which independently evokes dyspnea via carotid body output.

Clearly, however, patients without pulmonary disease also complain of dyspnea. These patients may have inadequate systemic oxygen delivery caused by either decreased oxygen-carrying capacity (e.g., anemia) or decreased cardiac output. They may complain of fatigue or weakness, but dyspnea can be the presenting complaint as well. The mechanism of dyspnea in these patients is less well defined. It may be due to a premature transition to anaerobic metabolism during exertion and subsequent lactic acidosis, which increases ventilation requirements and respiratory drive and thus elicits dyspnea. Patients with skeletal muscle abnormalities, such as myopathies or deconditioning, may also have a similar mechanism for their dyspnea. The premature lactic acidosis in this case, however, is due to an inefficient musculoskeletal system that requires supranormal oxygen delivery at only modest workloads.

This is an overly simplified approach to the pathophysiologic classification of dyspnea, since multiple factors are involved in the physiologic derangements associated with most disease states. For example, in emphysema, there are abnormal mechanics due to obstruction, as well as capillary bed destruction with subsequent hypoxemia and possibly pulmonary hypertension. These patients usually have a somewhat sedentary lifestyle and are deconditioned. The relatively common association of ischemic heart disease also complicates the problem.

In chronic heart failure, patients have inadequate cardiac output, which leads to dyspnea by the mechanisms described. However, they also have interstitial edema and pleural effusions, which worsen parenchymal and pleural compliance, respectively. The edema also impairs oxygenation through diffusion block. Chronic edema can also induce peri-capillary fibrosis, causing further mechanical and dead space abnormalities. Thus restrictive mechanics and hypoxemia, along with an inadequate cardiac output, further contribute to the dyspnea of chronic heart failure.

Patients with interstitial lung diseases have diffusion block and hypoxemia but commonly have a restrictive ventilatory defect that results from poor parenchymal compliance. In addition, the chronic hypoxemia and capillary bed remodeling that occurs in fibrosis can lead to both pulmonary hypertension and shunting across a foramen ovale, which further exacerbate hypoxemia and dyspnea.

A final salient example relates to pulmonary vascular diseases. Some patients have pulmonary hypertension and dyspnea related to hypoxemia. In addition, ventilation to under-perfused alveoli results in increased dead space. These patients can also have associated right ventricular dysfunction, which imposes cardiogenic limitations and further contributes to exertional dyspnea.

In many diseases, there is an independent contribution from other less well-defined modulators of dyspnea (see Figure 5-2). Pulmonary vascular "stretch" receptors may contribute to dyspnea perception in cases of pulmonary arterial or venous hypertension (e.g., pulmonary hypertension, heart failure). Pulmonary parenchymal receptors (J-receptors) seem to play a role in the dyspnea experienced by patients with interstitial fibrosis. Similarly, airway receptors appear to play a role in asthma. These afferent neural inputs independently modulate the perception of dyspnea and may explain the disproportionate dyspnea experienced by some patients with relatively mild physiologic derangements.

Despite the complicated and multifactorial pathophysiology of most causes of dyspnea, the history, physical examination, pulmonary function tests, and the chest x-ray can narrow the diagnostic possibilities and make a specific diagnosis in many cases. Despite the extensive list of possible diagnoses, the majority of the causes of chronic dyspnea are due to chronic obstructive pulmonary disease (COPD), asthma, interstitial lung disease, or cardiac dysfunction.

Clinical Features that Suggest a Specific Cause of Chronic Dyspnea

History

The diagnostic approach, like most problems in clinical medicine, initially involves a thorough history and physical. The clinician should explore specific characteristics of the symptom such as the time course, positional changes, exacerbating factors, and associated symptoms. Table 5-1 summarizes key historical features for some important causes of dyspnea.

TABLE 5-1
Key Differentiating Features of the History

Condition	Features
COPD	Sputum, exacerbated by smoking
Asthma	Intermittent, bronchodilator relief
Bronchiectasis	Copious sputum, hemoptysis, childhood or recurrent pneumonia, tuberculosis
Chest wall abnormalities	Congenital, previous empyema
Diaphragm abnormalities	Peripheral muscular weakness, orthopnea, history of neuromuscular disease
Interstitial lung diseases	Clubbing
Idiopathic pulmonary fibrosis	Slowly progressive dyspnea
Sarcoidosis	Arthralgias, rash, visual changes
Occupational diseases	Occupational exposure
Associated autoimmune diseases	Rash, arthralgias, dysphagia, Raynaud's phenomenon
Lymphangitic carcinomatosis	Lung, breast, or gastrointestinal cancer
Pulmonary vascular diseases	Primary and secondary pulmonary HTN
Chronic thromboembolic disease	Underlying pulmonary diseases; history or family
AVMs	history of thrombosis, obesity; platypnea,
Congenital (Osler-Weber-Rendu)	epistaxis, telangiectasias, liver disease
Cirrhosis	
Intra-cardiac shunts	Cyanosis, history of childhood murmur,
Congenital heart disease	pulmonary HTN
Patent foramen ovale	
Anemia	Bleeding, gastrointestinal symptoms
Cardiac ischemia	Exertional angina
Cardiomyopathies	Orthopnea, PND, edema, CAD
Deconditioning	Weight gain, prolonged inactivity

COPD, Chronic obstructive pulmonary disease; *HTN,* hypertension; *PND,* paroxysmal nocturnal dyspnea; *CAD,* coronary artery disease; AVMs, arteriovenous malformations.

Time course. The presence of intermittent dyspnea helps focus the differential diagnosis on etiologies such as asthma or cardiac ischemia. Other etiologies, especially COPD, can have acute exacerbations that result from either other superimposed processes (e.g., pneumonia) or progression of an underlying disease process (e.g., recurrent pulmonary embolism), but in general, these cause chronic progressive dyspnea. Nocturnal dyspnea may suggest asthma, either intrinsic or induced by gastroesophageal reflux, or congestive heart failure.

Position. Positional dyspnea also helps narrow the differential diagnosis. *Orthopnea,* defined as dyspnea with recumbency, most commonly implies chronic heart failure but also can be associated with COPD or states that affect normal diaphragmatic functioning such as ascites or pregnancy. Orthopnea occurring acutely on recumbency is associated with bilateral diaphragm dysfunction.

Platypnea, defined as dyspnea in the upright position that improves with recumbency, is commonly associated with orthodeoxia, or desaturation in the upright position. This dyspnea suggests that intra-pulmonary shunting is occurring at the lung bases and commonly occurs with congenital arteriovenous malformations or with cirrhosis. The upright position probably increases the shunt fraction and thus exacerbates hypoxemia and dyspnea.

Exacerbating factors. Dyspnea of most etiologies worsens with exertion. However, the dyspnea of exercise-induced asthma occurs after the activity ends. Dyspnea not associated with activity may suggest intrinsic or extrinsic (i.e., allergic or irritant induced) asthma or may be a clue to psychogenic causes. Other precipitating factors, such as seasonal or perennial allergies, cold exposure, or exercise, suggest asthma as well.

Associated symptoms. Associated symptoms of productive cough can be suggestive of chronic bronchitis or bronchiectasis, especially if copious or associated with hemoptysis. Dry cough, however, is somewhat non-specific and can be associated with many pulmonary or cardiac causes of dyspnea. Rheumatologic complaints (i.e., arthralgias, skin changes, Raynaud's phenomenon) may suggest a lung disease related to connective tissue disease. Patients with transient cardiac ischemia may complain of classic anginal symptoms. Chest tightness, however, also suggests a broader differential, including pulmonary hypertension or asthma.

Past medical history. The past medical history sometimes gives clues to the underlying diagnosis. For example, childhood eczema or atopy can suggest asthma. Previous severe or childhood pneumonias can suggest bronchiectasis. A history of empyema or hemothorax places the patient at risk for pleural fibrosis. In addition to a thorough cardiac and pulmonary disease history, the respiratory clinician should focus on underlying hepatic, rheumatologic, neuromuscular, and oncologic diseases, all of which have associated cardiopulmonary manifestations.

Social, family, and occupational history. Other vital clues are the smoking history, which raises the possibility of COPD. A negative smoking history, however, virtually excludes COPD, except in the rare case of familial emphysema. A family history of atopy or eczema suggests asthma. A personal or family history of

TABLE 5-2
Clinical Features that Suggest a Specific Cause of Chronic Dyspnea

Condition	Features
COPD	Hyperinflation, accessory muscle use, pursed-lip
Asthma	breathing, wheezing
Bronchiectasis	
Chest wall abnormalities	Anatomic defects, chest excursion
Neuromuscular abnormalities	Peripheral weakness, poor diaphragm excursion
Interstitial lung diseases	Coarse crackles
Idiopathic pulmonary fibrosis	
Sarcoidosis	Lymphadenopathy, eye and skin changes
Occupational diseases	
Associated autoimmune disease	Skin and joint changes
Pulmonary vascular disease	Loud P_2, ventricular heave, JVP, edema
Primary and secondary pulmonary HTN	Leg edema, venous stasis changes
Chronic thromboembolic disease	
Intra-cardiac shunts	Murmurs, clubbing
Congenital heart disease	
Patent foramen ovale	
Anemia	Pallor, ejection murmur
Cardiac ischemia	
Ischemic and non-ischemic cardiomyopathy	S_3, elevated JVP, fine crackles, edema

COPD, Chronic obstructive pulmonary disease; *HTN,* hypertension, *JVP,* jugular venous pulsation.

venous thrombosis may suggest chronic thromboembolic disease. A complete work history should also be taken to reveal risk factors for occupationally-induced interstitial lung diseases (e.g., asbestosis, silicosis, coal-worker's pneumoconiosis).

Physical Examination

The general physical examination may provide clues to the underlying diagnosis. Table 5-2 summarizes key physical examination features for some important causes of dyspnea. Significant abnormalities in respiratory rate and pattern should be observed. For example, patients with restrictive mechanics tend to have rapid, shallow breathing patterns. Pursed-lip breathing and accessory muscle use suggest COPD. Significant obesity sometimes suggests deconditioning. Inspection of the chest wall can diagnose an obvious anatomic defect at times, but more subtle abnormalities in chest wall movement and symmetry are often the only clue to underlying pleural fibrosis or effusion, for example. Poor diaphragmatic excursion is a clue to underlying neuromuscular diseases. An increased anteroposterior diameter is found with the hyperinflation of COPD. Auscultation may reveal wheezes to suggest airways obstruction, fine crackles to suggest pulmonary congestion, or coarse crackles to suggest interstitial fibrosis. Percussion may reveal the hyperresonance of emphysema or the dullness associated with pleural fibrosis or effusions.

A complete cardiac examination is essential to assess the patient with chronic dyspnea. Specifically, the clinician is looking for evidence for heart failure (laterally displaced point of maximal impulse, S_3, elevated jugular venous pulsation [JVP]), right ventricular hypertension (ventricular heave, murmur of tricuspid regurgitation, prominent P_2, elevated JVP, hepatomegaly), or valvular abnormalities.

The remainder of the examination should focus on the extremities for clubbing, edema, and evidence for associated rheumatologic and neuromuscular conditions.

The Current Case of Chronic Dyspnea

Applying this approach to the current case helps narrow the differential diagnosis. The patient's smoking history suggests COPD, but the lack of productive cough or exacerbations make this less likely. He has hypertension, diabetes, and a family history of coronary artery disease, which increase his risk for ischemic heart disease, but chest pain or symptoms of left heart failure (orthopnea, paroxysmal nocturnal dyspnea) are lacking.

On physical examination, the patient's mild obesity may suggest deconditioning. His cardiac examination, however, is consistent with pulmonary hypertension associated with mild right heart failure, manifested by the elevated JVP and peripheral edema. The physical examination does not, however, suggest a parenchymal process as the cause for the pulmonary hypertension, since there is no evidence for chronic obstructive or interstitial lung disease. The patient's leg edema and chronic venous stasis changes are non-specific and can be associated with left- or right-sided heart failure. However, left heart failure is not suspected because there is no S_3 or crackles on lung auscultation. This overall clinical presentation is consistent with an isolated pulmonary vascular disease such as pulmonary vasculitis, chronic thromboembolic disease, or primary pulmonary hypertension. The patient's age argues against primary pulmonary hypertension. The lack of associated rheumatologic symptoms makes pulmonary vasculitis less likely as well.

Diagnostic Testing in the Evaluation of the Patient with Chronic Dyspnea

Pulmonary function tests with arterial blood gas levels, as well as a chest x-ray, play an integral role in the diagnostic evaluation of chronic dyspnea. Unlike most clinical problems in medicine, these diagnostic tests are almost routine in the initial diagnostic approach to dyspnea.

Laboratory Evaluation

Basic laboratory evaluation is occasionally helpful for the diagnosis. For example, the complete blood count may reveal anemia as the cause of exertional dyspnea. Polycythemia is a clue to chronic hypoxemia of any cause. Other less specific abnormalities, such as pancytopenia or an elevated sedimentation rate, may suggest an associated connective tissue disease.

Pulmonary Function Tests

Although pulmonary function tests are fairly sensitive for most causes of dyspnea, the severity of abnormality does not necessarily correlate with the severity of the clinical symptoms. Evidence for obstructive lung disease or restrictive physiology is easily obtained from spirometry. Lung volume measurements may help confirm restrictive abnormalities found by spirometry. In addition, a decreased $DLCO_{corrected}$ is associated with many diseases that cause obstruction or restriction. However, an isolated abnormality of the $DLCO_{corrected}$ suggests an early interstitial process or pulmonary vascular disease.

Arterial blood gas levels can reveal unexpected hypoxemia, which suggests any of the etiologies associated with a gas exchange abnormality (see Box 5-1). Hypoxemia with hypercapnia suggests a ventilatory defect, either obstructive or restrictive. Severe hypoxemia, especially without hypercapnia or apparent lung disease, implies pulmonary vascular disease or shunt physiology (intra-cardiac shunt, arteriovenous malformations, or chronic air space diseases). Hypocapnia can be associated with many lung diseases, but is particularly associated with mild asthma, early interstitial lung disease, pulmonary vascular disease, and psychogenic causes.

Chest X-Ray

The chest x-ray also plays a central role in the diagnostic approach to dyspnea. Common patterns include hyperinflation with decreased vascularity and a small cardiothoracic ratio, which suggests COPD. Diffuse interstitial changes with diminished lung volumes suggest a restrictive interstitial process. The x-ray also may give clues to pulmonary vascular disease (e.g., enlarged pulmonary arteries), neuromuscular diseases (e.g., elevated hemidiaphragms with preserved lung parenchyma), pleural processes (e.g., effusions or fibrothorax), chest wall abnormalities (e.g., bony deformities), or heart failure (e.g., cardiomegaly with effusions and pulmonary venous congestion).

Even a normal chest x-ray can be helpful, especially if there are demonstrable physiologic abnormalities on pulmonary function testing. Obstructive spirometry with a normal chest x-ray most commonly suggests asthma, but the radiographic abnormalities associated with COPD, bronchiectasis, or upper airway obstruction may not be evident or may easily be missed on plain film. Restrictive spirometry with a normal x-ray classically suggests neuromuscular diseases; however, early interstitial lung disease also is sometimes not evident on plain x-ray. An isolated decreased $DLCO_{corrected}$, isolated hypoxemia, or isolated exercise desaturation with a normal x-ray suggests pulmonary vascular disease or early interstitial disease. In addition, cardiac abnormalities without overt heart failure (intermittent ischemia, valvular diseases, diastolic dysfunction) commonly have no radiographic abnormalities.

Electrocardiogram

The electrocardiogram (ECG) is most useful when it is abnormal, since it directs the diagnostic approach toward cardiac etiologies. Common useful findings include the presence of Q waves, which suggest previous infarction and possible ischemic cardiomyopathy. Left ventricular hypertrophy and axis deviation may suggest hypertensive heart disease and diastolic heart dysfunction. Right ventricular hypertrophy and right axis deviation suggest pulmonary hypertension.

Further Diagnostic Testing

When the history and physical examination are performed in conjunction with the basic test outlined and are unrevealing, more specific testing is sometimes necessary. Specific tests include methacholine challenge testing when asthma is suspected but difficult to objectively document. An echocardiogram may confirm or further delineate suspected cardiac abnormalities. It also is useful in assessing pulmonary artery pressure in cases of suspected pulmonary hypertension. Nuclear cardiac testing may help define the presence and extent of coronary artery disease. A $\dot{V}/\dot{Q}$ scan or spiral CT of the chest may confirm chronic thromboembolic disease. High resolution CT may be used to diagnose early interstitial disease (in patients with restrictive spirometry but no parenchymal abnormalities on plain x-ray) or bronchiectasis.

Integrative cardiopulmonary exercise testing may be useful if the etiology of dyspnea remains unclear despite extensive testing. Although the most involved of the tests, it provides the most information in terms of the underlying mechanism of the dyspnea and is very helpful in making a specific diagnosis in conjunction with the clinical impression. It is also useful in cases in which the severity of the dyspnea is out of proportion to objective measurements. This test can clarify the relative importance of abnormalities in cases of multifactorial dyspnea (e.g., COPD with cardiomyopathy, cardiopulmonary diseases with deconditioning, and so on).

Evaluation of Diagnostic Tests in the Current Case

Pulmonary function tests reveal a normal FEV_1/FVC ratio, suggesting that the mild decrease in FVC is not due to airway obstruction. The FVC, TLC, and RV are all slightly and proportionately decreased, suggesting mild restrictive physiology. The abnormal $D_{LCO_{corrected}}$ may be related to the underlying restrictive process. However, it is markedly abnormal and the clinician should consider a superimposed physiologic process. Arterial blood gas levels reveal a mild respiratory alkalosis with severe hypoxemia, supporting the gas exchange abnormality found on the D_{LCO}. The mild restriction is most likely a result of obesity, since it is not associated with any parenchymal, pleural, or chest wall abnormalities noted on physical examination or chest x-ray.

The severe hypoxemia is not likely due to the mild restriction of obesity and therefore requires an explanation. In such a case, the clinician should consider early interstitial disease, intra-cardiac shunt, or pulmonary vascular diseases. The high resolution CT scan was obtained to rule out an early interstitial process that may not have been visible on plain x-ray.

The normal CT scan narrowed the differential diagnosis to intra-cardiac shunt or a pulmonary vascular process. The results of the patient's physical examination suggested pulmonary hypertension and made a pulmonary vascular process more likely. Since he has no lung parenchymal abnormalities, this suggests an isolated pulmonary vascular process. As discussed, primary pulmonary hypertension is unlikely because of the patient's age, and the lack of associated rheumatologic or systemic symptoms made pulmonary vasculitis unlikely as well. Subsequently, a contrasted, spiral chest CT scan confirmed the diagnosis of chronic thromboembolic disease.

Pitfalls and Common Mistakes in the Assessment of the Patient with Chronic Dyspnea

Many diseases associated with chronic dyspnea are serious, and thus the clinician must be wary of common diagnostic mistakes. This is particularly important because many of these diseases are easily treatable or at least have specific therapies.

Firstly, the clinician should not automatically associate a historical clue or physical finding with a specific disease. For example, a history of smoking or cardiac disease alone does not suggest the underlying mechanism of dyspnea. Similarly, wheezing on examination commonly suggests asthma or COPD. However, the clinician should remember that differential diagnoses of dyspnea are much broader, and etiologies, such as tracheal stenosis, large airway tumors, or vocal cord disorders, can cause chronic dyspnea with wheezing.

Conversely, the clinician should not discount the presence of disease based on a lack of physical evidence. For example, as discussed, the finding of restrictive mechanics on pulmonary function tests with a normal chest x-ray does not rule out an interstitial lung process. Although this pattern usually suggests chest wall or neuromuscular disease, the chest x-ray can be normal in up to 10% of patients with interstitial lung diseases. The diagnosis of early interstitial lung disease is even easier to overlook when there is no associated restrictive abnormality or resting hypoxemia. In these cases, patients may only have exercise-induced desaturation and a mildly decreased D_{LCO}.

Similarly, the clinician should not discount the possibility of multifactorial dyspnea, especially when combined physiologic abnormalities are found. For example, the finding of obstructive abnormalities on spirometry should not preclude other common diseases (e.g., ischemic heart disease), particularly when the obstruction is relatively mild or especially if the clinical impression is suggestive of a second diagnosis.

The accuracy of our diagnostic tests requires critical assessment as well. The pulse oximeter, for example, has a range of error of 6% to 8%, and an even broader range with dark-skinned persons. Therefore a reading of 90% actually may represent a saturation of 86% to 94% and does not rule out significant hypoxemia. This was exemplified in our patient whose pulse oximeter reading of 90% represented a P_{O_2} of 56 mm Hg. In addition, since the pulse oximeter does not measure the P_{CO_2}, a patient may have significant chronic hypoventilation and still maintain a normal arterial saturation, especially while on supplemental oxygen. Arterial blood gas levels should therefore always be obtained if ventilatory abnormalities are suspected.

▼ SUMMARY

Chronic dyspnea has a complex, multifactorial pathophysiology, as well as a broad differential diagnosis. However, the history, physical examination, pulmonary function tests, and chest radiography, in combination with a pathophysiologic approach, can narrow the differential diagnosis quickly. Further diagnostic testing may be necessary to make a specific diagnosis but should be guided on clinical grounds.

▼ BIBLIOGRAPHY

Dyspnea: Mechanisms, assessment and management: a consensus statement. American Thoracic Society, *Am J Respir Crit Care Med* 159:321, 1999.

Epler GR, McLoud TC, Gaensler EA, et al: Normal chest roentgenograms in chronic diffuse infiltrative lung disease, *N Engl J Med* 298(17):934-939, 1978.

Guenard H, Gallego J, Dromer C: Exercise dyspnea in patients with respiratory disease, *Eur Respir Rev* 5:6-13, 1995.

Mahler DA, Horowitz MB: Clinical evaluation of exertional dyspnea, *Clin Chest Med* 15(2):259-269, 1994.

Manning HL, Schwartzstein RM: Pathophysiology of dyspnea, *N Engl J Med* 333(23):1547-1553, 1995.

O'Donnell DE, Bain DJ, Webb KA: Factors contributing to relief of exertional breathlessness during hyperoxia in chronic airflow limitation, *Amer Rev Respir Crit Care Med* 155:530-535, 1997.

Pratter MR, Curley FJ, Dubois J, et al: Cause and evaluation of chronic dyspnea in a pulmonary disease clinic, *Arch Intern Med* 149(10):2277-2282, 1989.

Schwartzstein RM: Approach to the patient with dyspnea, *Up to Date CD-ROM* June 22, 1999.

Stulbarg MS, Adams L: Manifestations of Respiratory Disease. In Murray JF, Nadel JA: *Textbook of respiratory medicine*, Philadelphia, 1994, WB Saunders, pp 511-524.

Sue DY, Wasserman K, Moricca B, et al: Metabolic acidosis during exercise in patients with chronic obstructive pulmonary disease, *Chest* 94:93-98, 1998.

Taguchi O, Kikuchi Y, Hida W, et al: Effects of bronchoconstriction and external resistive loading on the sensation of dyspnea, *J Appl Physiol* 71:2183-2190, 1991.

Widdicombe JG: Pulmonary and respiratory tract receptors, *J Exp Biol* 100:41-57, 1982.

CHAPTER 6

FATIGUE-ASSOCIATED DAYTIME SLEEPINESS

Patrick J. Strollo Jr.

Key Terms

▼ Daytime sleepiness
▼ Fatigue
▼ Insufficient sleep
▼ Obstructive sleep-disordered breathing (OSBD)

▼ Upper airway resistance syndrome
▼ Sleep apnea/hypopnea syndrome
▼ Narcolepsy
▼ Idiopathic hypersomnolence

▼ Obesity
▼ Nocturnal polysomnography (PSG)
▼ Multiple sleep latency test (MSLT)
▼ Sleep study

▼ THE CLINICAL PROBLEM

A 43-year-old man presents with a primary complaint of fatigue that interferes with his daytime performance. On closer questioning, he admits to falling asleep at his computer in mid-afternoon and being very drowsy when driving home from work. He states he knows he is "out of shape." He gradually has gained approximately 50 pounds over the past 10 years.

He has been told that he is a snorer and that the snoring gradually has gotten worse. He has occasionally awakened himself with a "snort." He is unsure whether he stops breathing at night. He falls asleep "as soon as his head touches the pillow."

He sleeps approximately 8 hours per night. His sleep frequently is interrupted by the need to get up to urinate. He feels tired when he awakens.

His past medical history is remarkable for a 20 pack-year smoking history, social alcohol consumption, and a history of hypertension. His hypertension has been treated with an angiotensin-converting enzyme (ACE) inhibitor.

On physical examination, he is 6 foot, 2 inches and 250 pounds. His body mass index (BMI) is 32 kg/m^2. His blood pressure is 150/92 in his right arm sitting. His nasal mucosa is slightly boggy. His oropharynx is crowded. His neck measures 42 cm at the cricothyroid membrane. His lungs are clear to auscultation and percussion. His cardiac examination is unremarkable, as was the remainder of the examination with the exception of moderate obesity. A chest x-ray and a spirometry are ordered because of the smoking history; both are normal.

What is the differential diagnosis for this patient's complaint of fatigue, and what is the most likely cause?

Differential Diagnosis of Fatigue-Associated Daytime Sleepiness

Box 6-1 lists the common and less common causes of fatigue associated with daytime somnolence. Fatigue associated with daytime sleepiness is an important complaint that requires careful assessment. Identifying true daytime sleepiness as opposed to fatigue alone is essential. Daytime sleepiness is associated with impaired daytime performance that can result in motor vehicle or industrial accidents affecting the patient as well as those around him. Proper diagnosis and treatment can improve quality of life substantially and, in some instances, can save a life.

Modern life has reduced the time allocated for adequate sleep. The most common cause of daytime sleepiness is a chronic decrease in the total sleep time, which results in an insufficient sleep syndrome. This syndrome should be explored in all patients who present with the complaint of daytime sleepiness.

Box 6-1
Differential Diagnosis of Fatigue-Associated Daytime Sleepiness

Common Causes	Less Common Causes
Insufficient sleep syndrome	Atypical depression
OSDB	Hypothyroidism
Narcolepsy	Acromegaly
Idiopathic hypersomnolence	Obesity/poor conditioning
	Chronic fatigue syndrome
	Chronic sinus congestion
	Drugs/alcohol use
	Restless legs syndrome

OSDB, Obstructive sleep-disordered breathing.

How much sleep does someone need? The requirement for sleep varies. One way to gain insight into an individual's sleep need is to ask the patient how long he or she sleeps in the absence of an alarm clock to induce awakening.

A variety of medical problems can result in daytime sleepiness in the absence of decreased total sleep time. Obstructive sleep-disordered breathing (OSDB) is common. This clinical problem affects approximately 5% of the middle-aged population. The clinical spectrum of OSDB includes the upper airway resistance syndrome and the sleep apnea/hypopnea syndrome. Occasionally, OSDB is associated with daytime hypercapnia and right ventricular failure (i.e., the pickwickian syndrome). The common feature is ventilatory-related arousals that result in sleep fragmentation and lead to daytime sleepiness (Figure 6-1).

Narcolepsy is much less common, affecting approximately 0.01% of the population. Recent data indicate that the mechanism of daytime sleepiness is related to hypocretin neurotransmission deficiency.

The mechanism of daytime sleepiness is unknown in idiopathic hypersomnolence. These patients do not experience cataplexy and do not have sleep-onset, rapid eye movement (REM) sleep on multiple sleep latency testing (see later section), both of which are characteristic features of narcolepsy.

A variety of other clinical conditions can present with daytime sleepiness. The prevalence of daytime sleepiness in these conditions is not well defined. However,

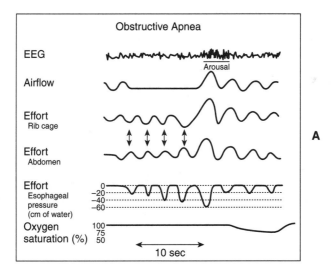

▼ **Figure 6-1**   Manifestations of upper airway closure. **A** depicts obstructive apnea. Increasing ventilatory effort is seen in the rib cage, the abdomen, and the level of esophageal pressure (measured with an esophageal balloon), despite lack of oronasal airflow. Arousal on the electroencephalogram (EEG) is associated with increasing ventilatory effort as indicated by the esophageal pressure. Oxyhemoglobin desaturation follows the termination of apnea. Note that during apnea, the movements of the rib cage and the abdomen (Effort) are in opposite directions *(arrows)* as a result of attempts to breathe against a closed airway. Once the airway opens in response to arousal, rib cage and abdominal movements become synchronous.   *Continued*

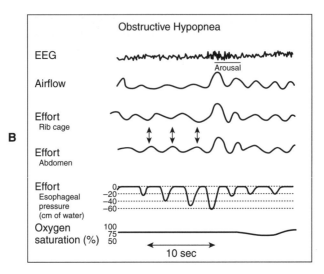

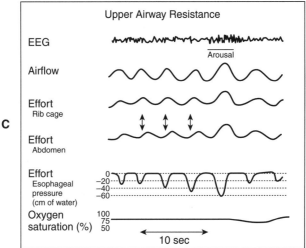

▼ **Figure 6-1, cont'd** **B** depicts obstructive hypopnea. Decreased airflow is associated with increasing ventilatory effort (reflected by the esophageal pressure) and subsequent arousal on the EEG. Rib cage and abdominal movements are in opposite directions during hypopnea *(arrows)*, reflecting increasingly difficult breathing against a partially closed airway. Rib cage and abdominal movements become synchronous after arousal produces airway opening. Oxyhemoglobin desaturation follows the termination of hypopnea. **C** depicts upper airway resistance. Asynchronous movements of the rib cage and abdomen and a substantial decrease in airflow are not seen. Arousal on the EEG is associated with increasing ventilatory effort due to increased airway resistance, as reflected by the esophageal pressure. There is no significant oxyhemoglobin desaturation. From Strollo PJ, Rogers RM: *N Engl J Med* 334:99-104, 1996.

establishing a proper diagnosis and instituting appropriate treatment can significantly improve daytime sleepiness (Table 6-1). Two of these conditions, chronic sinus congestion and the restless legs syndrome, deserve additional comment.

Chronic sinus congestion can result in prominent complaints of fatigue and may be associated with the upper airway resistance syndrome variant of OSDB. This

TABLE 6-1

Interpreting Signs and Symptoms in the Patient with Fatigue-Associated Daytime Sleepiness

Possible Causes	Mechanisms	Suggestive Clinical Features
Insufficient sleep syndrome	Decreased total sleep time	Normal examination History reveals less than 8 hours sleep per night
OSDB	Ventilatory-related arousals resulting in sleep fragmentation	Crowded oropharynx, retrognathia, snoring, observed apnea, upper body obesity, and/or hypertension
Narcolepsy	Hypocretin (orexin) neurotransmission deficiency	Sleep attacks, cataplexy, sleep paralysis, hypnagogic hallucinations
Idiopathic hypersomnolence	Unknown	Normal examination
Atypical depression	Unknown	Normal examination History reveals depressed mood, decreased libido, decreased appetite, anhedonia
Hypothyroidism	Decreased thyroid hormone	Decreased deep tendon reflexes, loss of lateral eyebrow hair, loss of hair over shins History reveals cold intolerance
Acromegaly	Increased secretion of growth hormone	Increased head circumference, large nose, tongue, hands, and feet
Obesity/poor conditioning	Elevated inflammatory cytokine levels (speculative)	Severe or morbid obesity
Chronic fatigue syndrome	Fragmented sleep not related to ventilatory arousals	Tender muscle trigger points to palpation
Chronic sinus congestion	Increased upper airway resistance leading to snoring and ventilatory arousals	Boggy nasal mucosa and/or nasal discharge History reveals evidence of perennial nasal congestion and post-nasal drip
Drugs/alcohol use	Fragmented sleep, overall depression of CNS	Alcohol: Rhinophyma, spider hemangiomas Drugs: Needle tracks
Restless legs syndrome	Leg movements resulting in sleep fragmentation and increased wake time after sleep onset	Normal examination History reveals increased urge to move legs, crawling sensation in calves Difficulty initiating and/or maintaining sleep due to leg discomfort

OSDB, Obstructive sleep-disordered breathing; *CNS,* central nervous system.

clinical problem frequently is overlooked. Treatment with non-sedating antihistamines and topical nasal steroids can favorably modify upper airway resistance. This relatively simple intervention can substantially improve complaints of fatigue and daytime sleepiness.

Restless legs syndrome is reported to be as common as OSDB. There is little objective evidence that these patients are sleepy during the day. More commonly, they report fatigue in association with insomnia. Occasionally the condition will result in increased wake time after sleep onset, causing insufficient sleep as a mechanism of daytime sleepiness.

Clinical Features that Suggest a Specific Cause of Fatigue-Associated Daytime Sleepiness

In this patient, the history and physical examination indicate that the specific cause of his fatigue associated with daytime sleepiness is OSDB (Table 6-1). He admits to falling asleep in sedentary situations such as working at his computer and driving. He awakens at night with a "snort" that corresponds with ventilatory arousals from sleep. He is able to fall asleep easily, suggesting increased sleep pressure, but awakens frequently to urinate. His sleep is not refreshing, suggesting chronic sleep fragmentation secondary to the ventilatory arousals.

The complaint of nocturia is a relatively common clinical finding in OSDB. Patients with untreated OSDB may have elevated atrial natriuretic peptide levels during sleep. This hormone is secreted by the atrium of the heart in response to increased atrial pressures. Pulmonary arterial vasoconstriction in response to the hypoxemia associated with the OSDB events (see Figure 6-1) precipitates the increase in the right atrial pressure, which frequently is a marker for severe OSDB in younger adults.

His past medical history is positive for smoking and hypertension and both are risk factors for OSDB.

The physical examination offers further support for a diagnosis of OSDB. The presence of moderate obesity (BMI = 32 kg/m^2), suboptimally controlled hypertension, a large neck, and a crowded oropharynx are all compatible with a diagnosis of OSDB.

Diagnostic Testing in the of Evaluation of Fatigue-Associated Daytime Sleepiness

Further diagnostic testing clearly is indicated in this patient. Evaluation of the patient's breathing during sleep allows the clinician to confirm the diagnosis of OSDB and to assess the severity of the problem. The number of OSDB events, the frequency and degree of hypoxemia, and the impact of these events on sleep architecture and continuity should be examined. Currently an attended, in-laboratory nocturnal polysomnogram (PSG) is the best way to accomplish such an evaluation.

If severe OSDB is unequivocally identified in the early portion of the overnight study, medical therapy with nasal continuous positive airway pressure could be initiated during the later portion of the PSG. This type of PSG is called a *split-night study*.

If the patient has less severe OSDB, a full diagnostic PSG may be required to establish a diagnosis. If there is no evidence of clinically significant OSDB present on the diagnostic PSG and insufficient sleep has been ruled out, an objective evaluation to exclude a non-pulmonary cause of excessive daytime sleepiness should be pursued.

This evaluation is best accomplished with a special laboratory study called the *multiple sleep latency test (MSLT)*. The MSLT evaluates the patient's propensity to fall asleep in five "naps" that are scheduled at 2-hour intervals during the day. Pathologic sleepiness can be confirmed if the mean sleep latency for the five naps is ≤5 minutes. If REM sleep is identified on at least two of the five naps in association with pathologic sleepiness, a diagnosis of narcolepsy should be considered. If there is no evidence of clinically significant OSDB and pathologic sleepiness is present without evidence of REM sleep, a diagnosis of idiopathic hypersomnolence should be considered.

Additional information may be helpful in conjunction with the MSLT. The patient should be asked to keep a "sleep diary" for the 2 weeks before the MSLT. This diary can help evaluate the amount of sleep the patient gets on a nightly basis. It is helpful to obtain a urine sample for illicit drugs at the time of the MSLT. Many sleep clinicians require a negative urine screen before initiating stimulant therapy if the history, PSG, and MSLT suggest that such treatment would be an appropriate intervention.

Finally, if there is clinical concern that an endocrine abnormality exists, hormonal assays to exclude hypothyroidism and/or acromegaly should be obtained. A clinical suspicion of acromegaly on the basis of the physical examination usually prompts further work-up. A diagnosis of hypothyroidism can be more elusive. Approximately 10% of patients referred for evaluation of OSDB have concomitant occult hypothyroidism.

Pitfalls and Common Mistakes in the Assessment of Fatigue-Associated Daytime Sleepiness

The three common pitfalls in evaluating patients with fatigue-associated daytime sleepiness are (1) the failure to obtain an adequate sleep history, (2) the type of monitoring used to evaluate breathing during sleep, and (3) not identifying and treating coexisting conditions that contribute to fatigue-associated daytime sleepiness.

As previously discussed, insufficient sleep is the most common cause of daytime sleepiness. If the patient is not carefully questioned regarding the amount of sleep obtained on a nightly basis, a diagnostic PSG and/or an MSLT may be inappropriately ordered. The resulting information may confuse the treating physician and lead to incorrect therapy.

Once insufficient sleep is excluded from the differential diagnosis, OSDB is unquestionably the most common cause of daytime sleepiness. Currently, the manner in which airflow and ventilatory effort are assessed varies widely. The American Academy of Sleep Medicine examined the evidence for establishing a diagnosis of OSDB and identified significant limitations in currently accepted monitoring techniques. The current community standard of using thermocouples to monitor airflow and piezoelectric belts to assess effort can substantially limit the ability to detect ventilatory arousals related to hypopneas or respiratory effort-related arousals (i.e., the upper airway resistance syndrome). These limits can lead to misdiagnosis and inappropriate treatment.

Finally, although it is intellectually satisfying to identify just one clinical problem causing daytime sleepiness, multiple, comorbid conditions may exist that contribute to the patient's impaired daytime function. Insufficient sleep, depression, endocrine abnormalities, obesity, chronic sinus congestion, and concomitant drug and/or alcohol abuse can all coexist with OSDB, and, if not addressed, result in an inadequate treatment effect.

▼ BIBLIOGRAPHY

Anonymous: Sleep-related breathing disorders in adults: recommendations for syndrome definition and measurement techniques in clinical research. The Report of an American Academy of Sleep Medicine Task Force, *Sleep* 22:667-689, 1999.

Chesson AL Jr, Ferber RA, Fry JM, et al: Practice parameters for the indications for polysomnography and related procedures, *Sleep* 20:406-422, 1997.

Nishino S, Ripley B, Overeem S, et al: Hypocretin (orexin) deficiency in human narcolepsy, *Lancet* 355:39-40, 2000.

Strohl KP, Redline S: Recognition of obstructive sleep apnea, *Am J Respir Crit Care Med* 154:279-289, 1996.

Strollo PJ, Rogers RM: Obstructive sleep apnea, *N Engl J Med* 334:99-104, 1996.

Strollo PJ: Sleep disorders in primary care. In Poceta JS, Mitler MM (editors): *Sleep disorders: Diagnosis and treatment*, Totowa, New Jersey, 1998, Humana Press.

Vgontzas AN, Bixler EO, Tan T, et al: Obesity without sleep apnea is associated with daytime sleepiness, *Arch Intern Med* 158:1333-1337, 1998.

CHAPTER 7

SOLITARY PULMONARY NODULE

Albert L. Rafanan
Atul C. Mehta

▼ Key Terms

▼ Lung cancer ▼ Hamartoma ▼ Popcorn calcification
▼ Granuloma ▼ Calcification ▼ Laminated calcification

▼ THE CLINICAL PROBLEM

A 65-year-old man presents with a newly detected solitary pulmonary nodule (SPN) on a chest x-ray obtained for a life insurance application. He is in good health and denies weight loss, fever, hemoptysis, cough, or night sweats. His past medical history is unremarkable. He was a heavy smoker (40 pack-years) but stopped smoking 15 years ago. He is a teacher and has no occupational exposure. He is from Cleveland and denies any recent travel. Physical examination is unremarkable.

The anteroposterior (AP) and lateral views of the chest x-ray show a 3-cm noncalcified SPN in the left lower lobe. A chest x-ray obtained 1 year ago was normal. Spirometry reveals a moderate obstructive ventilatory defect (forced expiratory volume in 1 second [FEV_1] = 1.9 L [60% predicted], forced vital capacity (FVC) = 3.15 L [95% predicted], and FEV_1/FVC = 0.6). The high resolution computed tomography (CT) scan confirms the presence of the noncalcified spiculated nodule. The hilar and mediastinal nodes are not enlarged.

What is the differential diagnosis for SPN? How should the work-up proceed?

Differential Diagnosis of a Solitary Pulmonary Nodule

SPN is defined as a distinct round or oval pulmonary lesion surrounded by aerated lung and not associated with areas of atelectasis or hilar enlargement (Figure 7-1). The incidental finding of an SPN on a routine chest film is common. Approximately 140,000 new cases of SPNs are detected annually in the United States. No consensus exists as to the upper limit of its size, although most experts agree that lesions larger than 3 cm be considered as pulmonary masses rather than SPNs. Pulmonary masses do not pose the same diagnostic dilemma as SPNs, since almost all (93% to 99%) are malignant.

Approximately 60% of SPNs detected by chest x-ray are benign; most (80%) are due to histoplasmosis, coccidiomycosis, or mycobacteria. Hamartomas account for 10% of benign SPNs. Most malignant lesions are from bronchogenic carcinoma, and the radiographic pattern often can suggest a specific cell type. For example, malignant peripheral nodules usually are adenocarcinoma or large cell carcinoma. Squamous or small cell cancers infrequently present as SPNs; rather, they occur within the bronchi and are more likely to cause atelectasis. Metastases from extrathoracic malignancies account for 10% to 30% of all malignant SPNs and are usually responsible for multiple nodules (Box 7-1).

Clinical Features that Suggest a Specific Cause for a Solitary Pulmonary Nodule

The challenge in evaluating the SPN lies in determining whether it is benign or malignant. Malignant SPNs are potentially curable with surgical resection. On the other hand, unnecessary surgical resection of a benign lesion can harm the patient. The initial evaluation includes a thorough medical history, physical examination, and careful review of current and old chest x-rays. Table 7-1 presents features of the solitary pulmonary nodule that may suggest a specific cause.

Advanced age increases the likelihood that an SPN is malignant. The chance for a malignant SPN is 65% for patients over 50 years old, whereas it is only 33% for younger patients. Smoking and a prior history of cancer increase the likelihood that the nodule is malignant. In patients with a history of extrathoracic malignancy, the likelihood of developing a second primary malignancy or a solitary metastasis is high; SPNs are malignant in 80% of such cases. The history regarding travel, place of residence, occupation, pets, and hobbies is also valuable in the evaluation of SPN. For instance, histoplasmosis is the most common cause of SPN among residents along the Ohio, Mississippi, and Missouri River Valley areas. Similarly, coccidiomycosis and tuberculosis would be the most likely etiologies in certain endemic areas.

The physical examination usually is normal in patients with SPN. Infrequently, the physical examination may be helpful in discovering an extra-pulmonary

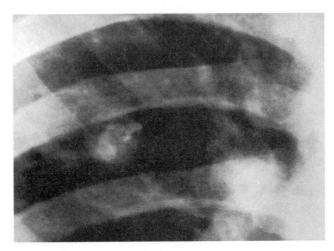

▼ **Figure 7-1** Chest x-ray of a solitary pulmonary nodule with a popcorn type of calcification. From Minai OA, Ahmad M: Solitary pulmonary nodule. In Bone RC, Campbell GD Jr., Payne D (editors): *Bone's atlas of pulmonary and critical care medicine*, Philadelphia, 1998, Williams and Wilkins.

Box 7-1
Common Causes of Solitary Pulmonary Nodules

Benign	Malignant
Granulomatous Infection	**Bronchogenic Carcinoma**
Coccidiomycosis	Adenocarcinoma: Bronchoalveolar
Histoplasmosis	cell carcinoma
Tuberculosis	Large cell
Atypical mycobacterial infection	Squamous cell
	Small cell
Pulmonary Arteriovenous Malformation	
	Solitary Metastasis
Bronchogenic Cyst	Head and neck tumors
	Breast cancer
Benign Tumors	Renal cell cancer
Hamartoma	Colon cancer
Fibroma	Germ cell
Lipoma	Thyroid
Lymphangioma	
Leiomyoma	**Bronchial Carcinoid Tumor**
Neurofibroma	Pulmonary sarcoma
	Non-Hodgkin's lymphoma
Wegener's Granulomatosis	Multiple myeloma (plasmacytoma)
Rheumatoid Nodule	
Sarcoidosis	
Amyloid	
Pulmonary infarction	
Pneumonitis	
Parasitic infection (Echinococcus cyst,	
ascariasis, dirofilariasis)	
Pulmonary hematoma	

TABLE 7-1
Clinical and Radiologic Features that Suggest a Specific Cause of a Solitary Pulmonary Nodule

Etiology	Clinical Features	Radiologic Features
Neoplasm **Bronchogenic carcinoma**	Older age; smoking history; prior history of lung cancer; paraneoplastic symptoms (weight loss, anorexia, malaise, clubbing, Eaton-Lambert syndrome)	Enlargement on serial chest x-rays; ill-defined, spiculated, lobulated, or umbilicated margins; absence of calcifications (eccentric deposition if present); predominantly upper lobes
Bronchoalveolar cell carcinoma	Usually asymptomatic with localized form; excessive amount of mucus production occasionally seen in advanced state	May have well-circumscribed margins; presence of "air bronchogram" on high resolution CT; can have indolent course over months or years, but transformation to diffuse form can occur rapidly
Carcinoid tumor	Peak incidence between 35-45 years; not associated with smoking; pulmonary symptoms (hemoptysis, cough, and often a localized wheeze) present in one third of patients, although clinically silent if tumor is located peripherally; rarely present with carcinoid syndrome unless metastatic	Well-defined and smooth margin; very slow growth rate; most common sites are the right upper and middle lobes and the lingula; can rarely calcify
Metastatic tumors	Usually does not have any pulmonary symptoms; extra-pulmonary symptoms may reveal primary site; prior history of extra-pulmonary malignancy	Smooth, well-defined margins; usually lower lobes; rarely calcify unless from chondrosarcoma or osteogenic sarcoma; presents usually as multiple nodules
Benign **Mycobacterium tuberculosis (tuberculoma)**	History of exposure; recent PPD conversion; nonspecific symptoms (cough, fever, weight loss, hemoptysis, etc); may be asymptomatic	Calcification is common; predilection for upper lobes (R >L); well-circumscribed margins (25% lobulated); associated with "satellite" lesions in 80%

CT, Computed tomography; *PPD,* purified protein derivative; *DVT,* deep vein thrombosis.

TABLE 7-1
Clinical and Radiologic Features that Suggest a Specific Cause of a Solitary Pulmonary Nodule—cont'd

Etiology	Clinical Features	Radiologic Features
Benign—cont'd *Histoplasma capsulatum* (histoplasmoma)	Endemic to river valleys of the midwestern and southern United States; nonspecific symptoms and most often asymptomatic	Commonly calcified; central type of calcification most common; laminated calcification diagnostic; smooth margins; more frequently in the lower lobes; associated with hilar, mediastinal, hepatic, or splenic calcification; "satellite" lesions are common
Coccidiodes immitis	Endemic to the lower Sonoran life zone; nonspecific symptoms and most often asymptomatic	Commonly cavitate with and often presents as a thin-walled cyst; calcify in come cases; well-defined margins; usually in upper lobes
Arteriovenous malformation	Associated with hereditary hemorrhagic telangiectasia in 40%-65% of cases; audible bruit over lesion site; can have clubbing and cyanosis	Rounded or serpiginous subpleural nodule with two feeding vessels (feeding artery and draining veins), pulsatile lesion under fluoroscopy; more common in lower lobes
Hamartoma	Usually asymptomatic; occurs more frequently in males than females (3:1); peak incidence in the sixth decade; uncommon before age 30	Calcification is present in 40%; "popcorn" type of calcification is diagnostic; presence of fat (-40 to -120 HU by high resolution CT); margins are sharply defined and may be lobulated or smooth; on occasion may demonstrate a rapid growth rate
***Aspergillus* sp.** (mycetoma, aspergilloma, or "fungus ball")	Hemoptysis in 45%-85% and usually minimal; rarely presents with constitutional symptoms; can be asymptomatic	Mass within a cavity outlined by an air crescent; movement of mass with change in position ("Monad's sign"); usually in upper lobe; does not calcify
Bronchogenic cyst	Peak incidence during third decade, more common in males and Yemenite Jews	Located most commonly near the hilum or mediastinum; lower lobe predilection; smooth margins; cyst contents may contain calcification; can cavitate if communication with bronchial tree occurs

Continued

TABLE 7-1
Clinical and Radiologic Features that Suggest a Specific Cause of a Solitary Pulmonary Nodule—cont'd

Etiology	Clinical Features	Radiologic Features
Benign—cont'd		
Pulmonary infarction	Dyspnea, pleuritic pain, unexplained hypoxemia, predisposing factors (recent surgery, hypercoagulability, injury or surgery involving the lower extremities or pelvis, congestive heart failure, immobility, pregnancy, cancer, prior episode of DVT, obesity, and contraceptives)	Pleural-based triangular density with apex directed toward the hilum (Hampton's hump); serial chest films demonstrate rapid shrinkage of the lesion
Rheumatoid nodule	Evidence of rheumatoid arthritis; nodules wax and wane in association with subcutaneous nodules and activity of rheumatoid arthritis	Nodule is dense and well circumscribed; may cavitate; usually lower lobes; peripheral subpleural areas

PPD, Purified protein derivative; *DVT,* deep vein thrombosis.

malignancy, increasing the likelihood that the SPN is a solitary metastasis. The findings of dermal and mucosal telangiectasia, hypoxemia, or embolic lesions also would suggest the possibility of pulmonary arteriovenous malformation as the cause.

The most important first step in evaluating the SPN is comparing the current chest x-ray with previous ones. An extra effort to obtain these films can spare the patient unnecessary interventions.

The volume doubling time of malignant pulmonary nodules is from 21 to 400 days. Since the SPN is a sphere (i.e., volume = $4/3 \pi r^3$), the nodule doubles in size when the diameter is increased by approximately 26%. Thus, if the nodule's diameter has increased by 25% in less than 20 days or if there is no growth over a 2-year period, the lesion is probably benign. However, accurately assessing the diameter can be difficult (especially for small nodules), so doubling time is infrequently relied on.

Nodule characteristics (size, calcification, and shape) are most useful in determining if the nodule is benign or malignant. The larger the nodule size, the greater the likelihood that it is malignant. For nodules greater than 2 cm in diameter, 80% will be malignant, whereas only 20% are malignant when the SPN is less than 2 cm. The presence of calcification increases the likelihood that the nodule is benign. Only about 10% of malignant SPNs show calcification. Furthermore, some specific patterns of calcification can help establish that the nodule is benign. Laminated, diffuse, central, or speckled calcifications are characteristic of granulomata

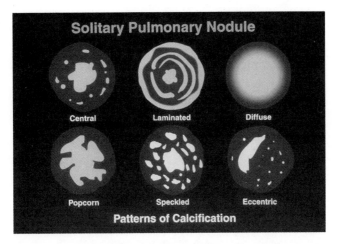

▼ **Figure 7-2**   Patterns of calcification. Central, laminated, diffuse, and popcorn type of calcification suggest a benign lesion. Speckled and eccentric patterns of calcification suggest a malignant lesion.

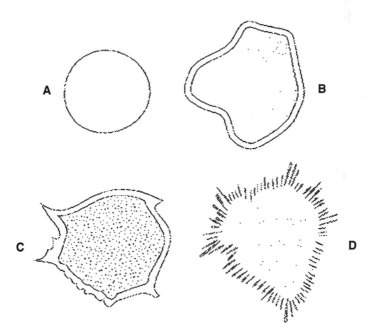

▼ **Figure 7-3**   Nodular margin patterns. Smooth and well-defined margins (**A** and **B**) are suggestive of a benign lesion. Lobulated (**C**) and spiculated (**D**) margins are suggestive of a malignant lesion. Adapted from Siegelman SS, Khouri NF, Leo FP, et al: *Radiology* 160:307-312, 1986.

(Figure 7-2). A "popcorn" type of calcification strongly suggests a hamartoma (see Figure 7-1). However, a stippled or eccentric calcification pattern does not establish a benign cause but rather raises the suspicion for malignancy. The presence of pleural retraction or a spiculated or lobulated nodule margin also makes the nodule more likely to be malignant (Figure 7-3).

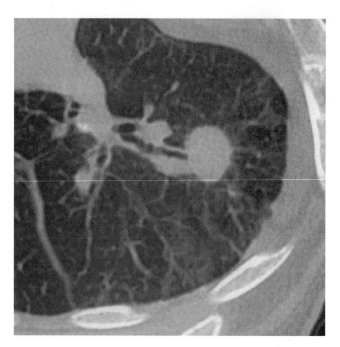

▼ **Figure 7-4**   Bronchus sign is a CT finding in which the bronchus leads directly to or is contained within a nodule or mass. From Mehta AC, Kathawalla SA, Choon-Chee C, et al: *J Bronchol* 2:315-322, 1995.

Diagnostic Testing in the Evaluation of the Patient with a Solitary Pulmonary Nodule

In evaluating the patient with an SPN, a high resolution CT is useful, especially if old films do not establish a stable appearance over at least 2 years. The CT provides greater anatomic detail of the nodule. Alternative diagnoses, such as rounded atelectasis, aspergilloma, or arteriovenous malformations, can easily be made with high resolution CT. The imaging of the pulmonary parenchyma and the mediastinum sometimes reveals synchronously occurring nodules or mediastinal nodes not visualized on chest x-ray. The presence of enlarged or calcified mediastinal lymph nodes along the drainage area may suggest cancer or granulomatous infection, respectively. The high resolution CT can also be used to measure fat and calcium density. Fat tissue in an SPN suggests a diagnosis of hamartoma. In addition, high resolution CT can evaluate for nodule location and a "bronchus sign" (i.e., a bronchus leading directly into a nodule) and may aid in selecting the next diagnostic step, which may be flexible bronchoscopy (FB) or percutaneous needle aspiration (PCNA) (Figure 7-4).

The probability of malignancy can be better assessed with a careful review of the medical history, physical examination, chest x-rays, and CT scan. On this basis, the SPN can be categorized into one of three groups: definitely benign, indeterminate, or high probability for malignancy. For definitely benign SPNs, no further work-up is necessary. An SPN with a high probability for malignancy benefits most from curative resection. For indeterminate nodules, there is no consensus as to what constitutes the best approach. Management options include observation, other noninvasive roentgenographic tests, biopsy with FB or PCNA, and resection.

TABLE 7-2
Factors that Influence the Yield of Bronchoscopy in the Evaluation of Solitary Pulmonary Nodules

Feature	Diagnostic Yield of Bronchoscopy (%)
Size of Nodule	
>2 cm	50-70
<2 cm	5-30
Bronchus Sign	
Positive	60
Negative	30
Location of Nodule	
Inner and middle third of the lung	60-70
Outer third of the lung	26-48
Pathology	
Primary lung malignancy	58-63
Metastatic lesion	28
Benign	12-38
Bronchoscopic Procedures	
Transbronchial biopsy	12-40
Brush	4-43
Wash	36-52
TBNA	28-65

TBNA, Transbronchial needle aspiration.

The probability of malignancy, comorbid illness, and lung function measurements usually dictate the tempo of further testing. More importantly, the patient's preferences regarding options helps determine the subsequent diagnostic work-up.

The following noninvasive radiographic techniques have been developed for evaluating indeterminate nodules:

1. The use of a CT reference phantom (a model constructed to simulate the chest configuration, nodule size, and location) can identify 3% to 55% of benign nodules.
2. Quantitative measurement of contrast enhancement during chest CT has been used to differentiate benign and malignant SPNs. An increase of greater than 20 Hounsfield units (HU) after contrast injection is a characteristic suggesting a malignant cause, with a sensitivity of 98% and a specificity of 73%.
3. Positron emission tomography (PET) imaging is able to identify malignant lesions with 93% to 97% sensitivity and 80% to 100% specificity.

Because these studies may produce false-positive and false-negative results, they are best used to support a clinical impression and to direct the next step. The true nature of most nodules cannot be confirmed without a definitive tissue biopsy. In such indeterminate lesions, biopsies can be obtained using FB, PCNA, video-assisted thoracotomy (VATS), or open thoracotomy.

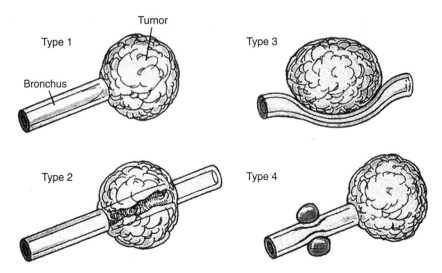

▼ **Figure 7-5** Tsuboi's classification of nodule-bronchus relationships. From Tsuboi E, Ikeda S, Tajima M, et al: *Cancer* 20:687-698, 1967.

**Box 7-2
Contraindications for Percutaneous
Needle Aspiration**

Solitary pulmonary nodule close to blebs or behind fissure
Bullous emphysema
Inability to hold breath
Bleeding diathesis
Severe pulmonary hypertension
$FEV_1 < 1$ Liter
Previous pneumonectomy

FB is most useful for large SPNs (>2 cm diameter) with a positive "bronchus sign" that is located in the central and middle third of the lung (Table 7-2). Overall, FB has a yield of 40% to 60%. Transbronchial needle aspiration (TBNA), in addition to regular bronchoscopic procedures, increases the diagnostic yield by approximately 25%. The "needle" is able to sample lesions inaccessible to the brush or the forceps, the so-called type III or IV Tsuboi SPN type lesions (Figure 7-5). Concomitant staging and diagnosis can be performed if a malignancy and enlarged lymph nodes are suspected by using the TBNA to sample mediastinal and hilar lymph nodes.

PCNA has a sensitivity of 75% to 97% for malignant lesions but only a 12% to 68% yield for benign lesions. Also, the technique is associated with a 25% to 30% rate of pneumothorax as compared to only 1% to 2% for bronchoscopy (Box 7-2). If FB, PCNA, or both fail to provide a diagnosis, surgical resection using VATS or conventional thoracotomy may be necessary.

Prospective observation may be an acceptable option in patients for whom the likelihood of malignancy is low (i.e., young nonsmoker with a small nodule) and for patients who decline further invasive procedures. Serial chest x-rays every 3 months for the first year, every 6 months for the second year, and yearly thereafter are recommended. Nodules not clearly seen by chest x-ray may require follow-up CTs.

In the current patient, several features suggest a high concern for malignancy: the patient's age, history of smoking, the nodule diameter and spiculated margin, and the lack of calcification or evidence that the nodule was present on prior chest x-rays. Because of this concern and the adequacy of his lung function for surgery, proceeding to surgical resection for both diagnosis and treatment of the SPN is a reasonable option.

Common Pitfalls in the Assessment and Treatment of a Solitary Pulmonary Nodule

As many as 10% to 20% of nodules detected by chest x-ray are artifacts or SPN mimics. Common SPN mimics include nipple shadows, soft-tissue tumors (e.g., neurofibromas), bony shadows (e.g., healed rib fracture), pseudotumor, round atelectasis, and pleural plaques. Careful review of both the AP and lateral views of the chest x-ray frequently picks out these SPN mimics without resorting to chest CT.

The failure to seek old chest films for comparison is a common pitfall. This oversight can lead to unnecessary procedures and risk to the patient. In some instances, a simple review of old chest x-rays can secure a benign diagnosis and end the work-up. An SPN that has been stable over the last 2 years or that has a doubling time less than 21 days is benign and will not need any other diagnostic tests. In the case of the enlarging nodule, work-up to resolution is warranted.

The concept of doubling time also is frequently misunderstood. Doubling time is the time it takes for a mass to double in volume. An SPN is approximately a sphere. The volume of a sphere is $4/3\ \pi r^3$ or $1/6\ \pi D^3$, where r = radius and D = diameter. Thus doubling of nodule size occurs when a 1-cm nodule increases by 3 mm in diameter or a 2-cm nodule by 5 mm (increase of diameter by about 26%). When the nodule doubles in diameter, it has actually increased by eightfold in volume.

▼ Bibliography

Jain P, Kathawalla SA, Arroliga AC: Managing solitary pulmonary nodules, *Cleve Clin J Med* 65:315-326, 1998.

Mehta AC, Kathawalla SA, Choon-Chee C, et al: Role of bronchoscopy in the evaluation of solitary pulmonary nodule, *J Bronchol* 2:315-322, 1995.

Midthun DE, Swensen SJ, Jett JR: Clinical strategies for solitary pulmonary nodule, *Ann Rev Med* 43:195-208, 1992.

Minai OA, Mehta AC, Ahmad M: Solitary pulmonary nodule. In Bone RC, Campbell GD Jr, Payne D (editors): *Bone's atlas of pulmonary and critical care medicine,* Philadelphia, 1998, Williams and Wilkins.

Siegelman SS, Khouri, NF, Leo FP, et al: Solitary pulmonary nodule: CT assessment, *Radiology* 160:307-312, 1986.

Stoller JK, Ahmad M, Rice TW: Solitary pulmonary nodule. *Cleve Clin J Med* 55:68-74, 1988.

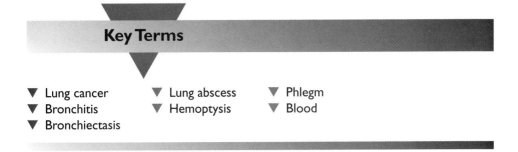

CHAPTER 8

HEMOPTYSIS

Robert Gerber
Raed A. Dweik

Key Terms

▼ Lung cancer   ▼ Lung abscess   ▼ Phlegm
▼ Bronchitis   ▼ Hemoptysis   ▼ Blood
▼ Bronchiectasis

▼ THE CLINICAL PROBLEM

A 50-year-old man with a remote smoking history (30 pack-years, quit 10 years ago) presents with complaints of fevers, chills, and cough productive of blood-streaked sputum of 1-week duration. He denies night sweats, shortness of breath, wheezing, decreased appetite, or weight loss.

His past medical history is significant only for an episode of pneumonia that did not require hospitalization approximately 5 years ago. He takes no medication and has no contributory family history. Physical examination reveals his nasopharynx and oropharynx to be clear with no associated lymphadenopathy. Auscultation of the chest is clear, and cardiac examination reveals no murmurs or gallops. The remainder of his physical examination is unremarkable. A chest x-ray reveals a normal cardiovascular silhouette and clear lung fields.

What is the differential diagnosis for this patient's hemoptysis, and how should the patient be managed?

Clinical Features of Hemoptysis

Symptoms referable to the respiratory tract are an extremely common reason for office visits. Hemoptysis is a common outpatient problem responsible for a significant number of pulmonary and thoracic surgery referrals every year.

Hemoptysis is defined as expectoration of blood from the lower respiratory tract (beneath the vocal cords). Minor hemoptysis usually is considered to be less than 15 to 20 mL/day and commonly resolves spontaneously. The range for *massive hemoptysis* is from greater than or equal to 100 mL in 24 hours to greater than 1 L in 24 hours. Massive hemoptysis also can be judged by its clinical consequences such as requiring hospitalization, the risk of airway occlusion from bleeding, laboratory evidence of blood loss, or even risk of death. In the context that the current patient has blood-streaked sputum, this chapter focuses on the diagnosis and management of minor hemoptysis, not massive hemoptysis.

Differential Diagnosis of Hemoptysis

When considering the etiology of minor hemoptysis, it is important to be familiar with the normal pulmonary circulation. The pulmonary arteries that supply the pulmonary parenchyma are but one of the circulatory systems in the chest. The pulmonary arteries are a low-pressure, high-flow system that receive the entire cardiac output. A second circulatory system within the chest is the bronchial arteries. There are usually only one or two per lung, and these originate from the aorta or intercostal arteries. The bronchial circulation is a high (systemic) pressure, low-flow system, which tends to be the major source of hemoptysis because it is more likely to be the source of the collaterals and the neovascularization that characteristically occurs in the setting of chronic infection or malignancy.

The most common causes of minor hemoptysis are bronchitis, bronchiectasis, bronchogenic carcinoma, and tuberculosis. Bronchitis and bronchiectasis together account for approximately 20% to 40% of cases of minor hemoptysis. Carcinoma accounts for another 20% of cases, including bronchogenic, metastatic (endobronchial tumors such as melanoma, cancers of the breast and colon, and renal origin cancers), and carcinoid tumors (particularly in the younger, non-smoking population), as well as Kaposi's sarcoma in human immunodeficiency virus (HIV)-positive patients. Box 8-1 also lists some of the less common causes of minor hemoptysis.

Evaluation of the Patient with Hemoptysis

The first step in evaluating any patient with hemoptysis is a thorough history and complete physical examination to confirm that the patient truly has hemoptysis and not epistaxis (bleeding from the nose) or hematemesis (bleeding from the gastrointestinal tract). Table 8-1 lists clues to help a clinician differentiate bleeding hemoptysis from epistaxis or hematemesis. A careful physical examination can reveal the source of bleeding if it originates from the nasopharynx or oropharynx.

Bronchiectasis is an abnormal, irreversible dilation of the airways that leads to chronic sputum production (Table 8-2). Predisposing factors for the development of bronchiectasis include infection (bacterial, viral, mycobacterial, or fungal), airway obstruction (either from mucus, foreign bodies, neoplasms, or obstructive

Box 8-1
Differential Diagnosis of Minor Hemoptysis

Common Causes	Less Common Causes
Bronchitis	Necrotizing pneumonia
Bronchiectasis	Lung abscess
Bronchogenic carcinoma	Bronchial adenoma
Tuberculosis	Broncholithiasis
	Endobronchial metastatic carcinoma
	Alveolar hemorrhage syndromes
	Wegener's granulomatosis
	Goodpasture's syndrome
	Systemic lupus erythematosus
	Mitral stenosis
	Congestive heart failure
	Pulmonary embolus
	Arteriovenous malformation
	Coagulopathy
	Thrombocytopenia
	Trauma (blunt or penetrating)
	Foreign body
	Iatrogenic (pulmonary arterial catheter insertion, bronchoscopy, etc)
	Idiopathic

TABLE 8-1
Differentiating True Hemoptysis from Epistaxis and Hematemesis

Symptoms	Hemoptysis	Hematemesis	Epistaxis
Cough	Common	Uncommon	Uncommon
Dyspnea	Common	Uncommon	Uncommon
Nausea, vomiting, abdominal pain	Uncommon	Common	Uncommon
Gurgling sensation in chest	May be present	Absent	Absent
Concomitant nasal bleeding	Absent	Absent	Usually present
Frothy secretions	May be present	Absent	Absent
Food particles	Absent	May be present	Absent
Mixed with sputum	Common	Uncommon	Uncommon
Color	Bright red	Dark, coffee grounds	Bright red
Coughed blood pH	Alkaline	Acidic	Alkaline

TABLE 8-2
Interpreting Signs and Symptoms in the Patient
with Minor Hemoptysis

Possible Causes	Mechanisms	Suggestive Clinical Features
Bronchitis	Bronchial artery erosion in the setting of chronic inflammation	Fever; purulent sputum without evidence of consolidation on examination; clear chest x-ray
Bronchiectasis	Bronchial arterial bleeding	Cough and purulent sputum; frequently worse in the morning (after a night of sleeping supine); wheezing and dyspnea during exacerbations; "tram lines" on plain chest x-ray; predominantly CT diagnosis
Bronchogenic carcinoma	Usually bronchial arterial bleeding due to ulceration of the tumor	History of smoking, cough; symptoms include those related to airway obstruction (such as wheezing and dyspnea), hoarseness (due to recurrent laryngeal nerve involvement), anorexia, weight loss
Tuberculosis	Usually bronchial artery bleeding; the dilated vessel is located in the wall of the cavity (Rasmussen's aneurysm)	Fever, usually late in the afternoon; night sweats; cough; anorexia and weight loss; infiltrates (in reactivation) characteristically in the apical or posterior segment of the upper lobes or the superior segment of the lower lobes
Wegener's granulomatosis (and other connective tissue diseases such as Goodpasture's syndrome, SLE)	Pulmonary circulation (alveolar hemorrhage)	Typical features include pulmonary infiltrates, recent drop in hematocrit, hypoxemia, renal dysfunction, and other features of the underlying disease
Mitral stenosis	Submucosal bronchial veins from congestion	Symptoms and signs of left ventricular failure (orthopnea, PND, lower extremity swelling); characteristic murmur
Pulmonary embolus	Pulmonary circulation (infarction)	Chest pain worse with coughing and deep breathing; dyspnea; tachycardia; tachypnea; hypoxemia; usually clear chest x-ray
Arteriovenous malformation	Both bronchial and pulmonary circulations	Bruit on chest examination; mucosal arteriovenous malformation in Osler-Weber-Rendu syndrome
Coagulopathy	Bronchial or pulmonary	Liver disease; receiving anticoagulants; low platelets; high PT, PTT

CT, Computed tomography; SLE, systemic lupus erythematosus, PND, paroxysmal nocturnal dyspnea, PT, protime; PTT, prothrombin time.

lung diseases such as chronic obstructive pulmonary disease [COPD] or alpha$_1$-antitrypsin deficiency), immunodeficiency states, and inherited defects such as immotile cilia syndrome or cystic fibrosis.

Bronchiectasis more commonly occurs in the lower lobes. Physical examination can reveal localized rhonchi or wheezing. The chest x-ray may be unremarkable in the early stages. Later, it may reveal "tram lines" indicative of thickened bronchial walls and peribronchial fibrosis.

Although this patient may be predisposed to developing bronchiectasis because of his prior history of pneumonia, this diagnosis is unlikely since his cough is not chronically productive and his chest x-ray is normal.

Bronchogenic carcinoma is currently the leading cause of cancer-related death in men and women in the United States. Symptoms from lung cancer can be non-specific. They can include hemoptysis, as well as other associated symptoms such as chest pain, dyspnea, and weight loss. Occasionally, the symptoms may be related to the location of the tumor, causing localized obstruction and distal atelectasis. This diagnosis needs to be considered, particularly in persons over the age of 50 with a history of smoking. However, his normal chest x-ray makes this diagnosis less likely in this patient.

Symptoms of tuberculosis commonly include fever, dyspnea, cough, hemoptysis, night sweats, and weight loss. The disease occurs more commonly as reactivation of a remote infection. Persons prone to reactivation include the elderly, diabetics, patients with renal failure, patients on immunosuppressive medications, and patients with acquired immunodeficiency syndrome (AIDS) or malignancy. When hemoptysis occurs, it usually is due to either cavitary disease or rupture of an aneurysm (Rasmussen's aneurysm) into an old tuberculous cavity. Hemoptysis also can be due to several complications from old tuberculous disease such as bronchiectasis, broncholithiasis, or an aspergilloma in a prior cavity. The diagnosis is made by history, chest x-ray, acid-fast stains on sputum, and ultimately culture. The diagnosis of tuberculosis in this patient is unlikely given his lack of constitutional symptoms and the normal chest x-ray.

Bronchitis currently is the most common cause of minor hemoptysis. Bronchitis is most commonly associated with respiratory viruses (such as rhinovirus, coronavirus, influenza, and adenovirus) but may also be caused by nonviral organisms such as *Mycoplasma pneumoniae* and *Chlamydia pneumoniae*. The symptoms of bronchitis depend on the severity but can include fever, chills, and cough (which is occasionally productive). The cough associated with bronchitis can be prolonged, especially in smokers and in some cases, can last several weeks. Physical examination is variable but can reveal rhonchi or wheezing, and the chest x-ray normally is clear. It is most likely that this patient has bronchitis, given the relatively short duration of symptoms and the normal chest x-ray.

Diagnostic Testing in the Evaluation of the Patient with Hemoptysis

In addition to the history and physical examination, appropriate radiographic and laboratory testing may help establish a diagnosis. A chest x-ray routinely is ordered, although 20% to 30% of patients with hemoptysis have a normal chest x-ray. In certain situations, other tests may be helpful such as a complete blood count, coagulation profile, and a urinalysis (in the case of a suspected pulmonary-renal syndrome). Further testing, such as a ventilation-perfusion scan in suspected pulmonary embolus or an echocardiogram (in cases of suspected mitral valve disease or pulmonary hypertension) can be useful. If these studies are unrevealing, consideration may be given to bronchoscopy or high resolution computed tomography (CT) scanning. There is some debate as to which should come next, but these two procedures can be thought of as complementary. Performing a high resolution CT scan first can be helpful for several reasons. First, the CT scan can serve as a guide for bronchoscopy and transbronchial biopsies. Second, the scan can also diagnose bronchiectasis, which is a diagnosis that cannot be made bronchoscopically. Finally, if cancer is the cause, it is unlikely to be missed by CT scan. One study reports that most tumors are stage III or greater by the time they cause hemoptysis.

The yield for bronchoscopy in the diagnosis of hemoptysis is low (less than 5%). The yield increases if the patient is a man over the age of 50, is an active or former smoker, and if the duration of hemoptysis is greater than 1 week. Bronchoscopy should be undertaken within 48 hours of the last episode of hemoptysis to maximize the chance of finding the source and the cause of the bleeding.

In the current patient, it would be appropriate to treat for presumed bronchitis. If the hemoptysis does not resolve, however, additional testing such as a high resolution CT scan (to evaluate the possibility of bronchiectasis from the prior pneumonia) and a bronchoscopy (for radiographically occult malignancy) would be appropriate.

▼ BIBLIOGRAPHY

Colice GL: Hemoptysis. Three questions that can direct management, *Postgrad Med* 100(17):227-236, 1996.

Dweik RA. Stoller JK: Role of bronchoscopy in massive hemoptysis, *Clin Chest Med* 20(1):89-105, 1999.

Dweik RA, Arroliga AC, Cash JM: Alveolar hemorrhage in patients with rheumatic disease, *Rheum Dis Clin North Am* 23:395-410, 1997.

Fishman AP: Approach to the patient with respiratory symptoms. In Fishman AP, editor: *Fishman's pulmonary diseases and disorders*, ed 3, New York, 1998, McGraw-Hill, pp 379-382.

Tasker AD, Flower CD: Imaging the airways. Hemoptysis, bronchiectasis and small airways disease, *Clin Chest Med* 20(4):761-773, 1999.

Weinberger SE: Etiology and evaluation of hemoptysis, *UpToDate* v 8.1, 2000.

CHAPTER 9

DIGITAL CLUBBING

Sunder Sandur

Key Terms

▼ Digital clubbing ▼ Neoplasm ▼ Chronic obstructive
▼ Liver disease ▼ Bronchiectasis pulmonary disease (COPD)
▼ Cystic fibrosis ▼ Cyanotic heart disease ▼ Emphysema

▼ THE CLINICAL PROBLEM

A 55-year-old man presents with worsening shortness of breath for the last 3 months. His exertional dyspnea dates to 2 years ago when he found it difficult to lift heavy weights for long periods. Over the last 3 months, his dyspnea has progressed so that he is unable to walk more than 50 yards or climb one flight of stairs. He reports pain in his hands and feet for the last 5 months, which he attributes to "arthritis." He denies cough, hemoptysis, fever or shaking chills, or weight loss. There is no history of tuberculosis exposure or prior pulmonary disease. He denies heartburn, dysphagia, jaundice, or alteration in bowel habits. There is no history of palpitations, chest pain, syncope, or ankle swelling.

He smokes 2 packs a day and has done so for 30 years. He denies alcohol use. His past history is notable for a negative TB test (PPD) 2 years ago, when he applied for a part-time job in a nursing home as a health aide. He takes no regular

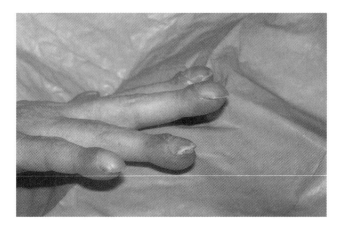

▼ **Figure 9-1** Digital clubbing revealing symmetric bulbous enlargement of the digital tips and beaking of the nails.

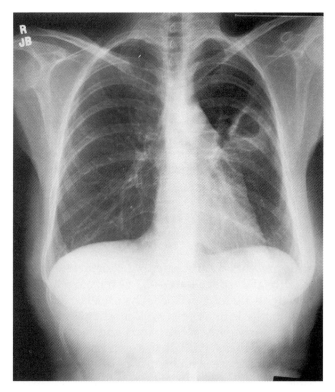

▼ **Figure 9-2** Anteroposterior (AP) chest x-ray revealing hyperexpanded lung fields, a normal cardiomediastinal silhouette, and a cavitary infiltrate in the right upper lobe.

medications. He is a factory machinist and denies occupational exposure to mineral dusts or asbestos.

On physical examination, his vital signs are pulse 90 and regular and blood pressure 130/80 mm Hg in his right arm while sitting upright. He seems comfortable. Examination of head, eyes, ears, nose, throat, and sinuses are normal. His neck reveals no evidence of lymphadenopathy, goiter, or jugular venous distension. His pulmonary examination reveals a hyperexpanded chest with scattered bilateral wheezes. Cardiac, abdominal, and neurologic examinations are unremarkable. His extremities are not cyanosed but reveal a symmetric bulbous enlargement of the digital segments of the digits of both hands with beaking of the nails (Figure 9-1). He has tenderness of both wrists to palpation without evidence of joint effusions. His legs also are tender along the shins but reveal no swelling or edema.

Laboratory tests include a normal complete blood count and electrolytes. His chest x-ray (Figure 9-2) reveals a normal cardiac silhouette, hyperexpanded lung fields, a cavitary infiltrate in the right upper lobe, and no pleural effusion.

What is the differential diagnosis for this patient's symptoms and abnormal digits?

Differential Diagnosis of Digital Clubbing

Clubbing, first described by Hippocrates some 2500 years ago, is characterized by broadening of the digits and shiny, abnormally curved nails. It can be graded in a five-step process:

Grade 1—Fluctuation and softening of the nail bed
Grade 2—Loss of the normal 15-degree angle between the nail and the cuticle
Grade 3—Accentuated convexity of the nail
Grade 4—Broadened terminal pulp of the digit
Grade 5—Shiny and glossy changes in the nail and adjacent skin with longitudinal striations in the nail.

Clubbing may occur as a consequence of hypertrophic osteoarthropathy (HOA), a clinical/radiologic syndrome characterized by digital clubbing, symmetric arthralgias of large joints, and periosteal proliferation of the long bones.

Several hypotheses have been proposed to explain the pathogenesis of digital clubbing. Tissue hypoxia, vagally mediated neural reflexes, and genetic factors have been implicated, as have several circulating factors, including growth hormone. These substances are thought to be normally inactivated by the lung and to act selectively on the digital microvasculature, causing vasodilation and increased blood flow. Serum tumor necrosis factor-alpha (TNF-α) is reported to be associated with digital clubbing. Recently, release of platelet-derived growth factor (PDGF) from impacted megakaryocytes and capillaries in the nail bed, promoting increased capillary permeability, fibroblastic activity, and smooth muscle hyperplasia, was proposed to cause digital clubbing. Tschoepe et al reported enhanced expression of P selectin (a surface marker of platelet activation) in finger-tip capillary blood compared with venous blood in normal subjects and in patients with Crohn's disease. Clubbing also has been found to correlate with smooth muscle proliferation in fibrotic lesions of open lung biopsy specimens in patients with idiopathic pulmonary fibrosis.

Clubbing has been described in many diseases (Box 9-1) that can be remembered using the acronym CLUBBING:

C: Cyanotic heart diseases, cystic fibrosis
L: Lung cancer, lung abscess, lung empyema, lung fibrosis, pulmonary arteriovenous malformations
U: Ulcerative colitis
B: Bronchiectasis
B: Benign mesothelioma
I: Infective endocarditis, idiopathic pulmonary fibrosis (IPF)
N: Neurogenic tumors
G: Gastrointestinal disease (i.e., regional enteritis, chronic liver disease)

Clubbing may be the presenting manifestation or may occur later in the disease course. The two forms of hypertrophic osteoarthropathy (HOA) are (1) primary HOA, an unusual autosomal dominant disease of puberty, and (2) secondary HOA, a more common form that is related to the previously mentioned diseases.

Tuberculous and purulent lung abscesses, bronchiectasis, and empyema were the most common causes of clubbing in the preantibiotic era. Today, lung cancer is by far the most common malignancy associated with clubbing. In a recent prospective study of digital clubbing among patients with lung cancer, clubbing was more frequent in patients with lung cancer that was not small cell (35%) than in small cell lung cancer (4%) and in women. Other cancers associated with clubbing or HOA include benign and pleural mesothelioma, mediastinal tumors, Hodgkin's lym-

---

Box 9-1
Differential Diagnosis of Digital Clubbing

Common Causes	Less Common Causes
Pulmonary	**Pulmonary**
Primary lung cancer	Sarcoidosis
Benign asbestos pleural disease	Hypersensitivity pneumonitis
Malignant mesothelioma	Pulmonary metastatic disease
Tuberculous or nontuberculous	Pulmonary arteriovenous malformations
Empyema	Pulmonary sarcoma
Bronchiectasis	Mediastinal tumors
Lung abscess	
Idiopathic pulmonary fibrosis	**Gastrointestinal**
	Achalasia of the esophagus
Cardiac	Esophageal adenocarcinoma
Subacute bacterial endocarditis	
Eisenmenger's syndrome	**Others**
Cyanotic congenital heart disease	Non-Hodgkin's lymphoma
	Mediastinal tumors
Gastrointestinal	
Ulcerative colitis	
Crohn's disease	
Chronic liver disease with cirrhosis	

phoma, thymoma, metastatic pulmonary neoplasms, and adenocarcinoma of the esophagus and stomach. Clubbing occurs in 30% of patients with benign pleural mesothelioma but is rare with malignant mesothelioma. Clubbing in patients with hypersensitivity pneumonitis is rare, except in a Mexican study by Sansores et al, who reported clubbing in 51% of patients with pigeon breeder's disease (PBD). The high frequency of clubbing in that series was thought to be due to a genetic predisposition to the disease and alterations in collagen metabolism similar to those observed in patients with IPF. There are reports of clubbing in association with sarcoidosis, pulmonary sarcomas, and secondary hyperparathyroidism.

Common clinical features of HOA include periostitis of long bones, symmetric arthralgias of large joints (usually knees, elbows, and wrists), and digital clubbing. Severe tenderness on lateral squeezing just above the joint such as the ankle or knee is a common sign. Significant periosteal proliferation of a long bone within a joint may cause a small joint effusion and mimic an active synovitis.

The patient presented here has clinical evidence of HOA with an abnormal chest x-ray. The differential diagnosis of an infiltrate in the right upper lobe with clubbing in a smoker is very limited. The leading contender in this case is primary lung cancer (most likely adenocarcinoma or large cell carcinoma). Small cell lung cancer is less likely because clubbing is unusual, and because it is unusual for small cell lung cancer to cause a peripheral nodule or mass. While pulmonary tuberculosis and hypersensitivity pneumonitis may present with finger clubbing and upper lobe infiltrates, they are less likely given the negative PPD and lack of exposure to foreign protein (i.e., pigeons).

Diagnostic Testing in the Evaluation of the Patient with Digital Clubbing

It must be emphasized that the work-up of patients with clubbing must begin with a good history (Table 9-1) that emphasizes the following:

1. Respiratory symptoms such as productive cough, dyspnea, hemoptysis, and sputum production
2. Cardiac symptoms such as cyanosis, syncope, palpitations, fever, chest pain, and decreased exercise tolerance
3. Gastrointestinal symptoms such as abdominal pain, nausea, vomiting, bloody diarrhea, and jaundice
4. Nonspecific symptoms such as fever, night sweats, anorexia, and weight loss

A personal history of cigarette smoking, alcohol intake, exposure to toxic fumes, exposure to persons infected to tuberculosis, and pigeon breeding also may be clinically significant.

In addition to the physical examination of the digits, large joints, and long bones, special attention should be paid to the presence of (1) tachycardia, heart murmurs, and cyanosis; (2) tachypnea, localized or generalized crackles, wheezes, rhonchi, dullness on percussion, decreased air entry, a barrel-shaped chest, and nicotine staining of the fingers; (3) an enlarged liver or spleen and evidence of chronic liver disease; and (4) evidence of lymphadenopathy and cachexia.

The most important test for patients with clubbing is the plain chest x-ray because some of these patients may be asymptomatic. Clubbing may precede symptoms

Possible Cause	Suggestive Clinical Features
Lung cancer	History of cigarette smoking, hemoptysis, mass on chest x-ray
Benign asbestos pleural disease	History of asbestos exposure (lag time <20 years), chest pain, cough, dyspnea, pleural effusion ± pleural plaques on x-ray
Malignant mesothelioma	History of asbestos exposure (lag time 20-40 years), age of onset >55 years, chest pain dominant symptom
	Other symptoms reflect local invasion (i.e., Horner's syndrome, constrictive pericarditis, and superior venacaval obstruction)
	Chest x-ray: Pleural effusion or mass-like pleural densities
	Open pleural biopsy is diagnostic
Empyema	Pneumonia with a persistent fever, enlarging infiltrate despite appropriate antibiotics
	Chest x-ray: Layering of fluid (early stages) or loculation (late stages)
	Pleural fluid—pus, transudate, Gram's stain positive for organisms, pH <7.2, glucose <40 mg/dL
Bronchiectasis	History of childhood infection, foreign body aspiration, or recurrent pulmonary infections with purulent sputum
	Fever, weight loss, focal auscultatory wheeze or crackles, asthma, hemoptysis, anemia, and sinusitis are features
	Chest x-ray: Areas of cystic radiolucency
	Computed tomography is diagnostic
	Cystic fibrosis, allergic bronchopulmonary aspergillosis, tuberculosis, and fungal infections affect the upper lobes
Lung abscess	History of slowly resolving/unresolving pneumonia, or post-obstructive pneumonia
	Symptoms similar to empyema
	Chest x-ray: Cavitary infiltrate with air fluid level
Idiopathic pulmonary fibrosis	Middle-aged patient with dyspnea, cough, and hypoxemia
	Bilateral "velcro" rales by auscultation
	Chest x-ray: Bilateral subpleural and basal pulmonary interstitial infiltrates
	CT more accurate
	Open lung biopsy diagnostic
Pulmonary arteriovenous malformation	Associated with hereditary hemorrhagic telangiectasia (20%)
	Mucocutaneous telangiectasia, hemoptysis, hypoxemia, cyanosis, and bruit over site of malformation
	Chest x-ray: Multiple oval or round, slow-growing lesions in the lower lobes
	Angiography is diagnostic
Subacute bacterial endocarditis	History of valve replacement, intravenous drug use, or recent dental work
	Common signs and symptoms: Fever, chills, "new" murmur, arrhythmia, anemia, splenomegaly, spider hemorrhages, "Roth" spots on fundi, and microscopic hematuria
	Blood cultures and ECG help diagnosis
Ulcerative colitis/ Crohn's disease	History of bloody diarrhea, weight loss, malabsorption, or bowel obstruction
	Associated with arthritis, uveitis, sclerosing cholangitis, erythema nodosum, and pyoderma gangrenosum
	Diagnosis by small bowel biopsy or colonoscopy

of neoplasm by months. The decision to order laboratory tests should be guided by the patient's clinical history and physical signs. Commonly employed tests include a complete blood count, electrolytes, fecal occult blood screen, electrocardiogram (ECG), and pulmonary function tests. Particularly challenging cases may require echocardiography and cardiac catheterization (to detect right-to-left shunts), sputum cytology, flexible bronchoscopy, chest computed tomography (CT) scans (to diagnose lung cancer), thoracentesis and closed pleural biopsy (to diagnose benign and malignant mesothelioma), liver biopsy (to diagnose primary biliary cirrhosis), and sigmoidoscopy or colonoscopy (to diagnose gastrointestinal malignancy or inflammatory bowel disease).

X-rays of long bones may be necessary to differentiate HOA from other inflammatory arthritides. Plain x-rays may reveal soft tissue swelling of the terminal digits and periosteal proliferation of long bones. The periosteal changes are observed in a bilateral, symmetric fashion, first along the distal third of the tibia and fibula, followed in frequency by the femur and ulna. The distal phalanges may undergo a distinctive bone remodeling process at the tips of the phalanges, adopting a hypertrophic "mushrooming" of the tuft or an osteolytic "whittling." CT and magnetic resonance imaging (MRI) of the bones are more sensitive than plain x-rays and may detect soft tissue abnormalities and widening or narrowing of the medullary bone.

Pitfalls and Common Mistakes in the Assessment and Treatment of Digital Clubbing

Because clubbing may be hereditary, its presence does not always imply disease. Also, clubbing should not be confused with "pseudoclubbing," which can be seen after digital trauma, hypothyroidism, and fungal infections of the nail. Periostitis due to infections may be mistaken for HOA. Inflammatory synovitis or unilateral synovial inflammation should not be confused with HOA, which is bilateral and nonerosive. Clubbing is not found in patients with tuberculosis, emphysema, and chronic bronchitis without coexisting lung cancer, lung abscess, bronchiectasis, or empyema. Finally, a history of asbestos exposure alone cannot be implicated as a cause of clubbing unless a benign asbestos pleural effusion or mesothelioma is present.

Treatment of Digital Clubbing

The management of clubbing centers around treatment of the primary cause because clubbing is a secondary phenomenon. Surgical resection of pulmonary neoplasms, correction of cardiac abnormalities, and liver transplantation have resulted in regression of digital clubbing. The pain of advanced clubbing may be managed by nonsteroidal antiinflammatory agents such as indomethacin or naproxen. Previous observations had suggested that colchicine could be used at a dose of 1 mg/day to reduce finger clubbing, albeit with frequent severe gastrointestinal side effects. A subsequent blinded study that compared surgery with colchicine 0.5 mg/day found no role for this drug in the treatment of digital clubbing. There also are a few reports of regression of clubbing after vagotomy, presumably due to neural mechanisms. More recently, growth hormone analogues such as somatostatin have caused a striking reduction in joint tenderness and clubbing in patients with lung cancer. Current hypotheses implicating platelet microthrombi, PDGF, and endothelial factors in the pathogenesis of clubbing have led to trials of growth factor analogues for treatment.

Prevention of Digital Clubbing

The most important preventive measure that patients can take is to shun cigarette smoking, which is a leading cause of lung cancer that is in turn the leading cause of digital clubbing. Control of alcohol intake and administration of hepatitis B immunization in pertinent populations may help to prevent liver-induced digital clubbing.

▼ BIBLIOGRAPHY

Altman RD, Tenenbaum J: Hypertrophic osteoarthropathy. In Kelly WN, Harris ED, Ruddy S, et al (editors): *Textbook of rheumatology*, ed 5, Philadelphia, 1997, WB Saunders, pp 1514-1520.

Anonymous: Is clubbing a growth disorder? *Lancet* ii: 848-849, 1990.

Bourke SJ, Banham SW, Carter R, et al: Longitudinal course of extrinsic allergic alveolitis in pigeon breeders, *Thorax* 44:415-418, 1989.

Braegger CP, Corrigan CJ, McDonald TT: Finger clubbing and tumor necrosis factor α. *Lancet* 336:759-760, 1990.

Davis GM, Rubin J, Bower JD: Digital clubbing due to secondary hyperparathyroidism, *Arch Intern Med* 150:452-454, 1990.

Dickenson CJ, Martin JF: Megakaryocyte and platelet clumps as the cause of finger clubbing, *Lancet* ii:1434-1435, 1987.

Dickenson CJ: The etiology of clubbing and hypertrophic osteopathy, *Eur J Clin Invest* 23:330-338, 1993.

Flavell G: Reversal of pulmonary hypertrophic osteoarthropathy by vagotomy, *Lancet* I:260-262, 1956.

Gallagher B, Cosgrove E: Finger clubbing, *Lancet* I:656, 1988.

Gilliand BC: Relapsing polychondritis and miscellaneous arthritis. In Wilson JD, Braunwald E, Isselbacher KJ, et al (editors): *Harrison's principles of internal medicine*, ed 12, New York, 1991, McGraw Hill, pp 1484-1490.

Kanematsu T, Kitaichi M, Nishimura K, et al: Clubbing of the fingers and smooth muscle proliferation in fibrotic changes in the lung in patients with idiopathic pulmonary fibrosis, *Chest* 105:339-342, 1994.

Leung R, Williams AJ: Indomethacin therapy for hypertrophic osteoarthropathy in patients with bronchogenic carcinoma, *West J Med* 142:345-347, 1985.

Loredo JS, Fedullo PF, Piovella F, et al: Digital clubbing associated with pulmonary artery sarcoma, *Chest* 109:1651-1653, 1996.

Matucci-Cerinic M: Response of hypertrophic osteoarthropathy to drugs inhibiting growth hormone, *J Rheumatol* 11:865, 1984.

Matucci-Cerinic M, Ceruso M, Lotti T, et al: The medical and surgical treatment of finger clubbing and hypertrophic osteoarthropathy. A blind study with colchicine and a surgical approach to finger clubbing reduction, *Clin Experimental Rheumatol* 9(suppl 7):67-70, 1992.

Matucci-Cerinic M, Fattorini L, Gerini G, et al: Colchicine treatment in a case of pachydermoperiostosis and acroosteolysis, *Rheumatol Int* 1988; 8:185-188.

Mc Gavin C, Hughes P: Finger clubbing in malignant mesothelioma and benign asbestos pleural disease, *Respir Med*, 92:692, 1998.

Pineda C: Diagnostic imaging in hypertrophic osteoarthropathy, *Clin Experimental Rheumatol* 10(suppl 7):27-33, 1992.

Rahbar M, Sharma OP: Hypertrophic osteoarthropathy in sarcoidosis, *Sarcoidosis* 7:125-127, 1990.

Sansores R, Salas J, Chapela R, et al: Clubbing in hypersensitivity pneumonitis: Its prevalence and possible prognostic role, *Arch Intern Med* 150:1849-1851, 1990.

Selman M, Montano M, Ramos C, et al: Lung collagen metabolism and the clinical course of hypersensitivity pneumonitis, *Chest* 94:347-353, 1988.

Shneerson JM: Digital clubbing and hypertrophic osteopathy: The underlying mechanisms, *Br J Dis Chest* 75:113-131, 1981.

Stoller JK, Moodie D, Schiavone WA, et al: Reduction of intrapulmonary shunt and resolution of digital clubbing associated with primary biliary cirrhosis after liver transplantation, *Hepatology* 11:54-58, 1990.

Sridhar KS, Lobo CF, Altman RD: Digital clubbing and lung cancer, *Chest* 114:1535-1537, 1998.

Tschoepe D, Schwippert B, Schumacher B, et al: Increased P-selectin (CD62) expression on platelets from capillary whole blood of patients with Crohn's disease, *Gastroenterology* 104:A1680, 1993.

West SG, Gilbreath RE, Lawless OJ: Painful clubbing and sarcoidosis, *JAMA* 246:1338-1339, 1981.

CHAPTER 10

BILATERAL PLEURAL EFFUSIONS

Howard Christie

Key Terms

▼ Congestive heart failure (CHF)
▼ Lymphoma

▼ Transudate
▼ Exudate
▼ Tuberculosis

▼ Systemic lupus erythematosus (SLE)
▼ Thoracentesis

▼ THE CLINICAL PROBLEM

A 60-year-old man presents with the complaint of increasing dyspnea on exertion (DOE) for the past 3 weeks. He states that he can hardly climb the stairs in his house without getting short of breath (SOB). He awakens during the night with SOB and cough and breathes more comfortably when he sits up. He has noticed some wheezing with exertion and some ankle swelling. He does bring up clear, frothy mucus but denies hemoptysis.

The patient is an active 40 pack-year smoker and drinks alcohol socially. His past medical history is significant for hypertension and hyperlipidemia. He is currently taking atenolol (Tenormin) 50 mg/day and lovastatin (Mevacor) 20 mg/day. Relevant family history includes heart disease and diabetes mellitus. He has been a school teacher for over 30 years and has always lived in Ohio.

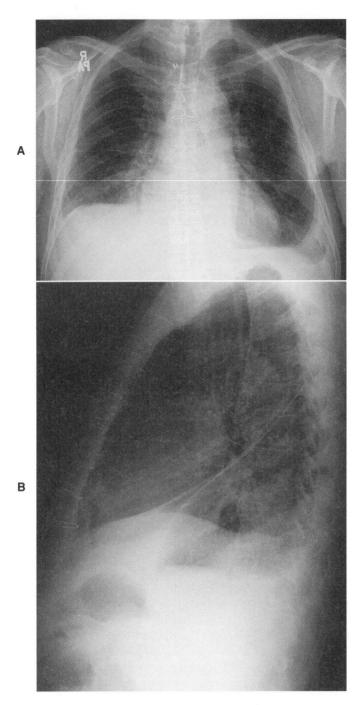

▼ **Figure 10-1** **A,** Anteroposterior (AP) chest x-ray showing bilateral pleural effusions with left ventricular enlargement and fluid in the lung fissures. **B,** Lateral chest x-ray demonstrating fluid in the major fissure and in the costophrenic sulcus.

Physical Examination

Physical examination reveals a mildly obese male, with slightly labored breathing. His blood pressure is 160/94, pulse 122, respirations 20, oximetry 92% on room air. The oropharynx is clear, nares patent, tympanic membranes within normal limits, pupils are equal, round, and reactive to light. Examination of his neck shows no bruits; jugular vein distension is 7 cm at 30 degrees; and thyroid is non-palpable. He has decreased bibasilar breath sounds with crackles and dullness to percussion at both bases.

Heart rate is tachycardic but regular, S_1 and S_2 normal, and no S_3 or murmur is heard. Soft bowel sounds are present; the liver edge is 2 cm below the costal margin, but no splenomegaly and no palpable masses are found. Extremities show 1+ lower extremity pitting edema; no cyanosis or clubbing is evident.

A chest x-ray shows an enlarged heart (17.5 cm width compared to 33 cm internal width of the chest on the film) with pulmonary vascular congestion and equal bilateral pleural effusions (Figure 10-1).

▼ Differential Diagnosis of Bilateral Pleural Effusions

The pleural space is composed of a thin layer of fluid that separates the lining of the lung (visceral pleura) from the lining of the inner chest wall (parietal pleura). Despite similar appearances, these membranes have significant differences. Only the parietal pleura is innervated, and although lymphatic networks are present in both, those in the parietal pleura have connections with the pleural space that serve to drain that area. Stomata or openings in the surface allow access to the pleural cavity to enable fluid removal.

The development of excess fluid in the pleural space is not normal and requires investigation. Fluid can be seen unilaterally or bilaterally. Gravity is responsible for the basal accumulation of the fluid and for its accumulation in the costophrenic angles. Radiographically, 175 mL of fluid may be visible on the frontal view, but as little as 5 mL may be seen on the lateral decubitus film.

Bilateral pleural effusions have many possible etiologies, but some causes are more common than others. Common causes include congestive heart failure (CHF), nephrotic syndrome, systemic lupus erythematosus (SLE), malignancy, and hepatic cirrhosis (Box 10-1). Whereas CHF may present with cardiomegaly, Kerley B lines on chest x-ray (indicating lymphatic thickening due to edema), and vascular redistribution, the other etiologies are favored when the heart size is normal.

CHF is the most common cause of bilateral pleural effusions. The definition of heart failure has evolved to encompass much more than simple "pump failure." Humoral and inflammatory changes are among the contributors to a continuum of clinical signs, which may initially be mediated by compensatory mechanisms (Table 10-1). These mechanisms may delay the development of the normally associated findings in CHF (e.g., edema, cardiomegaly). The appearance of pleural effusions associated with congestive failure is a later sign of left ventricular failure with elevated pulmonary artery occlusion pressure. This capillary pressure forces fluid into the interstitium and subsequently into the pleural space at a rate

Box 10-1
Differential Diagnosis of Bilateral
Pleural Effusions

Common Causes	Less Common Causes
CHF	Pancreatic disorders
SLE	Meig's syndrome
Malignancy	Asbestos-related disease
Nephrotic syndrome	Drug-induced disease
Hepatic cirrhosis	Constrictive pericarditis
	Dressler's syndrome
	Pneumonia

CHF, Congestive heart failure; *SLE*, systemic lupus erythematosus

TABLE 10-1
Interpreting Signs and Symptoms in the Patient with Bilateral
Pleural Effusions

Possible Causes	Mechanisms	Suggestive Clinical Features
CHF	Elevated hydrostatic pressure due to high pulmonary venous pressures with left ventricular dysfunction	Cardiomegaly on chest x-ray; paroxysmal nocturnal dyspnea; orthopnea; jugular vein distension; lower extremity edema; presence of S_3; bibasilar crackles
Malignancy	Impaired lymphatic drainage Direct tumor involvement Atelectasis via endobronchial obstruction Hypoproteinemia due to neoplasm	Hemoptysis; weight loss/fever/chills; metastatic signs/symptoms (e.g., skin nodules, bone fractures, palpable lymph nodes or masses) Chest x-ray: Normal heart size
Nephrotic syndrome	Hypoalbuminemia leading to decreased oncotic pressure Pulmonary embolism as complication	Anasarca; hypoalbuminemia; proteinuria; Chest x-ray: Normal heart size
SLE	Localized immune response	Pleuritic pain; SLE characteristics (e.g., malar rash, oral ulcers, arthralgias, etc) Chest x-ray: Normal heart size
Hepatic cirrhosis	Transfer of peritoneal fluid via lymphatics and diaphragmatic defects	Ascites/hepatomegaly; history of liver disease

CHF, Congestive heart failure; *SLE,* systemic lupus erythematosus.

exceeding the drainage capabilities of the lymphatics. An isolated left-sided pleural effusion is uncommon in CHF and should suggest consideration of other etiologies (e.g., pericardial disease, pancreatitis, and so on).

Nephrotic syndrome is characterized by proteinuria (>3 g/day) with edema, hyperlipidemia, and hypoalbuminemia. Urinary loss and some redistribution cause the decreased albumin. The resulting decrease in oncotic pressure is opposed by still normal hydrostatic pressure, a state that favors fluid leakage. As with congestive heart failure, the development of pleural effusions occurs at a later stage, usually after generalized edema is visible. Pulmonary emboli are a common complication of nephrotic syndrome and also must be considered as a cause of the effusion.

Pleural involvement may complicate SLE more than half the time, involving pleurisy and/or pleural effusions. Approximately half of SLE effusions are bilateral. Although the exact mechanism is uncertain in lupus, the effusions are likely due to a localized immune pleuritis. SLE resulting from drug therapy (e.g., hydralazine, procainamide, INH, phenytoin, and so on) can cause similar pleural reactions. Mixed connective tissue disease, a hybrid of SLE, scleroderma, and polymyositis also may present rarely with bilateral fluid.

After CHF, malignancies are the most common causes of pleural effusions in the elderly. Most commonly, malignant effusions are caused by lung cancer (36%) and breast cancer (25%) with smaller percentages a result of lymphoma (10%) and gastric and ovarian cancer. Several mechanisms may be responsible either directly or indirectly related to the neoplasm. According to Light, these include the following:

1. Direct pleural involvement producing increased pleural membrane permeability
2. Lymphatic obstruction by tumor
3. Endobronchial obstruction leading to atelectasis
4. Pneumonitis due to bronchial obstruction causing effusion
5. Effusion due to neoplasm-related hypoproteinemia

Therefore effusions may be malignant with direct tumor involvement as in the first example or paramalignant (negative cytology) if they are a secondary manifestation, as in bronchial obstruction. While unilateral effusions ipsilateral to the tumor are more common with both lung and breast cancer, bilateral effusions do occur. A series by Chernow and Sahn reviewed 96 patients with pleural metastases of various etiologies and found 31% had bilateral effusions. This included 5 of 27 lung cancers, 11 of 17 breast cancers, and 2 of 5 ovarian pregnancies. The five primary bronchogenic carcinomas all had contralateral lung involvement and hepatic metastases. Tertiary spread of tumor from liver metastases is thought to be one source of pleural involvement from breast cancer and cancer from below the diaphragm, and this is commonly bilateral.

Hepatic cirrhosis usually presents with a right-sided effusion but may be bilateral 15% of the time. Patients develop ascites from their underlying liver disease. The elevated peritoneal pressure pushes fluid through diaphragmatic defects and lymphatic channels into the pleural space. Hypoproteinemia also may play a role in this fluid transfer.

Bilateral pleural effusions are most commonly a result of CHF, nephrotic syndrome, SLE, malignancies, or cirrhosis, but they also may occur with several other conditions. Bilateral pneumonia may present with infiltrates and bilateral pleural effusions. Drug reactions may cause bilateral pleural effusions and must always be considered. Drugs implicated include nitrofurantoin (Macrodantin), dantrolene (Dantrium), bromocriptine (Parlodel), procarbazine (Natulan), and methysergide (Sansert). Constrictive pericarditis, Dressler's syndrome, pancreatic disorders, asbestos-related lung disease, and Meig's syndrome (e.g, pleural effusion associated with ovarian disease) may occasionally present with bilateral pleural effusions.

Clinical Features that Suggest a Specific Cause of Bilateral Pleural Effusions

The most common presenting symptoms of bilateral pleural effusions are dyspnea, cough, and chest pain. Dyspnea occurs because effusions reduce other lung volumes by taking up space in the thorax. They may even impair left ventricular filling if they become large enough, adding to the feeling of breathlessness. Cough may develop as a result of pleural inflammation or receptor stimulation in the compressed lung. Pleuritic chest pain, resulting from parietal pleural receptor inflammation, is another common complaint in patients with pleural effusions. Of course, dyspnea, cough, and chest pain either by themselves or in combination can herald many pulmonary and other diseases, so establishing a cause of pleural effusion requires much more than these common presenting symptoms.

Physical signs can suggest the diagnosis of pleural effusion, but they can neither establish the diagnosis nor determine the etiology of the effusion. In other words, examination may be able to uncover bilateral basilar abnormalities, but what they are (fluid versus mass versus thickening) would still be uncertain. Additionally, why the abnormalities are present requires even more investigation. Auscultation of the chest may reveal bibasilar, diminished, or absent breath sounds, depending on the size of the effusion. A friction rub may be heard with smaller accumulations. Dullness to percussion is evoked when spaces previously filled with air become consolidated or fluid-filled. Percussion is commonly used to determine the extent of the fluid and the site for thoracentesis after the diagnosis of pleural fluid is secure. Decreased vocal fremitus and "e" to "a" egophony are also signs on physical examination of consolidated (or airless) lung parenchyma due to local lung compression. None of these important physical findings, however, can accurately predict pleural effusion. Finally, tachycardia, tachypnea, and hypoxemia may be present but are not specific.

Despite the lack of specificity of these findings, there are some clinical features that can help narrow the differential diagnosis and guide treatment. The clinical problems of this patient suggest CHF as the likely etiology of the bilateral pleural effusions. The patient profile offers the first hints. This patient is 60 years of age, and CHF is the most common cause of effusion in patients over 50. This patient has previously diagnosed hypertension, which could predispose him to chronic left heart failure and subsequent acute episodes of CHF. The presence of hyperlipidemia and smoking increases the risk for atherosclerotic heart disease, which could lead to myocardial ischemia and ischemic cardiomyopathy.

The patient's history indicates night awakenings with SOB, which may be episodes of paroxysmal nocturnal dyspnea (PND). Usually occurring 2 to 4 hours after the beginning of sleep, PND is felt to result from the resorption of fluid leading to increased thoracic blood volume. Recumbency encourages resorption of the fluid. Normal respiratory depression during sleep along with increased bronchial secretions also may contribute to these episodes. The symptom of PND is commonly associated with left heart failure. This patient sleeps and breathes more comfortably in an elevated position, which is another feature suggesting CHF. This symptom, *orthopnea,* is a frequent complaint when heart failure leads to pulmonary edema, without the protective effect of gravity in the upright position. Additionally, this patient notes exertional wheezing that is more often associated with reactive airways disease in asthmatics but can be due to bronchospasm in heart failure, the so-called *cardiac asthma.* Finally, the patient's description of ankle swelling or lower extremity edema, although not a very specific indicator, may accompany significant left ventricular dysfunction.

The physical examination of this patient further supports the impression of CHF. Jugular vein distention (JVD) is an indicator of elevated right heart pressure, which may be due to left heart failure. Decreased breath sounds and dullness to percussion indicate consolidated airspace as previously discussed. Crackles or rales are adventitious breath sounds with several possible etiologies, one of which is the presence of fluid-filled airways in pulmonary edema. Similarly, an enlarged liver can be the product of fluid backing up from a failing right heart. Additionally, lower extremity edema as noted in the patient history, also can be a physical finding of poor right ventricular contraction.

In summary, this is a 60-year-old man with a history of hypertension who presented with DOE, wheezing, orthopnea, and PND. Examination revealed tachycardia, tachypnea, relative hypoxemia, blunted and adventitious bibasilar breath sounds, and lower extremity edema with JVD and hepatomegaly. Based on these data, the suspicion of a cardiac cause is high, although interstitial lung disease, pulmonary alveolar infiltrates, pulmonary hypertension, and hepatic disease remain possibilities. A chest x-ray is the next prudent step.

In this case, the chest film is crucial as it identifies the presence of bilateral pleural effusions as the cause of the abnormal chest examination. Additionally, the presence of cardiomegaly and pulmonary congestion virtually confirms CHF as the etiology, verifying the clinical impression. The presence of a normal-sized heart, in particular, would make it less likely that CHF is causing the effusions. Chakko et al found cardiomegaly in 87% of patients studied with chronic heart failure, while other radiographic signs such as fluid redistribution and interstitial edema were much less evident, even when the wedge pressure was high. Similarly, Badgett determined that cardiomegaly was the best radiographic indicator of decreased ejection fraction, but cautioned that the chest x-ray alone is not adequate to diagnose. The absence of any mass or infiltrate on the chest film makes a lung malignancy or infection less likely. Occasionally, pleural thickening or encapsulated fluid may appear as an effusion and requires a lateral decubitus chest film for clarification. Lying the patient on the side of the effusion allows free-flowing fluid to "layer out" in the dependent portion of the lung and appear as a column of fluid that tracks cephalad in the pleural space. In contrast, an opacity that is either pleural thickening or encapsulated fluid would not change in configuration with patient position change. A CT scan is not routinely done for pleural effusions but may be helpful when the character of pleural abnormalities is unclear from the plain x-ray.

The other more common causes of pleural effusions—nephrotic syndrome, SLE, and cancer—cannot be ruled out at this point, but there is no compelling evidence for any of them. Patients with nephrotic syndrome must, by definition, have proteinuria and often have anasarca. The diagnosis rests on laboratory evaluation to reveal proteinuria and hypoalbuminemia. SLE can present in various fashions, including skin rash and ocular and oropharyngeal abnormalities, but none of these was noted in this case. There are no signs of cancer in this patient (e.g., cachexia, pain, etc.), and the chest x-ray does not suggest a bronchogenic carcinoma. Malignancy remains a possibility, however, in an active smoker if therapy does not resolve the effusions.

The less common causes of bilateral pleural effusions also seem less likely in this patient. Meig's syndrome (pleural effusion associated with an ovarian tumor) can be eliminated in a male. Asbestos-related disease can be reasonably dismissed in the absence of exposure after careful and repeated questioning. The absence of a prior MI or cardiothoracic surgery eliminates Dressler's syndrome, and the absence of abdominal complaints makes pancreatic disorders unlikely. A chest x-ray without infiltrates in this patient presentation pushes pneumonia to the bottom of the differential.

Diagnostic Testing in the Evaluation of the Patient with Bilateral Pleural Effusions

Once the diagnosis of bilateral pleural effusions has been made, the next step is usually to sample and evaluate the fluid. This is done by thoracentesis both for diagnostic (what is this fluid?) and therapeutic (relieve dyspnea by fluid removal) purposes. Thoracentesis involves inserting a needle under local anesthesia through the posterior chest wall into the fluid and withdrawing adequate fluid for analysis. If the intent is therapeutic, up to approximately 1500 cc can be withdrawn at one time. This procedure can be complicated by pneumothorax in up to 20% of cases, along with pain at the site and cough. Reexpansion pulmonary edema is a hazard if too much fluid is withdrawn.

Fluid that is removed is sent for various analyses, depending on the clinical suspicion, but the first step always is to identify it as transudate or exudate (Box 10-2).

Box 10-2
Classification of Pleural Effusions as Transudates or Exudates

Transudates	Exudates
CHF	Malignancy (may be transudate)
Nephrotic syndrome	Pulmonary embolism (may be transudate)
Hepatic cirrhosis	Parapneumonic effusions
Atelectasis	Tuberculosis/fungal disease
Urinothorax	Connective tissue disorders
Peritoneal dialysis	Asbestos-related disease
Constrictive pericarditis	Drug-related disease
	Meig's syndrome
	Chylothorax
	Pancreatitis
	Dressler's syndrome
	Esophageal rupture

CHF, Congestive heart failure.

Transudates are fluid accumulations resulting from an imbalance in the pressures which usually maintain the normal fluid compartments. Oncotic pressure due to the presence of protein holds fluid within the vascular space opposed by hydrostatic pressure, which works to move fluid out of that space. The rate of fluid production is normally in balance with reabsorption by the parietal lymphatics. As a result, a small fluid volume normally occupies the pleural space. Alterations in this state, such as hypoalbuminemia (decreased oncotic pressure) or elevated venous pressures (elevated hydrostatic pressure), force fluid out of its normal space. If the rate of filtration is more than can be absorbed, excess pleural fluid is the result. In this scenario, the pleural lining remains intact with leakage occurring through the parietal stoma.

Exudates often result from inflammatory conditions in which the capillary membranes are violated and excess fluid crosses into the pleural space. Normal fluid drainage by the parietal lymphatics also may be impaired, most commonly due to blockage by malignancy. Exudative pleural fluid is characterized by elevated protein and/or lactic acid dehydrogenase (LDH) levels. Criteria proposed by Light distinguish transudates from exudates and are based on comparing pleural fluid protein and LDH levels to those values in serum as follows:

▼ Transudate	▼ Exudate
Pleural protein <0.5 serum protein	pleural protein >0.5 serum protein
AND	OR
pleural LDH <0.6 serum LDH	pleural LDH >0.6 serum LDH
AND	OR
pleural LDH <200 mg/dl	pleural LDH >200 mg/dl

While this method is very accurate, there have been cases of transudative effusions accompanying malignancy, so a determination that the fluid is a transudate may be reassuring but the clinician must remain vigilant, especially if treatment does not eradicate the fluid. Concomitant CHF, bronchial obstruction leading to atelectasis, or early mediastinal node development may result in transudative malignant effusions. The diagnosis of a transudate prompts a course of treatment of the underlying cause, while the diagnosis of an exudate requires further investigation to determine which of the many possible etiologies is most likely. Box 10-2 classifies effusions as transudate or exudate. (See Box 10-1 for common causes of bilateral effusions.) Of the transudates, only CHF, nephrotic syndrome, and cirrhosis commonly present as bilateral pleural effusions, placing them at the top of a differential for bilateral transudative effusions. If the fluid is exudative, the list of possibilities is more extensive. Malignancy and SLE are prime considerations when exudative bilateral pleural effusions are present, though asbestos-related effusions and pancreatic disorders are possibilities.

Although thoracentesis is generally the appropriate first step when a pleural effusion is discovered, a diagnostic tap can be deferred in patients for whom the overwhelmingly likely course is CHF. The patient presented here has obvious signs of heart failure and cardiomegaly on chest x-ray, which likely represent a transudative effusion due to left ventricular dysfunction. In this case, diuretics and inotropic agents could be administered on the strength of the strong clinical suspicion without performing a thoracentesis first. If the diagnosis of CHF is correct, such treatment would improve heart function and allow the fluid to clear. Lack of response to treatment would be an indication for pleural fluid analysis.

If thoracentesis is elected, fluid is withdrawn for analysis. Normal pleural fluid and transudative effusions are straw-colored but different colors can be important diagnostic clues. Red, bloody fluid may suggest various entities, including trauma, malignancy, pulmonary infarction or possibly SLE. White or milky fluid should suggest chylothorax. Yellow-green fluid is common with rheumatoid arthritis, while aspergillus infection may present as a black pleural effusion.

Beyond appearance, the fluid may subsequently be analyzed for components other than LDH and total protein. The pH of the fluid is important and is normally alkalotic, but the presence of bacteria can lead to lactic acid production causing the pH to be below 7.30. The pleural fluid glucose value is low in some exudative effusions (pneumonia, malignancy, tuberculosis, rheumatoid arthritis), with values less than 40 mg% indicating complicated effusions.

A pleural fluid white blood cell count greater than $1000/mm^3$ usually suggests an exudate, whereas counts greater than $10,000/mm^3$ are common with parapneumonic effusions and effusions due to malignancy, tuberculosis, pancreatitis, collagen vascular disease, and pulmonary infarction. The white blood cell differential count is more important in helping to establish the cause of an effusion. Granulomatous disease (e.g., tuberculosis) and malignancy may be associated with pleural fluid containing more than 50% lymphocytes. Mononuclear cell predominance may indicate malignancy or tuberculosis. Eosinophilia greater than 10% is commonly caused by blood or air in the pleural space, although benign asbestos effusions or drug-related effusions (dantrolene or nitrofurantoin) can cause eosinophilia.

Finally, a prevalence of polymorphonuclear leukocytes may occur in effusions due to pneumonia, pancreatitis, or other acute processes (e.g., abdominal abscess, pulmonary embolus). Specific tests, such as amylase (to evaluate pancreatic involvement), ANA (for lupus pleuritis), triglyceride levels and the presence of chylomicrons (for chylothorax characterization), and adenosine deaminase (for tuberculosis), are useful under the appropriate clinical circumstances. Gram stain and culture are required when infection is suspected, and cytology evaluation can help evaluate the presence of malignancy. If an etiology evades this work-up, a pleural biopsy may ultimately be useful to determine the cause of an exudative effusion, especially if there is a predominance of lymphocytes.

Pitfalls and Common Mistakes in the Assessment and Treatment of Bilateral Pleural Effusions

One pitfall is to confuse other causes of pleural abnormality on the chest radiograph with pleural effusion. Making this distinction is important to avert invasive procedures (e.g., thoracentesis) when there is no free-flowing fluid. Pleural processes that can be confused with effusions are loculated (or not free-flowing) effusions, pleural thickening or scarring (e.g., from prior inflammation), or pleural tumors. Loculated or encapsulated effusions are fluid collections surrounded by pleural adhesions and usually lack a meniscus sign (the appearance of a concave upper border where the fluid meets the chest wall on chest x-ray). The use of the lateral decubitus chest film can separate free fluid from loculated fluid. By filming the patient lying down or in the decubitus position, only free fluid will "layer out" along the dependent chest wall. A fluid width of >1 cm indicates that there is enough fluid to tap. Pleural thickening (from trauma, prior procedures, or asbestos exposure) and pleural masses would retain their original shape despite gravitational changes. Thus a lateral decubitus chest x-ray is the crucial first step to determine that the patient actually has free-flowing pleural fluid that can be analyzed.

Reaching the conclusion that heart failure is the etiology of bilateral pleural effusions is important because it leads to a decision to treat without undertaking thoracentesis and fluid analysis. Incorrectly diagnosing CHF, however, can lead to a delay in appropriate therapy. Although cardiomegaly (a cardiothoracic ratio on chest radiograph greater than 50%) should suggest left heart failure, it also can be erroneously diagnosed radiographically by a shallow inspiratory effort, or by a fat pad or in chest x-rays taken with the anteroposterior (AP) technique (the patient's back is against the film plate). In older patients, however, the manifestations of CHF are more subtle and CHF may be under-diagnosed. Thus heart failure can be both under- and over-diagnosed, and the presence of bilateral pleural effusions on chest x-ray must be correlated with other clinical and radiographic findings to correctly assess CHF.

Uncovering a transudate by pleural fluid analysis is usually a comforting discovery, but clinical suspicion should remain high in the appropriate circumstances. Malignancies can present with non-malignant or paramalignant effusions that may be transudates.

Finally, concomitant disease should not be overlooked in the search for the cause of pleural fluid. Malignancies can present in patients who also have heart failure. Drugs are frequently overlooked as a cause of pleural effusions.

▼ BIBLIOGRAPHY

Appel GB: Approach to patients with parenchymal renal disease. In Stoller JK, Ahmad M, Longworth DL (editors): *The Cleveland Clinic intensive review of internal medicine,* Baltimore, 1998, Williams & Wilkins.

Badgett RG, Mulrow CD, Otto PM, et al: How well can the chest radiograph diagnose left ventricular dysfunction? *J Gen Intern Med* 11:625-634, 1996.

Boggs DS, Kinasewitz GT: Review: pathophysiology of the pleural space, *Am J Med Sci* 309(1):53-59, 1995.

Chakko S, Woska D, Martinez H, et al: Clinical, radiographic, and hemodynamic correlations in chronic congestive heart failure: conflicting results may lead to inappropriate care, *Am J Med* 90:353-359, 1991.

Chernow B, Sahn SA: Carcinomatous involvement of the pleura: an analysis of 96 patients, *Am J Med* 63:695-702, 1997.

Joseph J, Sahn SA: Connective tissue diseases and the pleura, *Chest* 104:262-270, 1993.

Klein JS: Radiographic findings in chest disease. In Brant WE, Helms CA: *Fundamentals of diagnostic radiology,* ed 2, Baltimore, 1999, Williams & Wilkins.

Light RW: Diseases of the pleura, mediastinum, chest wall, and diaphragm. In George RB, Light RW, Matthay MA, et al (editors): *Chest medicine: essentials of pulmonary and critical care medicine,* Baltimore, 1995, Williams & Wilkins.

Light RW: *Pleural diseases,* ed 3, Baltimore, 1990, Williams & Wilkins.

Morelock SY, Sahn SA: Drugs and the pleura, *Chest* 116:212-221, 1999.

Ogirala RG, Azrieli FM: Thoracentesis and closed pleural biopsy. In Beamis JF, Mathur PN (editors): *Interventional pulmonology*, New York, 1999, McGraw-Hill.

Sahn SA: Diseases of the pleura and pleural space. In Baum GD, Crapo JD, Celli BR, et al (editors): *Textbook of pulmonary diseases*, Philadelphia, 1998, Lippincott-Raven.

Sahn SA: Pleural malignancies. In Bone RC, Dantzker DR, George RB, et al (editors): *Pulmonary and critical care medicine*, St Louis, 1997, Mosby.

Silver TM, Farber SJ, Bole GG, et al: Radiological features of MCTD and scleroderma—systemic lupus erythematosus overlap, *Radiology* 120:269-275, 1976.

Tresch D: The clinical diagnosis of heart failure in older patients, *J Am Geriatr Soc* 45:1128-1133, 1997.

Young JB: Overview of medical therapy in heart failure: the challenge of rational polypharmacy. In Balady GJ, Pina IL (editors): *Exercise and heart failure*, Armonk, NY, 1997, Futura Publishing.

CHAPTER 11

UNILATERAL RIGHT-SIDED PLEURAL EFFUSION

Howard Christie

Key Terms

- ▼ Congestive heart failure (CHF)
- ▼ Lymphoma
- ▼ Transudate
- ▼ Exudates
- ▼ Tuberculosis
- ▼ Pancreatitis
- ▼ Pulmonary embolism (PE)
- ▼ Systemic lupus erythematosus (SLE)

▼ THE CLINICAL PROBLEM

A 52-year-old woman presents complaining of right-sided chest discomfort for 3 to 4 days. She denies any injury to her chest or history of excessive movement. She describes the pain as dull, achy, and constant but says that it increases with deep breathing and coughing. She has had a dry, nagging cough for the last 2 weeks with some shortness of breath on exertion. She denies wheezing or hemoptysis. She has slept well, without orthopnea, but is more comfortable lying on her left side. There are no upper respiratory complaints, and she denies fever, chills, or sweats. She complains of slightly decreased appetite for 1 to 2 months with about an 8- to 10-pound weight loss. There is no dysphagia or hoarseness.

She is an active smoker with approximately 45 pack years but has no preexisting disease. Her last office visit was over 2 years ago, when hormone replacement therapy was started for menopause. Mammography and Papanicolaou's (Pap) test were negative at that time. She has never had a chest x-ray and denies prior pulmonary problems. Her family history is significant for hypertension and coronary artery disease. She is a housewife and has never worked outside the house. Her only travel is to Florida for winter vacation, and she is a lifelong Ohio resident. She has no pets. She takes Premarin 0.625 mg/day and Provera 5 mg/day.

She is thin and in no apparent distress. Her vital signs are blood pressure 132/86, pulse 100, respirations 16, and oxygen saturation as measured by oximetry (SpO_2) is 95% on room air. Her pupils are equal and reactive to light and accommodation. Her oropharynx is clear, her nares are patent, and her tympanic membranes are normal. She has no bruits, jugular vein distension, or palpable lymph nodes. Her thyroid is non-palpable. Her breath sounds are absent in the right base with dullness to percussion. Her breath sounds are clear on the left, and she has no wheeze or crackles. She has a regular heart rate and rhythm, normal S_1 and S_2, and no murmur. There are soft bowel sounds, no abdominal masses, and no hepatosplenomegaly. There is no cyanosis, clubbing, or edema, and there is 5/5 strength in all extremities. She has no skin rashes or lesions. Her breasts are symmetrical with no masses or discharge and no palpable axillary adenopathy.

A chest x-ray (Figure 11-1) shows a moderate right-sided pleural effusion. Heart size is normal, and the lung parenchyma is otherwise clear.

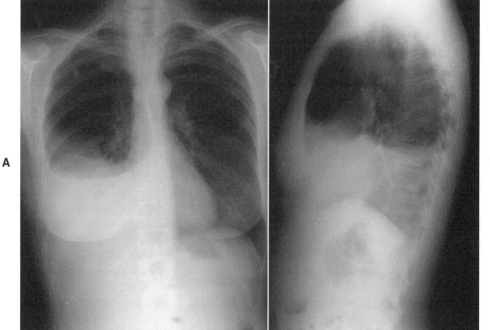

▼ **Figure 11-1** **A,** Anteroposterior (AP) chest x-ray of right-sided pleural effusion. **B,** Lateral chest x-ray of right-sided pleural effusion.

Differential Diagnosis of Unilateral Pleural Effusion

Etiologies of a unilateral pleural effusion are more diverse than those for bilateral effusions and include congestive heart failure (CHF) and other causes of bilateral pleural effusions. Common causes include malignancies, infection, pulmonary embolism (PE), atelectasis, and liver disease. Other etiologies are listed in Box 11-1. Right-sided effusions have more specific causes, but generally unilateral effusions are ipsilateral to the process causing them (i.e., liver disease causes right-sided fluid and pancreatic disease more commonly causes left-sided effusions).

CHF is the most common cause of bilateral pleural effusions in patients over 50 years of age and may also present as a unilateral pleural effusion with a 2:1 right-sided predominance. Left heart failure leading to elevated pulmonary venous pressure "squeezes" fluid into the interstitium. It can then enter the pleural space, which usually has lower pressure. As discussed in Chapter 10, this results from the alteration of hydrostatic and oncotic pressures, favoring the extravasation of microvascular fluid. Right heart failure alone, as evidenced by increased right atrial pressures, does not cause pleural effusions. A unilateral effusion may represent a point in time during which heart failure is progressing and perhaps leading to bilateral effusions.

Malignancy frequently causes pleural effusions, perhaps only slightly less often than CHF. Malignancy likely also ranks behind pneumonia as the leading cause of unilateral exudative effusions. Matthay et al reviewed 6 series that included 1868 patients and reported that 42% of effusions were linked to cancer. Lung cancer is the most common cause (36%), followed by breast cancer (25%), lymphoma (10%), and ovarian and gastric neoplasms. The most common primary tumor of the pleura is mesothelioma, which can present as effusion in its early stage. A unilateral effusion ipsilateral to the site of the lesion is most frequently seen with lung cancer and breast cancer, whereas bilateral effusions usually imply liver metastases.

Box 11-1
Differential Diagnosis of Unilateral Pleural Effusion

Common Causes	Less Common Causes
Malignancy (lung, breast, lymphoma, abdominal)	Iatrogenic causes (dialysis, line placement, esophageal perforation)
Infection (bacterial, fungal, TB)	Causes of chylothorax (trauma, lymphoma, LAM)
PE	Asbestos-related disease
CHF	Urinothorax
Connective tissue disorders (RA, SLE, Wegener's granulomatosis)	Drug-related disease (procainamide, amiodarone, nitrofurantoin, and others)
Hepatic cirrhosis	Pancreatitis
Atelectasis	Meig's syndrome
	Yellow nail syndrome
	Idiopathic

PE, Pulmonary embolism; *CHF*, congestive heart failure; *LAM*, lymphangioleiomyomatosis; *RA*, Rheumatoid arthritis; *SLE*, systemic lupus erythematosus.

A pleural effusion associated with malignancy may itself be malignant, para-malignant, or non-malignant. A malignant effusion results from direct pleural tumor invasion and often is identified by positive cytology on thoracentesis if there is mesothelial surface involvement. As noted, liver metastasis is commonly responsible for the development of pleural effusion from below the diaphragm, whereas a lung cancer primary spreads to the pleural space by pulmonary artery invasion and embolization. Lymphatic drainage compromised by tumor involvement also plays a role.

Paramalignant effusions do not result from direct tumor or metastatic involvement but are a secondary result of the malignancy. Common scenarios as grouped by Sahn include the following:

1. Local effect of tumor: Lymphatic obstruction, bronchial obstruction (pneumonia/atelectasis)
2. Systemic effect of tumor: PE, decreased plasma oncotic pressure
3. Result of therapy (chemotherapy/radiation)

Finally, a pleural effusion may be non-malignant but coincident with the discovery of the malignancy. This may be due to CHF or infection, for example, and must be appropriately identified to initiate correct treatment because it may have significant prognostic implications.

Infection is a common cause of unilateral pleural effusion, with ipsilateral effusions due to bacterial pneumonia being the most common exudative effusion. In an early study, Light et al found that 44% of 203 patients with acute bacterial pneumonia had pleural fluid. The combination of capillary permeability due to inflammation along with impaired lymphatic drainage is the etiology of parapneumonic effusions. These may be uncomplicated (pleural fluid pH >7.20, glucose >40 mg/dL) or may develop into complicated effusions (pleural fluid pH <7.20, glucose <40 mg/dL), if treatment is inadequate or delayed. This delay results in loculated fluid and/or empyema. A scheme of seven classifications has been proposed by Light ranging from an insignificant effusion (<10 mm thick on a lateral decubitus x-ray) in class 1 to complex empyema (frank pus, multiple locules) in class 7 with recommended treatment plans for each.

In addition to bacteria, *Mycobacterium tuberculosis* (TB) may present indolently or acutely with a pleural effusion often being a component. It is almost exclusively unilateral, although with no right or left predilection. Whereas pleural involvement with TB is believed to be present in about 7% of cases, this number can be higher in other countries such as Spain (about 25%). Pleural involvement is seen with both primary and reactivation TB and may result from direct extension, hematogenous spread, or by the rupturing of a subpleural focus of *M. tuberculosis* into the pleural space. Other infectious etiologies are also possible for unilateral pleural effusion including actinomycosis, nocardia, various fungal agents, parasites, and viruses.

PE presents with a unilateral pleural effusion almost half the time. Accompanying radiographic abnormalities may coexist, however, such as atelectasis, infiltrate, oligemia, or pleural-based opacity. Fluid analysis may yield varying results, since increased vascular pressures due to embolic obstruction can cause transudative fluid. Capillary leakage from infarction more commonly causes an exudate.

Various connective tissue disorders may manifest with pleural effusion. Systemic lupus erythematosus (SLE) can present equally with either bilateral or unilateral effusions, but rheumatoid arthritis (RA, 5% of cases) and Wegener's granulomatosis (5% to 55%) produce predominantly unilateral fluid. Although the etiologies remain unclear, local immune injury is suspected in RA, whereas infarction due to pleural vasculitis is a proposed mechanism in Wegener's granulomatosis.

With the exception of CHF and occasionally embolism, the preceding effusions are exudative. Hepatic hydrothorax, a transudative effusion, occurs in 4% to 6% of patients with cirrhosis of the liver and no primary pulmonary disorder. These are mainly right-sided, although they may present bilaterally approximately 17% of the time. Ascitic fluid passing through diaphragmatic defects into the pleural space is the likely mechanism.

Atelectasis is another cause of usually transudative unilateral pleural effusions. It most commonly presents after abdominal/thoracic surgery, since deep breathing is inhibited as a result of inactivity or inadequate pain management. Atelectasis can also be a component of a paramalignant effusion resulting from a tumor-obstructed bronchus. In atelectasis, the separation of the lung and chest wall is accentuated, which causes increased negative pleural pressure, allowing fluid to more easily enter the pleural space. Surgery by itself is a common cause of pleural effusion, with a 50% frequency in abdominal surgery and a universal appearance in lung transplant.

There are many additional causes of unilateral pleural effusions including iatrogenic causes such as peritoneal dialysis (usually right-sided), asbestos-related disease, causes of chylothorax (trauma, lymphoma, lymphangioleiomyomatosis), urinothorax (ipsilateral to obstructed kidney), Meig's syndrome (more commonly right-sided), and pancreatitis (predominantly left-sided). Drug-induced pleural effusions are less common than drug-induced pulmonary parenchymal disease but must be considered especially when procainamide and hydralazine have been used. Other drugs associated with pleural effusion include amiodarone, bromocriptine, methysergide, nitrofurantoin, dantrolene, and several chemotherapeutic agents (e.g., methotrexate, busulfan, bleomycin).

Despite appropriate use of x-rays and laboratory analysis, the cause of the pleural effusion remains unknown (idiopathic) in 20% of cases. Fortunately, most idiopathic effusions follow a benign course.

Clinical Features that Suggest a Specific Cause of Unilateral Pleural Effusion

Chapter 10 discussed the common presenting signs and symptoms for bilateral pleural effusions, which are dyspnea on exertion, cough, and chest pain (although not all need to be present). These symptoms are similar for unilateral pleural effusions. A small, unilateral effusion may even be an incidental radiographic finding in an asymptomatic patient. Physical examination also reveals similar abnormalities to bilateral effusions, but the contrast with a normal lung may be apparent. Decreased or absent breath sounds on auscultation, dullness to percussion, decreased vocal fremitus, and perhaps a friction rub all signal abnormality, especially when compared to the contralateral lung examination.

TABLE 11-1
Interpreting Signs and Symptoms in the Patient with Unilateral Pleural Effusion

Possible Causes	Mechanisms	Suggestive Clinical Features
Malignancy	Impaired lymphatic drainage; direct tumor involvement; atelectasis versus endo-bronchial obstruction; hypoproteinemia due to neoplasm	Hemoptysis; weight loss, fever, chills, sweats; metastatic signs/symptoms (e.g., skin nodules, bone fractures, stroke) Chest x-ray: Normal heart size
Infection	Capillary permeability due to inflammation with impaired lymphatic drainage	Fever/chills/sweats; discolored sputum/hemoptysis; accompanying alveolar infiltrate; positive PPD
PE	Increased vascular pressure secondary to emboli and capillary leakage secondary to infarction	Embolic precursors (e.g., post-operative state, travel, oral contraceptives); pleuritic chest pain; acute onset of symptoms; syncope; hemoptysis Chest x-ray: Accompanying pleural density
CHF	Elevated hydrostatic pressure due to high pulmonary venous pressures due to LV dysfunction	Paroxysmal nocturnal dyspnea; orthopnea; jugular vein distension; lower extremity edema; presence of S_3; bibasilar crackles Chest x-ray: Cardiomegaly
Connective tissue disorders	Localized immune response	Pleuritic chest pain; SLE/RA characteristics Chest x-ray: Normal heart size
Hepatic cirrhosis	Transfer of peritoneal fluid via lymphatics and diaphragmatic defects	Ascites/hepatomegaly; history of liver disease
Atelectasis	Airway collapse secondary to hypoinflation, airway obstruction	Post-operative state; evidence of airway obstruction; obesity

PPD, Purified protein derivative; PE, pulmonary embolism; CHF, congestive heart failure; LV, left ventricular; RA, rheumatoid arthritis; SLE, systemic lupus erythematosus.

Although a specific diagnosis of pleural effusion depends on the results of a thoracentesis, there may be specific clinical features that can narrow the differential diagnosis (Table 11-1). The clinical problem presented in this case suggests malignancy as a prime consideration. The patient is over 50 years of age and is an active smoker with a 45 pack-year history. Passive and active smoking are believed to be responsible for up to 90% of all lung cancers and up to 45% of all cancers in general. This patient also complains of decreased appetite and weight loss.

A series by Sahn and Chernow of patients with pleural carcinomas showed that the most common presenting symptoms were dyspnea (51%), cough (43%), weight loss (32%), and chest pain (26%), all of which are present in this patient. It should be noted, however, that 23% of the 96 patients in this series were asymptomatic. Also, several different primary cancer sites were represented, including lung, breast, ovarian, and stomach cancer. This patient has not had health maintenance screening in over 2 years, making breast and pelvic tumors possible etiologies. The fact that there is no discrete nodule or mass apparent on the chest x-ray does not rule out either pulmonary or non-pulmonary primary sites of malignancy.

Although malignancy is strongly suspected in this patient, it is important to consider the evidence for or against other causes of pleural effusion. CHF can be excluded in this patient with no known heart disease, no physical signs of heart failure on physical examination, and no cardiomegaly on chest x-ray. The patient is on no drugs known to cause effusion and has not had surgery. There is no evidence for atelectasis. Asbestos exposure was not elicited in the patient history. A normal liver and the absence of ascites make hepatic hydrothorax unlikely.

Several other etiologies require consideration as the cause of this right-sided effusion. Whereas there are no overt signs or symptoms of a connective tissue disorder, effusion can develop before the onset of the articular disease, so RA cannot be excluded. Similarly, nothing points directly toward infection as the cause, yet pneumonia can present insidiously with only headache or cough. The absence of obvious parenchymal infiltrate makes bacterial pneumonia very unlikely in this case. Tuberculous infections, however, may present just with cough and chest pain and only with pleural effusion from 38% to 63% of the time. Although this patient has no known exposures, either by occupation, lifestyle, or travel, and her PPD (purified protein derivative) status is unknown, the possibility of tuberculosis (TB) must be evaluated. Although there are no ascites or palpable masses on physical examination, abdominal or pelvic abnormalities (such as in Meig's syndrome) cannot be ruled out in this post-menopausal woman.

Finally, PE is a cause of unilateral pleural effusion that must always be considered. Chest pain (59%), dyspnea (78%), and cough (43%) were frequent symptoms in a review of patients with PE in the National Heart, Lung, and Blood Institute Prospective Investigation of Pulmonary Embolism Diagnosis (PIOPED). The current patient presents with all three symptoms, which puts PE in the differential diagnosis. Unilateral pleural effusion can be the radiographic finding in PE, although atelectasis or pulmonary parenchymal changes are also often present.

In summary, this 52-year-old woman with a 45 pack-year smoking history presents with a right-sided pleural effusion with dyspnea, chest pain, cough, and weight loss. She has no comorbidities but has not undertaken any recent health maintenance activities. Based on this presentation, malignancy of unknown primary (lung versus breast versus abdomen), PE, connective tissue disorder, and infection, especially TB, must be considered as the major possible causes.

Diagnostic Testing in the Evaluation of the Patient with Unilateral Pleural Effusion

Evaluating a unilateral pleural effusion is similar to evaluating bilateral pleural effusions. The presence of fluid versus mass should be assessed with a lateral decubitus chest x-ray (Figure 11-2). If the presence of adequate fluid is confirmed, thoracentesis is done for diagnostic and if necessary, therapeutic purposes. The determination of transudate or exudate is made using Light's criteria as outlined in

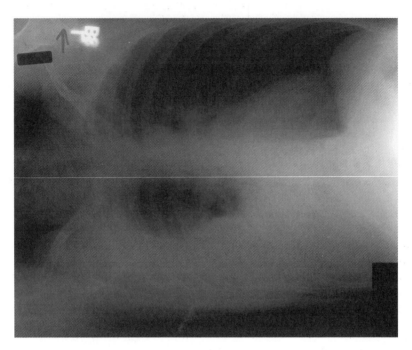

▼ **Figure 11-2** Right lateral decubitus chest x-ray that confirms the presence of right-sided pleural effusion. Note the fluid layers along the entire right pleural space when dependent.

Chapter 10. The differential diagnosis of a transudate is less extensive than for an exudate, although both malignancy and PE can present with transudates. Therefore, in some cases, suspicion of these entities must remain high despite the results of a thoracentesis.

Thoracentesis can be highly suspicious for malignancy or can be confirmatory. Although a malignant effusion can be serous or bloody, a grossly bloody tap with a red cell count >100,000 points toward cancer. Pleural fluid with low pH and glucose may also be malignant, but these findings are also possible with a complicated parapneumonic effusion, rheumatoid pleurisy, TB, and esophageal rupture. Significant lymphocytes (>50%) may also be associated with carcinoma, but TB and lymphoma cannot be excluded. The presence of malignant cells on cytologic examination can secure the diagnosis. This is an important finding because a malignant effusion indicates inoperability for cure and carries a poor prognosis. Unfortunately, the diagnostic yield in a tap is quite variable, primarily due to the presence of paramalignant effusions. Pleural biopsy may be indicated if this initial evaluation is non-diagnostic, but clinical suspicion remains high.

PE remains high on the differential diagnosis for this patient and like malignancy, it can present as either a transudate or an exudate. Whether to further pursue a clot depends on the degree of clinical suspicion. Does the patient have any prior history of embolic disease? Has she recently been immobilized as in a post-operative situation or a prolonged car, bus, or plane ride? Does she use birth control pills?

If PE remains a possibility, a ventilation-perfusion ($\dot{V}/\dot{Q}$) scan is the next recommended step. Recently, spiral computed tomography (CT) proved effective for visualizing emboli in main, lobar, and segmental pulmonary arteries. Evaluation beyond this depends on the results of the preliminary scanning. Further evaluation involves anticoagulation when the scan result is high probability or perhaps lower extremity ultrasound and pulmonary angiography when $\dot{V}/\dot{Q}$ scan is equivocal. A D-dimer assay value of <500 µg/L may also be helpful to exclude.

The connective tissue disorders, primarily RA and SLE, can be diagnosed by pleural fluid with appropriate clinical findings. Low pleural pH and glucose levels, along with an elevated pleural fluid rheumatoid factor (>1:320), are characteristic of RA effusion. Giant and elongated macrophages on cytologic examination support the diagnosis. LE cells in pleural fluid are very specific for lupus pleuritis, as is a pleural fluid antinuclear antibody (ANA) titer >1:160 or an ANA titer in the pleural fluid that exceeds the serum value.

Infectious causes of a pleural effusion can be suggested in several ways. In the correct clinical setting, the presumptive diagnosis of an uncomplicated parapneumonic effusion is made if the effusion and the accompanying infiltrate clear with appropriate antibiotic therapy. The appearance of pus on thoracentesis confirms empyema and requires a chest tube. A positive acid-fast bacillus (AFB) smear or culture establishes the diagnosis of TB, but fluid cultures are positive only between 23% and 86% of the time. Initial PPDs may be negative in one third of the patients ultimately proven to have tuberculous effusions. Increased lymphocytes (greater than 90% to 95%) suggest TB, but ultimately a pleural biopsy may be necessary to establish the diagnosis. The combination of fluid and tissue evaluations is diagnostic in 90% to 95% of cases.

Pitfalls and Common Mistakes in the Assessment and Treatment of Unilateral Pleural Effusion

As previously noted for bilateral effusions, the clinician must be sure that an effusion is present. Physical examination cannot clearly separate fluid from a mass or pleural thickening. The anteroposterior (AP) and lateral chest films also may not definitively diagnose the presence of fluid. Loculated or encapsulated fluid may be difficult to appreciate on upright films. The lateral decubitus chest x-ray may be crucial in determining whether a thoracentesis should be attempted. Chest CT scanning may be necessary to ultimately characterize the pleural abnormality.

Separating fluid as a transudate versus exudate is an important first step, but it is not conclusive. Malignancy and PE are two important diagnoses usually thought of as having exudative effusions, but they can present with transudates.

PE is a frequently overlooked clinical entity and must always be considered in searching for the etiology of pleural fluid. Pleural disease may occasionally precede the onset of rheumatologic symptoms, so that diagnosis of an underlying collagen vascular disease should not be dismissed if no specific evidence is present. Comorbid illness and drugs must always be considered when searching for the cause of a pleural effusion.

A negative PPD does not eliminate tuberculosis as a cause of the pleural effusion, as it can subsequently become positive. Whereas TB is usually considered in a younger patient, it may be overlooked in patients over 50 years of age.

▼ Bibliography

Alberts WM, Salem AJ, Soloman DA, et al: Hepatic hydrothorax, *Arch Intern Med* 151:2383-2388, 1991.

American Thoracic Society. The diagnostic approach to acute venous thromboembolism: clinical practice guidelines, *Am J Respir Crit Care Med* 160:1043-1066, 1999.

Beckett WJ: Epidemiology and etiology of lung cancer, *Clin Chest Med* 14:1-15, 1993.

Chernow B, Sahn SA: Carcinomatous involvement of the pleura: an analysis of 96 patients, *Am J Med* 63:695, 1977.

Ferrer JS, Munoz XG, Orriols RM, et al: Evolution of idiopathic pleural effusion: a prospective, long-term follow-up study, *Chest* 109:1508-1513, 1996.

Good JT, King TE, Antony VB, et al: Lupus pleuritis: clinical features and pleural fluid characteristics with special reference to pleural fluid antinuclear antibodies, *Chest* 84:714-718, 1983.

Joseph J, Sahn SA: Connective tissue disease and the pleura, *Chest* 104:262-270, 1993.

Judson MA, Handy JR, Sahn SA: Pleural effusion following lung transplantation: time course, characteristics and clinical implications, *Chest* 109:1190-1194, 1996.

Kinasewitz GT: Pleuritis and pleural effusions. In Bone RE, Dantzker DR, George RB, et al (editors): *Pulmonary and critical care medicine*, St. Louis, 1997, Mosby.

Light RW: A new classification of parapneumonic effusion and empyema, *Chest* 1098:299, 1995.

Light RW, Girard WM, Jenkinson SG, et al: Parapneumonic effusions, *Am J Med* 69:507-512, 1980.

Matthay RA, Coppage L, Shaw C, et al: Malignancies metastatic to the pleura, *Invest Radiol* 25:601-619, 1990.

McAdams HP, Erasmus J, Winter JA: Radiologic manifestations of pulmonary tuberculosis, *Radiol Clin N Amer* 33(4):655-678, 1995.

Morehead RS: Tuberculosis of the pleura, *South Med J* 91:631-636, 1998.

Morelock SY, Sahn SA: Drugs and the pleura, *Chest* 116:212-221, 1999.

Sahn SA: Pleural malignancies. In Bone RE, Dantzker DR, George RB, et al (editors): *Pulmonary and critical care medicine*, St. Louis, 1997, Mosby Co.

Sahn SA: The pleura: State of the art, *Am Rev Respir Dis* 138:184-234, 1988.

Valdes L, Alvarez D, San Jose E, et al: Tuberculous pleurisy: a study of 254 patients, *Arch Intern Med* 158:2017-2021, 1998.

Watanakunakorn C, Bailey TA: Adult bacteremic pneumococcal pneumonia in a community teaching hospital 1992-1996: a detailed analysis of 108 cases, *Arch Intern Med* 159:1965-1971, 1997.

Weiner-Kronish JP, Matthay MA, Callen PW, et al: Relationship of pleural effusion to pulmonary hemodynamics in patients with congestive heart failure, *Am Rev Respir Dis* 132:1253-1256, 1985.

Weiss JM, Spodick DH: Laterality of pleural effusion in chronic congestive heart failure, *Am J Card* 53:951, 1984.

Wilson JE, Bynum LJ: Characteristics of pleural effusions associated with pulmonary embolism, *Arch Intern Med* 136:159-162, 1976.

CHAPTER 12

PLATYPNEA

Paul A. Lange

Key Terms

- ▼ Platypnea
- ▼ Orthodeoxia
- ▼ Hepatopulmonary syndrome
- ▼ Intra-cardiac shunting
- ▼ Intra-pulmonary vascular dilatations
- ▼ Right-to-left shunt
- ▼ Cirrhosis
- ▼ Liver disease

▼ THE CLINICAL PROBLEM

A 35-year-old man with cirrhosis presents with a 6-month history of progressive shortness of breath and dyspnea on exertion. He reports that his shortness of breath is worse when he is standing or sitting upright and that the sensation of breathlessness improves when he lies flat. He denies any problems with cough, sputum production, wheezing, or hemoptysis. He has noticed increasing abdominal girth over the last several weeks but no significant change in the degree of his lower extremity edema.

He quit smoking 10 years ago. He denies any history of asthma, emphysema, or chronic bronchitis. He has no history of deep venous thrombosis or pulmonary embolism. He has had no recent thoracic surgery. He denies any history of a heart murmur or congenital heart disease.

Past medical history is significant for cirrhosis due to hepatitis B confirmed by liver biopsy. He takes Lasix, Aldactone, and lactulose.

His vital signs are blood pressure 110/60 mm Hg in his right arm sitting, pulse 100, respiration 18, weight 190 lbs. His pupils are equal, round, and reactive. He has mild scleral icterus; his ears, nose, and throat are otherwise unremarkable. His neck is supple and without adenopathy. There is no jugular venous distension, and his thyroid is not enlarged. His lungs are clear to auscultation and percussion. His heart is tachycardic with normal S_1 and S_2 and without significant murmurs, gallop, or rubs. His abdomen is distended, mildly tympanic, soft, and not tender to palpation. Ascites is noted by fluid wave. Liver and spleen are not palpable. There are some prominent capillaries noted over the abdomen. Numerous spider angiomata are present. Clubbing is present in the extremities. There is no significant cyanosis or edema. He is alert and oriented to person, place, and time. Cranial nerves II through XII are grossly intact. There are no tremors, and there is no asterixis.

Complete blood count is normal except for hemoglobin of 17.3 gm/dL and hematocrit of 49.0%. Electrolytes are normal. AST, ALT, and bilirubin levels are mildly elevated. The prothrombin time is 20.0 sec. The international normalized ratio (INR) is 2.0.

Spirometry shows no evidence of airflow obstruction. Lung volumes as measured by the helium dilution method demonstrate a total lung capacity (TLC) of 85% predicted. His diffusing capacity for carbon monoxide (DLCO) is 65% predicted. A chest x-ray is normal.

Supine room air arterial blood gas levels are pH 7.48, $PaCO_2$ 27 mm Hg, and PaO_2 52 mm Hg. The calculated alveolar-arterial oxygen difference is 62.6 mm Hg. Arterial blood gases performed sitting upright are pH 7.50, $PaCO_2$ 24 mm Hg, and PaO_2 44 mm Hg.

What is the differential diagnosis for this patient's shortness of breath that is exacerbated by sitting upright, and what is the most likely cause?

The Differential Diagnosis of Platypnea

Dyspnea is defined as the subjective feeling of breathlessness. A history of positional dyspnea may help identify the precise cause of the dyspnea. *Platypnea* (literally "flat breathing") is dyspnea induced in the upright position and relieved by recumbency. Platypnea is often associated with *orthodeoxia*, defined as a decline in arterial saturation in upright posture that improves with recumbency. The most common causes of platypnea (Box 12-1) include intra-cardiac shunts, pulmonary vascular shunts, and hepatic cirrhosis. Other less common causes of platypnea are parenchymal lung disease such as severe chronic obstructive pulmonary disease (COPD), interstitial fibrosis, pulmonary embolism (PE), and adult respiratory distress syndrome (ARDS).

The precise mechanism of both platypnea and orthodeoxia is unknown. Stated simply, platypnea results from an increased right-to-left shunt either at the interatrial level or the pulmonary vascular level when one assumes an upright posture. Most cases of right-to-left shunting through a patent foramen ovale or atrial septal defect are attributed to a pressure gradient in which the right atrial pressure exceeds that of the left atrium, forcing open a patent foramen ovale. However, platypnea and orthodeoxia have been observed in patients with normal right-sided pressures.

Putative mechanisms for positional shunting include transient right-to-left pressure gradients, altered compliance of the right atrium, preferential flow from the in-

Box 12-1
Differential Diagnosis of Platypnea

Common Causes	Less Common Causes
Intra-Cardiac Shunt (Right-to-Left)	**Conditions Resulting in Worsening $\dot{V}/\dot{Q}$**
Without overt lung disease: Patent	**Mismatch in Upright Position**
foramen ovale, atrial septal defect	COPD
With lung disease: Post-pneumonectomy,	ARDS
obstructive lung disease, after RV	Lower lobe pneumonia
myocardial infarction	PE
Intra-Pulmonary Shunt (Right-to-Left)	
AVM, Osler-Weber-Rendu syndrome	
Hepatopulmonary Syndrome	

$\dot{V}/\dot{Q}$, Ventilation/perfusion; *COPD*, chronic obstructive pulmonary disease; *ARDS*, adult respiratory distress syndrome; *PE*, pulmonary embolism; *RV*, right ventricular; *AVM*, arteriovenous malformation.

ferior vena cava, and respiratory factors such as variable intra-thoracic pressure. However, any lung disease that affects predominately the basal segments of the lung can worsen ventilation/perfusion mismatch when an erect or sitting position is assumed. In the absence of liver disease, platypnea most commonly occurs in patients with inter-atrial communications (patent foramen ovale or atrial septal defect) and a recent history of major pulmonary disorder such as pneumonectomy, pulmonary embolism, or right ventricular infarction (Table 12-1).

Patients with chronic liver disease have dyspnea and hypoxemia for many reasons. Mild hypoxemia is a frequent feature of chronic liver disease. It occurs in approximately one third of all patients and is multifactorial (pleural effusions, reduced lung volumes, and obstructive lung disease). More severe hypoxemia (PaO_2 <60 mm Hg) is less common with cirrhosis alone and is unusual without associated cardiopulmonary disease.

In the absence of independent lung disease, severe hypoxemia in the setting of liver disease strongly suggests the possibility of the hepatopulmonary syndrome. The hepatopulmonary syndrome is defined as the triad of liver disease, an increased alveolar-arterial oxygen difference (>20 mm Hg) while breathing room air, and evidence of intra-pulmonary vascular dilatations. Intra-pulmonary capillary and pre-capillary vascular dilatations range in size from 15 to 500 μm in diameter and are the defining feature of the hepatopulmonary syndrome.

The following three mechanisms are believed to contribute to the gas exchange abnormalities seen in patients with the hepatopulmonary syndrome:

1. Ventilation-perfusion ($\dot{V}/\dot{Q}$) mismatch
2. Intra-pulmonary shunt
3. Limitation of oxygen diffusion

$\dot{V}/\dot{Q}$ mismatching results from overperfusion of alveolar units that are normally ventilated. Increased perfusion is the result of intra-pulmonary vascular dilatations at the lung bases and a hyperdynamic circulatory state.

TABLE 12-1
Interpreting Signs and Symptoms in the Patient with Platypnea

Possible Causes	Mechanisms	Suggestive Clinical Features
Patent foramen ovale or atrial septal defect	Variable right-to-left shunting augmented by upright posture; follows a physiologic insult, resulting either in right-to-left pressure gradient across the interatrial septum, a derangement of atrial anatomy so that the flow into the right atrium is preferentially directed across the septum rather than across the tricuspid valve, or a decrease in RV compliance favoring flow from right to left	Post-pneumonectomy, PE, endomyocardial disease, RV myocardial infarction, right atrial myxoma
AVM	Increased blood flow through lung bases in upright position with resultant increased shunt (right-to-left)	Osler-Weber-Rendu syndrome (hereditary hemorrhagic telangiectasia), epistaxis, and GI bleeding
Hepatopulmonary syndrome	Preferential perfusion of intra-pulmonary vascular dilations (perfusion-diffusion impairment)	Chronic liver disease, cirrhosis, ascites, increased markings on chest x-ray at the lung bases
COPD	Upright posture exacerbates ventilation-perfusion mis-match; predominantly basilar lung disease; small airway closure causing air trapping at lung bases from premature closure	Airway obstruction on pulmonary function tests

PE, Pulmonary embolism; *RV,* right ventricular; *AVM,* arteriovenous malformation; *GI,* gastrointestinal bleeding; *COPD,* chronic obstructive pulmonary disease.

Physiologic studies have shown that diffusion limitation is rare in patients with hepatopulmonary syndrome. Whereas intra-pulmonary shunt is characterized by a lack of response to supplemental oxygen, patients with hepatopulmonary syndrome typically respond to oxygen more than would be expected with true anatomic shunts. This mechanism has been called diffusion-perfusion impairment and relates to the mechanism of hypoxemia associated with intra-pulmonary vascular dilatations seen in patients with hepatopulmonary syndrome (Figure 12-1). Because the capillary is dilated, oxygen molecules from adjacent alveoli cannot diffuse to the center of the dilated vessel to oxygenate hemoglobin in red blood cells at the center of the stream. However, supplemental oxygen provides enough driving pressure to partially overcome this relative perfusion defect.

Orthopnea ("straight-up breathing") is defined as dyspnea that develops in the recumbent position and is relieved by elevation of the head. The patient with orthopnea

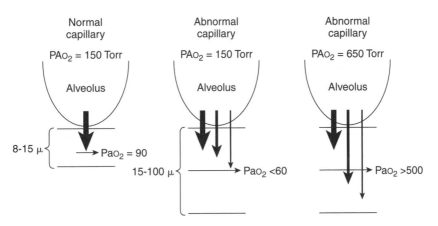

▼ **Figure 12-1**   Diagram of capillary level pulmonary vessel abnormality in chronic liver disease. Driving pressure of PaO$_2$ is depicted by arrows. From Krowka MJ, Cortese DA: *Mayo Clin Proc* 62(3): 164-173, 1987.

generally elevates his or her head and chest on several pillows to prevent nocturnal breathlessness (paroxysmal nocturnal dyspnea). Orthopnea is a common complaint in patients with pulmonary edema (congestive heart failure [CHF]), diaphragmatic dysfunction, advanced obstructive airway disease, and tracheal collapse. In left heart failure, orthopnea occurs from the redistribution of blood from the lower extremities into the chest. In severe obstructive airway disease, changes in gravitational forces that occur in the supine position may provoke dyspnea. A recumbent position causes a shift of abdominal contents toward the chest cavity, interfering with diaphragmatic movements. Neuromuscular disease can cause weakness and paralysis of the diaphragm and other respiratory muscles. Orthopnea may be the earliest symptom in patients with diaphragmatic weakness. Orthopnea is a relatively reliable marker for left ventricular failure, whereas the dyspnea associated with chronic lung disease or musculoskeletal disorders is typically less aggravated by lying flat.

Trepopnea ("twisted breathing") is a variation of orthopnea in which patients complain of dyspnea while lying on their side. Trepopnea may be seen in patients with both pulmonary and cardiac disease. Specifically, trepopnea occurs in patients with unilateral parenchymal lung disease, unilateral pleural effusions, unilateral airway obstruction, and after lung resection as a consequence of interatrial shunt. Trepopnea also has been observed in patients with CHF, most commonly when they lie with their right side down for reasons that are unclear. Usual causes of trepopnea include atrial myxoma and metastatic carcinoma with invasion into the right atrium and mesothelioma.

Clinical Features that Suggest a Specific Cause of Platypnea

In the present patient, clinical features point toward a liver-related cause of his platypnea and hypoxemia. This patient has chronic liver disease due to hepatitis B as manifested by ascites, coagulopathy, and elevated liver function tests. He has impaired gas exchange, platypnea, and orthodeoxia.

As discussed above, the clinical triad of liver disease, hypoxemia, and intra-pulmonary vascular dilatations characterizes the hepatopulmonary syndrome. Portal hypertension appears to be an essential element in the pathogenesis of the syndrome, but the degree of hypoxemia appears unrelated to the severity of liver disease. Most patients with the hepatopulmonary syndrome have cirrhosis due to various causes, and 15% of patients with cirrhosis have the hepatopulmonary syndrome.

Patients with hepatopulmonary syndrome exhibit characteristic signs and symptoms of lung and liver dysfunction. Most patients will present with complications of chronic liver disease such as gastrointestinal bleeding, esophageal varices, ascites, and splenomegaly. Associated classic pulmonary features include digital clubbing, cyanotic nail beds or lips, cutaneous spider angiomata, platypnea, and orthodeoxia. Dyspnea was the presenting symptom in 18% of patients in one series. Patients may complain of symptoms of breathlessness and platypnea for several years before the syndrome is recognized. Platypnea and orthodeoxia are common. In one large series, orthodeoxia was observed in 88% of patients with hepatopulmonary syndrome.

Chest x-rays may show decreased lung volumes, pleural effusions, and increased interstitial markings. A more characteristic pattern seen in patients with the hepatopulmonary syndrome is increased basilar interstitial and vascular markings. These markings are thought to be due to intra-pulmonary vascular dilatations. Pulmonary function testing commonly shows a reduction D_{LCO} with normal lung volumes and expiratory flow rates unless there is concomitant parenchymal lung disease.

Diagnostic Testing in the Evaluation of the Patient with Platypnea

When clinical features suggest the possibility of the hepatopulmonary syndrome, arterial blood gases should be sampled in the supine and upright positions while the patient breathes room air. The position of the patient is important in interpreting arterial blood gas results and should be documented at the time of sampling. Standing accentuates hypoxemia in patients with the hepatopulmonary syndrome, and if possible, the patient should be screened in this position. Because hyperventilation and respiratory alkalosis are common in patients with cirrhosis and may mask subtle arterial oxygenation abnormalities, measurement of the Pa_{O_2} should be accompanied by calculation of the alveolar-arterial oxygenation gradient (PA_{O_2}), as follows:

$$PA_{O_2} = PI_{O_2} - 1.25\,(Pa_{CO_2})$$

where $PI_{O_2} = FI_{O_2}$ (PB $-$ 47, PB = barometric pressure [mm Hg]). An abnormal alveolar-arterial oxygenation gradient corrected for age (normal = [2.5 + 0.21(age)]) indicates an oxygenation abnormality. If arterial oxygenation and alveolar-arterial gradients are normal, then the hepatopulmonary syndrome is excluded. If abnormal arterial blood gas measurements are detected, then further evaluation is warranted. This approach allows recognition of orthostatic changes in oxygenation but does not identify the location of the right-to-left shunt (i.e., intra-cardiac versus intra-pulmonary). Contrast-enhanced echocardiography or tilt table contrast echocardiography can differentiate the location of the shunt.

The 100% oxygen shunt study is frequently used in patients suspected of having hepatopulmonary syndrome to distinguish "functional" shunting (characterized by significant improvement in the PaO_2 while inspiring 100% oxygen) from "anatomic" shunting (characterized by little improvement in the PaO_2). Patients with hepatopulmonary syndrome may have either type of shunt so that a normal 100% oxygen shunt study does not exclude the hepatopulmonary syndrome. In performing a shunt study, the patient inspires pure oxygen through a tight-fitting mask.

The shunt fraction is calculated by using the following formula:

$$Qs/Qt = ([PAO_2 - PaO_2] \times 0.003) \div ([PAO_2 - PaO_2] \times 0.003) + 5$$

where Qs and Qt refer to shunt and total flow and PAO_2 and PaO_2 refer to the alveolar and arterial partial pressures of oxygen. Shunt fractions greater than 5% are abnormal, although the shunt fraction can be overestimated in individuals with the hepatopulmonary syndrome because the true arteriovenous oxygen content difference may be lower than the value (5 mL%) assumed in the equation. Although a PaO_2 that increases to less that 150 mm Hg on 100% oxygen has been proposed as a feature of significant anatomic shunting, the prognostic and therapeutic significance of this measurement remains undefined in patients with hepatopulmonary syndrome.

A chest x-ray identifies potentially reversible causes of hypoxemia such as pneumonia, large pleural effusions, and CHF. In the hepatopulmonary syndrome, the chest x-ray commonly is normal, but increased interstitial markings at the bases of the lungs may be observed and are often mistaken for interstitial fibrosis rather than vascular distension.

Pulmonary function tests are important to determine if intrinsic lung disease is present, but abnormal pulmonary function tests do not exclude the possibility of coexistent hepatopulmonary syndrome. Approximately 50% of cirrhotic patients have mild restrictive abnormalities, commonly due to ascites or pleural effusions. A decrease in the D_{LCO} is also seen in approximately 5% of non-smoking patients with severe liver disease but may occur as an isolated abnormality in 15% of patients with normal alveolar-arterial gradients and otherwise normal pulmonary function tests.

Two-dimensional contrast echocardiography is the most sensitive and commonly employed test to detect intra-pulmonary vasodilatation in patients suspected of having hepatopulmonary syndrome. This technique uses agitated saline or indocyanine green to produce microbubbles with intense echo reflections because of the distinct acoustic impedance relative to blood. Microbubbles traversing normal pulmonary capillaries are small enough to dissolve before reaching the left atrium, whereas larger bubbles traversing dilated pulmonary capillaries do not dissolve and can be visualized in left heart chambers. Screen studies and preliminary reports found the prevalence of post-contrast echocardiograms to range from 5% to 47% in pre-transplant cirrhotic patients. In addition, contrast echocardiography allows the distinction of intra-cardiac and intra-pulmonary shunting and provides information on ventricular and valvular function. Contrast echocardiography may be positive in cirrhotic patients with normal arterial blood gases, presumably reflecting a degree of intra-pulmonary vasodilatation insufficient to alter gas exchange.

Radionuclide lung perfusion scanning also is used to detect intra-pulmonary shunting. If a shunt is present, a percentage of intravenously injected, technetium-labelled, macroaggregated albumin particles (range: 20 to 90 μm) passes through lungs that have capillary dilation and lodge in the brain and kidneys. Unlike the echocardiogram, the calculation of a "shunt fraction" bypassing the lungs allows for quantification of intra-pulmonary shunting. Disadvantages of this technique as a screening study are that intra-pulmonary and intra-cardiac shunting cannot be distinguished, and no information on cardiac function is obtained. Lung scanning is also less sensitive for the hepatopulmonary syndrome than contrast-enhanced echocardiography.

Since pulmonary angiography (an invasive diagnostic test) is not sensitive for detecting intra-pulmonary vasodilatations, it has a limited role in evaluating patients with the hepatopulmonary syndrome. In patients known to have the hepatopulmonary syndrome, the following types of angiographic findings have been described: (1) type 1—a diffuse "spongiform" appearance of pulmonary vessels during the arterial phase of injection and (2) type 2—small discrete arteriovenous communications. Pulmonary angiography may be useful in patients with type 2 lesions and severe hypoxemia because embolization of the vascular dilatations may improve oxygenation.

Pitfalls and Common Mistakes in the Assessment of Platypnea

Because platypnea is an under-recognized symptom, clinicians may neglect to inquire about breathlessness on standing up. Having elicited a history of platypnea, clinicians should consider the hepatopulmonary syndrome and evaluate for liver disease, and, if present, for intra-pulmonary shunt.

Another pitfall is over-reliance on pulse oximetry for detecting hypoxemia. Although pulse oximetry is simple and noninvasive and can be useful for detecting desaturation on standing, shortcomings include its inaccuracy in patients with jaundice and the insensitivity to small variations in Pao_2 values. Furthermore, the alveolar-arterial oxygen gradient cannot be determined by pulse oximetry.

▼ BIBLIOGRAPHY

Herregods MC, Timmermands C, Frans E, et al: Diagnostic value of transesophageal echocardiography in platypnea, *J Am Soc Echocardiog* 6:324-327, 1993.
Lange PA, Stoller JK: The hepatopulmonary syndrome, *Ann Intern Med* 122:521-529, 1995.
Nacht A, Kronzon I: Intracardiac shunts, *Crit Care Clin* 12:295-319, 1996.
Robin ED: An analysis of platypnea-orthodeoxia syndrome including a "new" therapeutic approach, *Chest* 112:1449-1451, 1997.
Seward JB, Hayes DL, Smith, et al: Platypnea-orthodeoxia: Clinical profile, diagnostic workup, management, and report of seven cases, *Mayo Clin Proc* 59:221-231, 1984.
Smeenk FW, Postmus PE: Interatrial right-to-left shunting developing after pulmonary resection in the absence of elevated right heart pressures: Review of the literature, *Chest* 103:528-531, 1993.

CHAPTER 13

CHRONIC HYPERCAPNIA

Lynn T. Tanoue

Key Terms

▼ Hypercapnia
▼ Alveolar hypoventilation

▼ Chronic obstructive
   pulmonary disease (COPD)

▼ Hypoventilation
▼ Respiratory control

▼ THE CLINICAL PROBLEM

A 65-year-old man presents with a complaint of chronic sputum production and dyspnea on exertion. He reports a daily morning cough that produces 2 to 3 teaspoons of white sputum for many years. He has episodes when his sputum turns yellow or green, at which point he generally seeks medical attention and often is given antibiotics. He also reports that he has noticed decreasing exercise tolerance over the last year, particularly with effort such as climbing stairs or carrying bags of groceries. He denies chest pain, a history of heart disease, weight loss, or hemoptysis. His history is notable for smoking 1½ packs/day for the past 50 years. He is on no medications except for lorazepam, which he uses for anxiety.

On physical examination, blood pressure is 130/74 in both arms, pulse is 80, and respiratory rate is 24. Head, ears, eyes, neck, and throat examinations are negative. There is no jugular venous distension. Examination of the chest is notable for increased chest diameter and hyperresonance to percussion. The lung examination shows a prolonged expiratory phase with low-pitched rhonchi throughout.

Cardiac and abdominal examinations are unremarkable. There is no ankle edema. The neurologic examination is benign. The laboratory examination at the initial visit shows hemoglobin, hematocrit, white blood cell count, and platelets all within normal limits.

Chest x-ray demonstrates large lung zones with a small cardiac silhouette. There are no acute infiltrates. His arterial blood gas results are pH 7.38, $Paco_2$ 48 mm Hg, Pao_2 65 mm Hg, HCO_3^- 30, Sao_2 92%.

Pulmonary function test results are as follows:

	▼ Actual	▼ % Predicted
Total lung capacity (TLC)	6.99 L	128
Functional residual capacity (FRC)	4.97 L	164
Residual volume (RV)	4.67 L	238
Vital capacity (VC)	2.31 L	66
RV/TLC	183%	
Forced expiratory volume in 1 second (FEV_1)	0.75 L	29
FEV_1/FVC	35%	
$FEF_{25\% \text{ to } 75\%}$ (forced expiratory flow)	.27 L/sec	10
$FEF_{50\%}$	0.24 L/sec	5

What is the differential diagnosis for this patient's complaints, and what is the most likely cause of his hypercapnia?

Differential Diagnosis of Chronic Hypercapnia

Chronic hypercapnia, defined as a sustained increase in $Paco_2$ exceeding 45 mm Hg, is generally associated with chronic alveolar hypoventilation. Alveolar hypoventilation may result from disturbances in any aspect of breathing (Box 13-1). Diseases of the lung itself are the most obvious causes of hypercapnia. Chronic obstructive pulmonary disease (COPD) may be the most common cause, but airway obstruction at any level, including upper airway obstruction from obstructive sleep apnea and tracheal disease, may also cause persistent carbon dioxide (CO_2) elevation. Parenchymal lung disease, particularly advanced interstitial lung disease, may cause severe alveolar hypoventilation.

Patients with normal lungs may also develop chronic hypercapnia. Abnormalities in ventilatory control may range from central neurologic abnormalities including stroke or malignancy, impairment in respiratory drive such as primary alveolar hypoventilation or obesity-hypoventilation syndrome, metabolic disturbances such as severe thyroid deficiency, drugs causing central respiratory depression including narcotics and sedatives, and metabolic abnormalities such as hypokalemia, hypophosphatemia, and hypomagnesemia. Chest cage abnormalities such as severe kyphoscoliosis may contribute to alveolar hypoventilation. Neuromuscular disorders including myasthenia gravis, amyotrophic lateral sclerosis, polio, muscular dystrophy, diaphragmatic paralysis, cervical spine injury, or Guillain Barré syndrome may also result in hypercapnia. Thus it is important to recog-

Box 13-1
Differential Diagnosis of Hypercapnia

Common Causes	Less Common Causes
Airway Obstruction	**Airway Obstruction**
Lower airway: COPD	Upper airway: Tracheal stenosis or other tracheal
Upper airway: Obstructive	obstruction, tonsillar hypertrophy
sleep apnea	
	Neuromuscular Disorders
Parenchymal Lung Disease	Muscular dystrophy, myasthenia gravis, poliomyelitis,
Severe interstitial lung disease	ALS, Guillain-Barré syndrome, cervical spinal cord
Any disease resulting in destruction	injury, diaphragmatic paralysis
or loss of large amounts of lung	
parenchyma	**Impaired Ventilatory Drive**
	Severe thyroid deficiency
Impaired Ventilatory Drive	Metabolic derangements: Hypokalemia, hypophos-
Obesity-hypoventilation syndrome	phatemia, hypomagnesemia
Drugs: Narcotics, sedatives	Primary alveolar hypoventilation
	Chest cage abnormalities
	Kyphoscoliosis

COPD, Chronic obstructive pulmonary disease; *ALS,* amyotrophic lateral sclerosis.

nize that a disturbance at any level of respiration, from neural input to muscular effort to the lung itself, can result in chronic alveolar hypoventilation and CO_2 elevation.

Pathophysiology of Hypercapnia

CO_2 is a product of normal metabolism. Blood carries foodstuffs to the tissues and oxygen with which to oxidize them. The major products of this metabolism are carbon dioxide, water, heat, and high-energy phosphate bonds. CO_2 can be carried in the blood in the following forms: (1) physically dissolved CO_2 (approximately 5% of total CO_2), (2) CO_2 bound to proteins as carbamino compounds (approximately 5% of total CO_2), and (3) CO_2 in the form of bicarbonate ion (approximately 90% of total CO_2). Ultimately, acid-base balance is achieved by respiratory excretion of CO_2 through the lungs and renal regulation of bicarbonate. In the normal steady state, CO_2 production by tissues is equal to CO_2 elimination by the lungs, and thus hypercapnia does not occur.

Hypercapnia does occur in many clinical settings in which the above balance is upset. The pathophysiology of hypercapnia can be divided into the following four major categories (Table 13-1):

1. Disturbances in gas exchange occurring in the lungs
2. Alterations in CO_2 production
3. Abnormalities in the respiratory "pump"
4. Abnormalities in ventilatory control or respiratory "drive"

TABLE 13-1
Interpreting Signs and Symptoms in the Patient
with Chronic Hypercapnia

Possible Causes	Mechanisms	Suggestive Clinical Features
Lower airway obstruction (COPD)	Gas exchange abnormalities High dead space ventilation $\dot{V}/\dot{Q}$ mismatching	Examination consistent with hyperinflated lungs; history of chronic bronchitis, tobacco use PFTs: Airway obstruction, hyper-inflation, air trapping
Parenchymal lung disease	Gas exchange abnormalities $\dot{V}/\dot{Q}$ mismatching	Examination consistent with inter-stitial lung disease Chest x-ray: Small lung zones with interstitial markings PFTs: Restrictive ventilatory defect
Neuromuscular diseases	Abnormalities in the respiratory pump and/ or impaired respiratory drive	History and examination support-ive of neurologic disease Chest x-ray: Small lung zones without abnormalities PFTs: Restrictive ventilatory defect
Narcotic or sedative overuse	Impaired ventilatory drive	History suggestive of drug-induced problem Chest x-ray: Small lung volumes without parenchymal abnormality
Metabolic derangements Hypothyroidism, hypokalemia, hypophosphatemia, hypomagnesemia	Abnormalities in the respiratory pump and/ or impaired respiratory drive	History and examination sug-gestive of hypothyroidism; laboratory examination show-ing appropriate abnormality Chest x-ray: Normal to small lung volumes without parenchymal abnormality
Chest cage abnormalities	Abnormalities in the respiratory pump	Examination consistent with kyphoscoliosis, thoracoplasty, or other chest cage abnormality
Diaphragmatic weakness	Abnormalities in the respiratory pump	Presence of paradoxical breathing

PFTs, Pulmonary function tests.

Disturbances of Gas Exchange in the Lungs

Lung disease of the airways or interstitium may contribute to hypercapnia. Adequate gas exchange depends on adequate alveolar ventilation. Obstructive airway disease and interstitial lung disease may both decrease alveolar ventilation. In such situations, total minute ventilation may be normal or even increased; in other words, dead space ventilation increases. Additionally, ventilation-perfusion ($\dot{V}/\dot{Q}$) matching may be disturbed. Patients with chronic obstructive pulmonary disease (COPD) usually have $\dot{V}/\dot{Q}$ mismatching at baseline. In steady state, such patients often have increased total minute ventilation, which compensates for the mismatching. In mild to moderate disease, CO_2 is maintained at normal levels by this increased work. However, in severe disease or in the setting of acute illness superimposed on baseline $\dot{V}/\dot{Q}$ abnormality from moderate disease, patients may not be able to sustain a high enough minute ventilation and thus may develop hypercapnia.

Alterations in Carbon Dioxide Production

An average person produces approximately 200 mL of CO_2 per minute. Changes in metabolism can result in increases in CO_2 production. Fever, inflammation, increased physical activity, and infection all result in increased CO_2 production. People who have normal lungs and normal respiratory apparatus will increase alveolar ventilation to match this increase in CO_2 production and thus do not develop hypercapnia. However, patients who have abnormalities at any level of respiration (ventilatory control, neuromuscular status, abnormal lungs, etc) may not be able to increase ventilation appropriately. Hypercapnia may occur in such situations.

Abnormalities in the Respiratory "Pump"

Respiratory muscle fatigue, diaphragmatic abnormalities, and structural abnormalities in the spine or chest cage may all contribute to an ineffective respiratory "pump." Alveolar ventilation depends on adequate expansion of the lungs, which is affected by the strength of the respiratory muscles and the shape of the lung "bellows." Electrolyte disturbances, especially hypokalemia and hypophosphatemia, can contribute to respiratory muscle weakness, and, in severe cases, can precipitate hypercapneic respiratory failure. Poor diaphragmatic contraction, either related to neuromuscular disease or sometimes to phrenic nerve injury, may likewise contribute to respiratory failure. Abnormal structure of the chest cage, as may occur with severe kyphoscoliosis, may predispose to respiratory muscle fatigue and decreased muscle strength due to chronic malposition of both chest wall muscles and diaphragm.

In patients with severe airflow obstruction and hyperinflation, the diaphragm may be operating at a mechanical disadvantage. In this situation, the diaphragm is often in a lower, flatter position than normal. Because of this flattening, the transpulmonary pressure developed for any given diaphragmatic contraction is less than if the diaphragm were in its usual domed position. Furthermore, in a lung diseased by airways obstruction, greater pressure changes are required to produce a given change in volume. Thus diaphragmatic fatigue can be a significant issue in patients with severe COPD. Clinical signs of this include "paradoxical breathing," in which the abdomen moves inward instead of outward with inspiration. Paradoxical breathing is usually a sign of severe diaphragmatic weakness or fatigue.

Abnormalities in Ventilatory Control

Regulation of breathing is largely automatic even though the muscles of the respiratory system have no intrinsic pacemaker. Voluntary control during activities such as sniffing, coughing, singing, breath-holding, etc, occur frequently, but breathing is largely involuntary.

The control of breathing involves complex interactions between multiple sites. Centers regulating the rate of breathing, rhythmic respiration, and neural input to respiratory muscles are known to exist in the brainstem. These centers may maintain rhythmic breathing even in the absence of higher cortical input. Control of breathing is also regulated by the lung itself. Receptors in the lung respond to stretch of smooth muscle from lung distension as well as to inhalation of chemical or particulate irritants (stretch and irritant receptors) and also can be activated by an increase in pulmonary interstitial fluid (J receptors).

Fluctuations in oxygenation, carbon dioxide levels, and acid-base balance are sensed by chemoreceptors. Peripheral chemoreceptors include carotid bodies, usually located at the bifurcation of the common carotid arteries, and aortic receptors. These receptors are affected by changes in the chemical balance of the blood. Central chemoreceptors are located in the medulla and appear to be influenced by the chemical composition of both blood and cerebral spinal fluid. The interaction of all these various centers of breathing allow the respiratory system to respond to both acute and chronic changes induced by an enormous variety of intrinsic and environmental changes, including exercise, altitude, hypoxia, inflammation, acute and chronic illness, and metabolic derangements, among others. Abnormalities at any level of this complex apparatus can result in abnormal respiration. Such abnormalities may be subtle if a person is stable, but may become pronounced and obvious in the setting of superimposed stresses.

Clinical Features that Suggest a Specific Cause of Hypercapnia

In the current case, the clinical picture is consistent with COPD. The patient's history confirms a diagnosis of chronic bronchitis. His examination suggests the presence of large hyperinflated lungs, which is corroborated by the chest x-ray as well as his physiologic testing. The pulmonary function study is consistent with severe obstructive airway disease with hyperinflation and air trapping. His decreasing exercise tolerance is likely explained by the severe airways obstruction. In all likelihood, this patient's disease is related to his long history of tobacco use.

Thus in this case the hypercapnia seen on arterial blood gas testing is due to disturbance of gas exchange related to the patient's underlying COPD. In all likelihood, this particular patient has severe $\dot{V}/\dot{Q}$ mismatching related to the presence of emphysema and chronic bronchitis. The pathophysiology of his respiratory abnormality would include high minute ventilation with high dead space ventilation and relatively low alveolar ventilation.

Diagnostic Testing in the Evaluation of the Patient with Hypercapnia

As with most medical illnesses, the most important initial diagnostic evaluation of the patient with hypercapnia is a careful history and physical examination. The differentiation between the four major categories of pathophysiologic reasons for hypercapnia should be made by the patient's history, corroborated by supportive physical findings. In most cases, the history and physical examination will define the major categories outlined in Box 13-1 and Table 13-1. Further diagnostic evaluation of patients with hypercapnia will usually include chest x-ray, arterial blood gas testing, and pulmonary function testing. Patients with COPD, interstitial lung disease, or other parenchymal pulmonary abnormalities may have suggestive radiographic findings. Patients with chest cage abnormalities should have been identified on physical examination, but the chest x-ray may be helpful, for example, in assessing severity of the degree of scoliosis.

Arterial blood gas testing aids in determining the severity of hypercapnia and in assessing pH and whether there is accompanying hypoxia. In cases where lung disease is present, the degree of hypoxia, as well as hypercapnia, reflects the severity of the underlying disease. In contrast, patients who have normal lungs but who have alveolar hypoventilation because of neuromuscular disease or impaired ventilatory drive may have hypercapnia without hypoxia; that is, the alveolar-arterial oxygen difference will be normal. Pulmonary function testing may be helpful in defining obstructive from restrictive disease. Obstructive diseases are largely confined to asthma, emphysema, chronic bronchitis, and severe bronchiectasis, whereas the differential diagnosis of a restrictive ventilatory defect is considerably broader. Patients with interstitial lung disease, neuromuscular disorders, impaired ventilatory drive, and chest cage abnormalities may all have a restrictive defect on pulmonary function testing.

The clinician should have a reasonable grasp of the pathophysiologic cause of hypercapnia once the history, physical examination and above evaluation are done. Further diagnostic evaluation should be more specifically directed thereafter by the results of this initial assessment.

Assessment of Therapy for Hypercapnia

The current patient has COPD with features of chronic bronchitis and emphysema. The presence of hypercapnia and hypoxia indicates that his disease is severe. This is supported by pulmonary function testing showing a severe obstructive pattern with hyperinflation and air trapping. In this patient, therapeutic interventions might include bronchodilators and mucociliary agents. An assessment of whether there is any reversibility to his airways obstruction (i.e., spirometric measurement of FEV_1 and FVC after inhaled bronchodilator) might be useful, as some patients with COPD have a significant reversible component that can be effectively treated with medications more commonly used for asthma. Such medical interventions may result in improved exercise tolerance and quality of life. Objective measurements may show improvement in FEV_1 and also improvements in ventilation (as measured by $PaCO_2$) and oxygenation (as measured by PaO_2 or SaO_2). Patients with COPD also may benefit from non-pharmacologic interventions such as pulmonary rehabilitation. Pulmonary rehabilitation may not result in any changes in physiologic testing such as spirometry, but patients often demonstrate improved exercise tolerance and quality of life.

It is always important to look for factors other than the primary disease that may be affecting a patient's clinical status. In the case being discussed, the patient had been prescribed a benzodiazepine for anxiety. It would be important to assess how this sedative might be contributing to any central respiratory depression in this patient with very impaired lung function and hypercapnia.

Pitfalls and Common Mistakes in the Assessment and Treatment of Hypercapnia

Perhaps the most common pitfall clinicians make in the assessment of hypercapnia is failing to recognize that its causes can be so varied. In many cases, the assumption is mistakenly made that hypercapnia must represent a problem of the lungs itself, neglecting other potential causes of alveolar hypoventilation. As already described, these involve a wide range of diseases, including neurologic disorders, muscular abnormalities, disturbances of central respiratory drive, and problems with the lung bellows. Published series of causes of chronic hypercapnia do indicate that lung disease, primarily COPD, is indeed the cause of the majority of cases of hypercapnia. However, one cannot assume that lung disease is always the culprit. Inattention to historical detail or an inadequate physical examination may cause delay in correct diagnosis.

In the assessment of hypercapnia, the clinician must also pay careful attention to determining the acuity of the rise in CO_2. Patients with chronic CO_2 retention develop metabolic compensation for their respiratory acidosis. Acid-base balance in this setting occurs via renal compensatory mechanisms. Generation of HCO_3^- in the kidney is induced by the presence of hypercapnia. Over days to weeks, the presence of a respiratory acidosis will result in a compensatory metabolic alkalosis, the end result of which is a blood pH that ranges from slightly acidemic to normal. In contrast, patients with acute respiratory acidosis developing over hours will not have had adequate time for renal compensation to occur. These patients will have hypercapnia with acidemia, the severity of which will be determined by the severity of CO_2 retention. Thus clinicians should not view Pa_{CO_2} in isolation. Evaluation of the pH obtained with the arterial blood gas is an important and critical part of interpretation of the acuity or chronicity of alveolar hypoventilation.

▼ BIBLIOGRAPHY

Glauser FL, Fairman P, Bechard D: The causes and evaluation of chronic hypercapnia, *Chest* 91:755-759, 1987.

Miner AH: *Respiratory physiology,* ed 3, New York, 1993, Raven Press.

Strumpf DA, Millman RP, Hill NS: The management of chronic hypoventilation, *Chest* 98:474-480, 1990.

Weinberger SE, Schwartzstein RM, Weiss JW: Hypercapnia, *N Engl J Med* 321:1223-1231, 1989.

CHAPTER 14

COMMUNITY-ACQUIRED PNEUMONIA

David L. Longworth

Key Terms

▼ Community-acquired pneumonia

▼ Tuberculosis
▼ Pneumococcus

▼ Community-acquired legionella

▼ THE CLINICAL PROBLEM

During the summer a 53-year-old man presents in the emergency room with a 2-day history of fever to 103° F, chills, headache, and a cough productive of scant blood-tinged yellow sputum. He reports that these symptoms have come on gradually over the preceding 48 hours, after a fishing trip on Lake Erie. He is an accountant, has never smoked, has no underlying lung disease, and denies other travel or ill contacts. He reports mild shortness of breath.

His past medical history is notable for a myocardial infarction 3 years ago, mild compensated congestive heart failure (CHF), hypercholesterolemia, and hypertension. His medications include atenolol, digoxin, furosemide, and lovastatin. He has not received pneumococcal vaccine. He is married, has a pet cat, and denies HIV risk behaviors.

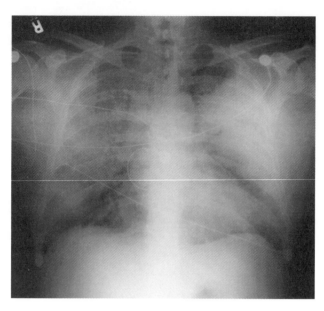

▼ **Fig. 14-1.** Dense left upper lobe and patchy right upper lobe infiltrates are evident on this anteroposterior (AP) chest x-ray.

On physical examination, his vital signs include a temperature of 103.1° F, blood pressure 135/86 mm Hg, pulse 90, and respirations 32. His chest is clear to auscultation and his heart sounds are normal and without murmurs or gallops. He has no hepatosplenomegaly or rash, and his sensorium is clear. His neck is supple and the remainder of the examination is normal.

His leukocyte count is 13,500 cells/mm³, hemoglobin 14.5 g/dL, platelet count 140,000/mm³, serum sodium 125 mmol/L, glucose 110 mg/dL, and blood urea nitrogen 40 mg/dL. A chest x-ray discloses right upper lobe and left upper lobe infiltrates (Figure 14-1). An electrocardiogram (ECG) demonstrates normal sinus rhythm and evidence of a remote anterolateral myocardial infarction, unchanged from a tracing a year previously. A room air blood gas discloses a resting PaO_2 of 58 mm Hg, PCO_2 25 mm Hg, and pH 7.34.

What is the most likely diagnosis and the most likely causes? What further tests are indicated? Should the patient be admitted to hospital, and how should he be treated?

Differential Diagnosis of Community-Acquired Pneumonia

The acute onset of fever, productive cough, and a new pulmonary infiltrate should suggest the diagnosis of community-acquired pneumonia. Other less common causes of fever, cough, and a new lung infiltrate include pulmonary embolism with infarction and CHF in the setting of a large anterior myocardial infarction, both of which may be accompanied by hemoptysis but generally not purulent sputum. There is no history of chest pain to suggest cardiac ischemia and no risk factors or physical findings suggestive of pulmonary embolism. The chest x-ray is inconsistent with heart failure, and the ECG does not disclose ischemic changes. Patients

Box 14-1
Differential Diagnosis of Community-Acquired Pneumonia

Common Causes	Less Common Causes
Streptococcus pneumoniae	Gram-negative bacilli
Legionella species	Fungi
Blastomyces dermatitidis	Histoplasma capsulatum
Haemophilus influenzae	Mycobacterium tuberculosis
Mycoplasma pneumoniae	Pneumocystis carinii (underlying HIV)
Chlamydia pneumoniae	Coxiella burnetti (Q fever)
Moraxella catarrhalis	Chlamydia psittaci (psittacosis)
Viruses	Viruses
Influenza	Adenovirus
Respiratory syncytial virus	Parainfluenza viruses
	Rhinovirus

with occult obstructing endobronchial malignancies may sometimes present with post-obstructive pneumonia that mimics community-acquired pneumonia. There is no history of smoking to suggest this diagnosis, and the presence of bilateral infiltrates would be atypical.

Aspiration pneumonia can present with fever, cough, and a new pulmonary infiltrate, but this usually occurs in the setting of recognized aspiration events, loss of consciousness (e.g., due to seizures or syncope) predisposing to aspiration, or in neurologically impaired individuals who lack a gag reflex. None of these predisposing historical features or events is present in this patient.

The microbial differential diagnosis of community-acquired pneumonia is summarized in Box 14-1. Common causes include *Streptococcus pneumoniae* (also called the pneumococcus), *Legionella* species, *Mycoplasma pneumoniae*, *Chlamydia pneumoniae*, *Haemophilus influenzae*, *Moraxella catarrhalis*, and viruses such as influenza, respiratory syncytial virus, and adenovirus. *Staphylococcus aureus* is a less common though occasional cause of community-acquired pneumonia in winter months following influenza. Uncommon causes of community-acquired pneumonia include gram-negative bacilli (although alcoholics have a predilection for *Klebsiella pneumoniae*), fungal pathogens, and *Mycobacterium tuberculosis*. *Pneumocystis carinii* may present as a community-acquired pneumonia in patients with unrecognized human immunodeficiency virus infection, although the cough is rarely productive and hemoptysis is unusual. Polymicrobial aerobic-anaerobic bacterial pneumonia is an uncommon cause of community-acquired pneumonia, and generally occurs in the setting of aspiration, seizures, or loss of consciousness. In up to 50% of patients with community-acquired pneumonia, no microbiologic diagnosis is established despite vigorous attempts.

The microbial differential diagnosis of community-acquired pneumonia varies depending on the age of the patient, the season of the year, the presence of underlying diseases, the epidemiologic setting, and the gravity of the illness. In young adults with milder illnesses not requiring hospital admission, *M. pneumoniae*, *C. pneumoniae*, and viruses are the most common pathogens. These organisms are also the most common in institutional settings such as military barracks and schools when outbreaks of pneumonia occur. In older individuals and those sick enough to require hospitalization, *S. pneumoniae, Legionella* species, *H. influenzae,* and other bacteria are the most frequent pathogens. In patients with multilobar pneumonias requiring intensive care unit support, legionellosis and pneumococcal disease are the most likely considerations.

Clinical Features of Community-Acquired Pneumonia

The history and physical examination are very important in the evaluation of the patient with suspected community-acquired pneumonia. The clinical syndrome of community-acquired pneumonia has classically been divided into typical and atypical presentations as summarized in Table 14-1. This distinction is based on the clinical presentation and likely microbiology. "Typical" community-acquired pneumoniae often presents with the sudden onset of fever, shaking chills, and a productive cough, sometimes with hemoptysis. Pulmonary symptoms predominate from the outset. This syndrome has been associated with bacterial pathogens such as the pneumococcus and *H. influenzae.*

The chest x-ray typically shows lobar consolidation. By contrast, "atypical" community-acquired pneumonia is more often gradual in onset with constitutional symptoms predominating at the outset. Pulmonary symptoms may be minor initially, and the cough is often non-productive. Relative bradycardia, defined as a heart rate less than 100 in the presence of fever and in the absence of beta blockade or intrinsic conduction system disease, may be associated.

Pathogens associated with atypical presentations include *Legionella* species, *M. pneumoniae, C. pneumoniae, Coxiella burnetti* (the agent of Q fever), *Chlamydia psittaci* (the cause of psittacosis), and viruses. The chest x-ray classically discloses patchy infiltrates. Recent studies have questioned the utility of distinguishing "typical"

TABLE 14-1
Typical Versus Atypical Community-Acquired Pneumonia

Feature	Typical	Atypical
Clinical presentation	Sudden onset, productive cough, rigors common, respiratory symptoms predominate at outset, relative bradycardia less common	Gradual onset, dry cough, rigors less common, constitutional symptoms may overshadow respiratory symptoms initially, relative bradycardia more common
Common pathogens	*Streptococcus pneumoniae* *Haemophilus influenzae* *Staphylococcus aureus* *Klebsiella pneumoniae*	*Legionella* species *Mycoplasma pneumoniae* *Chlamydia pneumoniae* *Coxiella burnetti* *Chlamydia psittaci* Viruses
Chest x-ray	Lobar consolidation	Patchy infiltrates

from "atypical" presentations, since typical pathogens can occasionally present with atypical presentations and vice versa. Nevertheless, the distinction can be helpful at the bedside in those with classic presentations and suggestive epidemiologic exposure histories. In the present patient, the presentation is most consistent with an atypical pathogen, given the gradual onset of symptoms over 48 hours, the predominance of constitutional symptoms at the outset, the minimally productive cough, and the patchy infiltrates on chest radiography.

In addition to distinguishing typical from atypical presentations, the history in the patient with suspected community-acquired pneumonia should explore a number of features which may provide a clue to the etiologic agent, as summarized in Box 14-2 and Table 14-2. The age of the patient is important. *Mycoplasma* and chlamydial pneumonias are more common in young adults, whereas typical bacterial pathogens occur more frequently in older individuals.

The place of acquisition should be determined, and a residence, travel, and exposure history should be obtained. For example, a patient who presents with acute pneumonia after travel to the desert in the Southwestern United States might have pulmonary coccidioidomycosis or the hantavirus pulmonary syndrome. A resident of the upper Midwest who presents with pneumonia after a canoe trip on a river with beaver dams might have blastomycosis. A military recruit who lives in a barracks and who presents with atypical pneumonia in an outbreak setting may have *Mycoplasma* or *Chlamydia* pneumonia. Finally, a patient who presents with pneumonia after exposure to fresh water (as occurred in the current patient) or to a construction site may have legionellosis.

An occupational history is also very important. Acute pneumonia in an abattoir worker or sheep farmer should suggest the possibility of Q fever pneumonia. Pneumonia in a health care worker should prompt consideration of tuberculosis. A construction worker who presents with pneumonia following inhalation of dust and dirt at an excavation site could have histoplasmosis, blastomycosis, legionellosis, or even inhalational aspergillosis.

The season of the year when the patient presents is also very important. *M. pneumoniae* and *Legionella* species often produce "summer pneumonias," whereas in-

---

Box 14-2
Essential Historical Considerations in the Patient with Community-Acquired Pneumonia

Age of the patient
Place of acquisition
Residence, travel, and exposure history
Occupation
Season of the year
Underlying diseases
Medications

TABLE 14-2
Specific Clues on History and Physical Examination in Patients with Community-Acquired Pneumonia

Clues	Associated Pathogens
Historical Clue	
Fresh water exposure	Legionella species
Construction or excavation site exposure	Legionella species, Histoplasma capsulatum,* Blastomyces dermatitidis,*Aspergillus species
Travel to Southwestern US or San Joaquin Valley	Coccidioides immitis
Outbreaks in institutional settings (military barracks, dormitories, nursing homes)	M. pneumoniae, C. pneumoniae, Mycobacterium tuberculosis
HIV risk behavior	P. carinii, S. pneumoniae, H. influenzae, Mycobacterium tuberculosis
Loss of consciousness	Polymicrobial aspiration
Animal Exposure	
Parakeets	Chlamydia psittaci
Chickens, pigeons	Histoplasma capsulatum
Beavers	Blastomyces dermatitidis
Sheep (birthing)	Coxiella burnetti
Occupational Clue	
Health care worker	Mycobacterium tuberculosis
Abattoir worker	C. burnetti
Physical Examination Clue	
Relative bradycardia†	Atypical pathogens
Splenomegaly	C. burnetti, Chlamydia psittaci, Histoplasma capsulatum
Nuchal rigidity	S. pneumoniae
Absent gag reflex	Polymicrobial aspiration
Fetid breath	Mouth anaerobes
Bullous myringitis	M. pneumoniae
Erythema multiforme	M. pneumoniae
Erythema nodosum	Mycobacterium tuberculosis, Histoplasma capsulatum, C. pneumoniae
Hoarseness	C. pneumoniae

*In the appropriate geographic locales. Histoplasmosis is endemic in the Ohio and Mississippi river valleys. Blastomycosis is endemic in the upper midwestern and southeastern US.
†Heart rate less than 100 beats per minute in the presence of fever and in the absence of beta blockade or intrinsic cardiac conduction system disease.

fluenza and complicating staphylococcal pneumonias are diseases of winter months. The present patient presented in the summer months.

The presence of underlying illnesses and a medication history should be ascertained. Splenectomized patients are at risk for overwhelming pneumonia with encapsulated organisms such as *S. pneumoniae, H. influenzae,* and *Neisseria meningitidis.* The presence of risk behaviors for human immunodeficiency virus infection should suggest the possibility of *Pneumocystis carinii* pneumonia as the presenting manifestation of the acquired immunodeficiency syndrome (AIDS). Patients receiving immunosuppressive medications are at risk for opportunistic pathogens not commonly considered in healthy patients with community-acquired pneumonia.

Findings on the physical examination may also, on occasion, suggest the etiologic diagnosis or differential diagnosis as summarized in Table 14-2. Chest examination is rarely helpful in this regard, although the finding on examination or chest x-ray of a large associated pleural effusion is more suggestive of a bacterial pathogen. Relative bradycardia should suggest an atypical pathogen. Community-acquired pneumonia accompanied by new onset splenomegaly should suggest psittacosis, Q fever, or disseminated histoplasmosis. Bullous myringitis and erythema multiforme may be seen with *M. pneumoniae* but are uncommon with other pathogens. Erythema nodosum may be seen with mycobacterial or fungal pneumonias. An absent gag reflex or fetid breath should suggest the possibility of a polymicrobial mixed aerobic-anaerobic aspiration pneumonia. Nuchal rigidity should suggest pneumococcal pneumonia with meningitis. Encephalopathy may be associated with overwhelming bacterial pneumonia and legionellosis. Cranial neuropathies and cerebellar findings are rare complications of mycoplasmal pneumonia.

Diagnostic Testing in the Evaluation of Suspected Community-Acquired Pneumonia

In patients with suspected community-acquired pneumonia, the initial assessment should focus on establishing the diagnosis, assessing risk factors for morbidity and mortality, and determining the need for hospital or intensive care unit admission. A chest x-ray should be performed in those in whom the diagnosis is suspected. The presence of a new infiltrate suggests the diagnosis, with the caveat that other non-infectious processes such as heart failure and pulmonary embolism may produce infiltrates. On occasion, the chest x-ray may be normal in the initial hours or in dehydrated patients with community-acquired pneumonia. In such individuals, repeating the film 12 to 24 hours later following hydration may disclose the presence of an infiltrate.

Risk factors associated with increased morbidity and mortality in patients with community-acquired pneumonia are summarized in Table 14-3. Most of these factors can be quickly ascertained at the bedside by history, physical examination, and some simple laboratory testing. A prognostic scoring system has been developed by Fine and others that accurately predicts mortality and the need for subsequent hospital admission as shown in Tables 14-3 and 14-4. In this system, points are assigned for age and the presence of specific comorbidities, physical findings, and screening laboratory test abnormalities. These points are then totaled to calculate a risk score, which stratifies the likelihood of mortality and the need for subsequent hospitalization if the patient is not initially admitted. Despite these data, the decision to admit patients to hospital for suspected community-acquired pneumonia is ultimately a clinical one, and physician judgment should always take precedence over algorithmic scoring systems. For example, a hypoxic patient, irrespective of the total Fine score, virtually always merits hospital admission. Physicians should exercise great caution in not admitting patients to hospital who have multiple risk factors for morbidity and mortality.

In the current patient, the Fine score would be calculated as follows. He is 53 years of age; 53 points would be assigned. His evaluation is notable for a history of

TABLE 14-3
Risk Factors for Morbidity and Mortality in Patients with Community-Acquired Pneumonia and Fine Score

Risk Factor	Fine Score (Points)
Demographics	
Advancing age	Males: 1 point per year
	Females: 1 point per year − 10
Comorbidities	
Neoplasia	+30
Chronic liver disease	+20
CHF	+10
Chronic renal disease	+10
Cerebrovascular disease	+10
Physical Findings	
Respiratory rate greater than or equal to 30/min	+20
Systolic BP <90 mm Hg	+20
Altered mentation	+20
Temperature greater than or equal to 104° F or less than 95° F	+15
Heart rate greater than or equal to 125/min	+10
Diagnostic Tests	
Arterial pH <7.35	+30
BUN >30 mg/dL	+20
Pao$_2$ <60 mm Hg	+10
Pleural effusion	+10
Serum sodium <130 mmol/L	+10
Glucose >250 mg/dL	+10
Hematocrit <30%	+10

Adapted from Fine MJ, Auble TE, Yealy DM, et al: *N Engl J Med* 336:243-250, 1997.
CHF, Congestive heart failure; *BP,* blood pressure; *BUN,* blood urea nitrogen.

TABLE 14-4
Morbidity and Mortality in Patients with Community-Acquired Pneumonia Stratified by Fine Score

Fine Class	Fine Score (Points)	Mortality (%)	Subsequent Admission Rate (%)
I*	—	0.1	5.1
II	<or = 70	0.6	8.2
III	71 + 90	2.8	16.7
IV	91-130	8.2	20.0
V	>130	29.2	0

Data from Fine MJ, Auble TE, Yealy DM, et al: *N Engl J Med* 36:243-250, 1997.
*Class I patients were 50 years of age or less, had no malignancy, CHF, cerebrovascular disease, renal disease, or liver disease, and had none of the following abnormalities: altered mentation, pulse ≥125, respiratory rate ≥30, systolic BP <90, temperature <95° F or ≥104° F.

Box 14-3
Indications for Admission to ICU in Patients with Community-Acquired Pneumonia

Significant hypoxemia
Need for intubation and mechanical ventilation
Hemodynamic instability
Significant cardiac, hepatic, or renal failure
Acute alteration in mental status

TABLE 14-5
Guidelines for Microbiologic Testing in Patients with Community-Acquired Pneumonia: Recommendations of the Infectious Disease Society of America (IDSA) and American Thoracic Society (ATS)

	Inpatients		Outpatients	
	IDSA	**ATS**	**IDSA**	**ATS**
Blood cultures	Yes	Yes	No	No
Sputum Gram's stain	Yes	No	Optional	No
Sputum culture	Yes	No	No	No

CHF (+10), respiratory rate of 32 (+20), BUN 40 mg/dL (+20), PaO$_2$ 58 mm Hg (+10), and pH 7.34 (+30). His total Fine score is 53 + 10 + 20 + 20 + 10 + 30 = 143. His risk of mortality exceeds 25%, and he should be admitted to the hospital and possibly to the intensive care unit (ICU). Indications for ICU admission are summarized in Box 14-3; his hypoxemia would make him a potential candidate.

Guidelines regarding the indications for selected microbiologic studies in patients with community-acquired pneumonia have been published by the Infectious Disease Society of America (IDSA) and the American Thoracic Society (ATS) and are summarized in Table 14-5. In patients well enough to be managed as outpatients, a sputum Gram's stain, sputum culture, and blood cultures are not mandatory. In hospitalized patients, blood cultures should be obtained, although they are positive in only 10% of patients. The utility of sputum Gram's stain and culture is debated, but these tests should be obtained if feasible. Serologic tests for *Legionella* species, *M. pneumoniae, Chlamydia* species, and selected other pathogens should be obtained when the history or physical findings suggests specific etiologic diagnoses, although serologies are often only helpful retrospectively and should not be relied on to direct empiric therapy.

The legionella urinary antigen test is usually positive within 3 days of symptom onset in patients with *Legionella pneumophila* serogroup 1 infection, which causes 80% of cases of legionellosis in the United States. This test may remain positive for up to 1 year but may be extremely helpful in the appropriate setting if positive. A negative test does not exclude legionellosis due to other strains of *L. pneumophila* or species of *Legionella.*

In hospitalized patients with community-acquired pneumonia, molecular diagnostic techniques such as DNA probes and PCR may be helpful in selected clinical settings when applied to respiratory secretions in search of *Legionella, Chlamydia, Mycoplasma,* and *Mycobacterium tuberculosis.* Direct fluorescent microscopy of sputum is positive in about 40% of patients with legionellosis and should be obtained in patients with a compatible illness.

Bronchoscopy is rarely indicated in patients with community-acquired pneumonia, although it should be considered in critically ill patients, especially if already mechanically ventilated. HIV testing should be performed after appropriate informed consent in patients with a history of intravenous drug use, blood transfusion, homosexual contact, or heterosexual promiscuity.

Patients with sizeable pleural effusions should undergo diagnostic thoracentesis to exclude the presence of empyema, which would require tube thoracostomy drainage. Sampled fluid should be sent for cell counts with differential, glucose, protein, lactate dehydrogenase (LDH), pH, Gram's stain, routine cultures, and mycobacterial and fungal stains and cultures when indicated by the history and clinical presentation.

The present patient is admitted to hospital and is transferred to the intensive care unit because of worsening hypoxemia. Blood cultures are sent, and he is able to produce a sputum specimen, which on Gram's stain, demonstrates many polymorphonuclear leukocytes, few epithelial cells, and no organisms. A direct fluorescent antibody test on sputum for *Legionella* is negative. Because of the severity of his illness, an acute serum specimen is collected and held for further serologic testing, to be compared with convalescent serologies in the event a microbiologic diagnosis is not established. A *Legionella* urinary antigen is sent.

Assessment of the Effect of Therapy

Antimicrobial chemotherapy is the cornerstone of treatment for community-acquired pneumonia, but supportive care is essential, especially in critically ill patients requiring hospital or intensive care unit admission. Careful attention to adequate oxygenation. and hydration is imperative.

Recommendations regarding antimicrobial therapy have been published by several professional organizations, including the American Thoracic Society and the Infectious Diseases Society of America. These recommendations deal with both empiric and pathogen-specific therapy; recommendations regarding empiric therapy are stratified by severity of illness and the need for hospitalization and are influenced by patient-specific modifying factors that suggest specific microbial etiologies (Box 14-4 and Table 14-6).

In most instances, the cause of community-acquired pneumonia may not be evident initially, although, in patients with a compelling sputum, Gram's stain with many polymorphonuclear leukocytes, few contaminating epithelial cells, and a predominant organism, empiric therapy may be appropriately directed against the specific pathogen. In patients such as the present one with many polymorphonu-

Box 14-4
Empiric Therapy in Patients with Community-Acquired Pneumonia

Outpatients	Hospitalized Patients
Preferred	**General Medicine Ward**
Macrolides (erythromycin, clarithromycin or azithromycin)	β-lactamase + macrolide or fluoroquinolone alone
Fluoroquinolones (levofloxacin, sparfloxacin, grepafloxacin)	Alternative: Cefuroxime with or without a macrolide, or azithromycin alone
Doxycycline	**Intensive Care Unit**
	Erythromycin, azithromycin, or a fluoroquinolone *plus*
Modifying Patient Factors	cefotaxime, ceftriaxone, or a β-lactamase inhibitor
Age 17-40: Doxycycline	Modifying patient factors
Aspiration event: Amoxicillin-clavulanate	Aspiration: β-lactamase inhibitor alone *or* fluoroquinolone plus either clindamycin or
Suspected PCN-resistant pneumococcus: Fluoroquinolone	metronidazole
	PCN allergic: Fluoroquinolone with or without clindamycin
	Structural lung disease
	Anti-pseudomonal penicillin *or*
	Carbapenem *or*
	Cefepime + macrolide *or*
	Fluoroquinolone + aminoglycoside

Table 14-6
Pathogen-Specific Therapy in Community-Acquired Pneumonia

Organism	Preferred Therapy
Streptococcus pneumoniae	
PCN MIC <0.1	PCN, amoxicillin
PCN MIC 0.1-1	Amoxicillin
	Cefotaxime or ceftriaxone
	Fluoroquinolone
PCN MIC >2	Vancomycin
	Fluoroquinolone
Additional Pathogens	
Haemophilus influenzae	Ceftriaxone or cefotaxime
Mycoplasma pneumoniae	Macrolide
Legionella species	Macrolide
Chlamydia pneumoniae	Macrolide *or* doxycycline

PCN MIC, Penicillin minimal inhibitory concentration.

clear leukocytes and no organisms on sputum Gram stain, atypical pathogens such as *Legionella* species should be suspected.

Most patients with community-acquired pneumonia who receive appropriate therapy respond within several days. Response to therapy is defined as defervescense, resolution of leucocytosis, improvement of cough and sputum production, and improvement in constitutional symptoms and overall sense of well-being. In critically ill patients who require ICU admission, response to appropriate therapy may be more delayed, especially in those with overwhelming *Legionella* infection. Such individuals may require 7 to 10 days of appropriate therapy before a clinical response is evident. In patients with less severe illnesses, including outpatients, clinical improvement should be evident within 72 hours of initiation of appropriate antimicrobial chemotherapy. Failure to improve over this time frame should raise several differential diagnostic concerns, including a pathogen not covered by the antimicrobial regimen, an undrained empyema, or an occult obstructing endobronchial lesion in heavy smokers with unilobar disease.

The current patient was treated with high-dose erythromycin plus ceftriaxone. On day 3 of his hospitalization, he began to improve clinically, although improvement in his chest x-ray was not apparent for several more days. His *Legionella* urinary antigen returned positive and a diagnosis of Legionnaire's disease was made. Ceftriaxone was discontinued, and he completed a 3-week course of erythromycin and did well. He was converted to oral therapy and discharged from hospital on day 7 and received the remainder of his therapy as an outpatient.

Pitfalls and Common Mistakes in the Assessment and Treatment of Community-Acquired Pneumonia

There are potential pitfalls in both the evaluation and management of patients with community-acquired pneumonia. The elderly individual with community-acquired pneumonia may lack the classic history of fever and cough. It has been estimated that up to 25% of older individuals with pneumonia may have a normal body temperature at presentation and may exhibit only altered mental status. The leukocyte count may be normal or even low in elderly patients with community-acquired pneumonia. Thus the clinician must have a high index of suspicion for the diagnosis in such individuals.

Immunocompromised hosts, such as those receiving corticosteroids or cancer chemotherapy, may also lack the classic features of community-acquired pneumonia. In addition, the microbial differential diagnosis in such patients is broader and includes opportunistic pathogens, such as *P. carinii*, reactivation tuberculosis, and fungal pathogens. In immunocompromised hosts who present with pneumonia, bronchoscopy is often indicated so as to define the microbiology and guide subsequent antimicrobial chemotherapy.

Although the Fine score is quite helpful in estimating mortality risk, blind reliance on a calculated score should never override physician judgment regarding the need for hospital admission. Hypoxic patients should always be hospitalized. In addition, individuals who are apt to be non-compliant or who lack adequate support in the home setting may be candidates for hospitalization irrespective of Fine score.

In most circumstances, the microbiologic diagnosis is not confirmed at the time therapy is initiated and thus an empiric regimen is chosen. Once a microbiologic diagnosis is established, however, it is appropriate to tailor the antibiotic regimen to cover the specific pathogen. Decisions in this regard should take into consideration the spectrum of activity of an agent, along with issues of efficacy, tolerability in the individual patient, and cost. In general, an agent with the narrowest spectrum, fewest side effects, and least cost should be employed. For example, in a patient with penicillin-susceptible *S. pneumoniae* pneumonia, penicillin is appropriate therapy and would be preferred to the more expensive and broader-spectrum macrolides (such as azithromycin and clarithromycin) and fluoroquinolones.

In assessing the response to therapy, it is important to emphasize that radiographic improvement may lag behind clinical improvement. Thus the decision to switch from intravenous to oral therapy in hospitalized individuals and the timing of hospital discharge should be made on clinical rather than radiographic grounds.

▼ BIBLIOGRAPHY

Ailani RK, Agastya G, Mukunda BN, et al: Doxycycline is a cost effective therapy for hospitalized patients with community-acquired pneumonia, *Arch Intern Med* 159:266-270, 1999.

Bartlett JG, Breiman RF, Mandell LA, et al: Community-acquired pneumonia in adults: Guidelines for management, *Clin Infect Dis* 26:811-838, 1998.

Bartlett JG, Mundy LM: Current concepts: Community-acquired pneumonia, *N Engl J Med* 333:1618-1624, 1995.

Cassiere HA, Fein AM: Duration and route of antibiotic therapy in community-acquired pneumonia: Switch and step-down therapy, *Semin Respir Infect* 13:36-42, 1998.

Fang GD, Fine M, Orloff J, et al: New and emerging etiologies for community-acquired pneumonia with implications for therapy. A prospective multicenter study of 359 cases, *Medicine* 69:307-316, 1990.

Fine MJ, Auble TE, Yealy DM, et al: A prediction rule to identify low-risk patients with community-acquired pneumonia, *N Engl J Med* 336:243-250, 1997.

Fine MJ, Smith MA, Carson CA, et al: Prognosis and outcomes of patients with community-acquired pneumonia: A meta analysis, *JAMA* 275:134-141, 1996.

Leeper KV Jr: Severe community-acquired pneumonia, *Semin Respir Infect* 11:96-108, 1996.

Marrie TJ: Community-acquired pneumonia, *Clin Infect Dis* 18:501-513, 1994.

Marrie TJ: Community-acquired pneumonia in adults: Epidemiology, etiology, treatment, *Infect Dis Clin North Am* 12:723-740, 1998.

Meeker DP, Longworth DL: Community-acquired pneumonia: An update, *Cleve Clin J Med* 63:16-30, 1996.

Niederman MS, Bass JB Jr, Campbell GD, et al: American Thoracic Society guidelines for the initial management of adults with community-acquired pneumonia: Diagnosis, assessment of severity, and initial antimicrobial therapy, *Am Rev Respir Dis* 148:1418-1426, 1993.

Stout JE, Yu VL: Legionellosis, *N Engl J Med* 337:682-687, 1998.

CHAPTER 15

PLEURITIC CHEST PAIN

Bipin D. Sarodia
James K. Stoller

▼ Key Terms

▼ Chest pain
▼ Pulmonary embolism (PE)
▼ Pneumonia
▼ Pleuritis

▼ Empyema
▼ Myocardial infarction (MI)
▼ Pericarditis

▼ Gastroesophageal reflux disease (GERD)
▼ Esophageal spasm
▼ Pleural effusion

▼ THE CLINICAL PROBLEM

A 54-year-old man presents with severe chest pain 5 days after total hip replacement. The pain is localized to the right lower chest without any radiation. It started suddenly after he woke up, which was about 2 hours ago. The pain is severe, sharp, and unrelated to change in posture but worse on deep inspiration. It is associated with shortness of breath at rest, mild cough, and scanty white sputum with red streaks. He also complains of diaphoresis, dizziness, and a feeling of anxiety. He denies fever, nausea, vomiting, anorexia, weight loss, headache, weakness, or palpitations.

He denies any lung or heart disease in the past. He has had arthritis of the hips and knees for many years. The pain was severe and not controlled adequately with non-steroidal analgesics. He underwent right total hip replacement 5 days ago without any immediate complications. Otherwise, he has been healthy throughout his life and is not on any medication other than analgesics. During the current hospitalization, he did not receive any medication other than analgesics, sedatives, and anesthetic agents. He has no known drug or food allergy. He smokes 1 pack/day and has consumed a can of beer daily over the last 30 years.

On physical examination, his temperature is 99.8° F orally, pulse 120, respiration 30, and blood pressure 98/48 mm Hg. Pulse oximetry reveals an oxygen saturation of 93% on room air. He is uncomfortable with rapid shallow breathing and moderate respiratory distress. Examination of the nose and throat is unremarkable. Neck examination reveals no jugular venous distension. Lung examination reveals a few crackles with slightly diminished breath sounds and dullness over the right lower chest posteriorly. A "crunchy" to-and-fro sound is heard with inspiration and expiration just above the area of dullness. The surgical wound over the right hip is clean without any redness or discharge. The remainder of his physical examination is unremarkable, including his legs.

Laboratory tests including a complete blood count and electrolytes are normal, except the white blood cell count of 16,000/mm^3 with 80% neutrophils and 12% lymphocytes. Arterial blood gas values (ABG) on room air show pH 7.46, Paco$_2$ 32 mm Hg, Pao$_2$ 74 mm Hg, and oxygen saturation 94%. The chest x-ray reveals a small peripheral triangular infiltrate in the right lower lobe with blunting of the right costophrenic angle and otherwise clear lungs with a normal cardiac silhouette. Electrocardiogram (ECG) reveals sinus tachycardia, with an S wave in lead I, and a Q wave and inverted T wave in standard lead III but is otherwise unremarkable.

What is the differential diagnosis and the most likely cause of this patient's chest pain?

Differential Diagnosis of Chest Pain

Acute chest pain is a common symptom caused by diseases affecting various organ systems including the pulmonary, cardiovascular, gastrointestinal, and musculoskeletal systems, or it may be psychogenic. Chest pain can be an important indicator of a life-threatening disease. The most common causes of acute chest pain include myocardial ischemia or infarction (MI), pneumonia, empyema, pulmonary embolism (PE), gastroesophageal reflux disease (GERD), esophageal spasm, and muscular or skeletal pain. Less common causes of chest pain include abdominal diseases like cholecystitis, pancreatitis, gastritis, colitis or diverticulitis, psychogenic causes, and a pre-eruptive phase of herpes zoster along the course of a nerve (i.e., a dermatomal distribution). Common and less common causes of chest pain are reviewed in Box 15-1.

Chest pain may be classified into pleuritic (i.e., pain that worsens on deep inspiration, coughing, sneezing, or moving) and non-pleuritic pain. Acute pleuritic chest pain is most commonly caused by acute pleurisy (secondary to pneumonia, PE, pulmonary infarction, or viral pleurisy), pneumothorax, pericarditis, thoracic cage or muscular pain, and rheumatoid arthritis or connective tissue disease. In young adults, one series suggested that the most common causes of acute pleuritic pain of unclear cause (after exclusion of obvious causes such as pneumococcal pneumonia, uremia, pericarditis, and chest wall pain) are viral or idiopathic pleurisy (53%), PE (21%), infectious pneumonitis (18%), and miscellaneous causes (8%), including bronchial asthma, sickle cell crisis, tuberculosis, pancreatitis, ruptured aortic aneurysm, and fractured rib.

Box 15-1
Differential Diagnosis of Chest Pain

Common Causes	Less Common Causes
Cardiovascular	
Myocardial ischemia (angina pectoris) or MI; coronary atherosclerosis	Myocardial ischemia (angina pectoris) or MI: Coronary vasospasm, coronary arteritis, coronary dissection, cocaine induced, Prinzmetal's angina, hyperthyroidism, severe anemia, paroxysmal tachydysrhythmias
Aortic dissection*	Mitral valve prolapse
Aortic valvular stenosis or regurgitation	Myocarditis, cardiomyopathy, ventricular hypertrophy
	Inflammatory pericarditis†: Infectious (viral, tuberculous, Lyme disease), autoimmune diseases, uremia, neoplastic, radiation therapy, drug toxicity, inflammation of myocardium or lung; primary pulmonary hypertension; syndrome X
Pulmonary	
Pneumonia†	Traumatic pleuritis
Empyema†	Pleuritis due to collagen vascular diseases
Spontaneous pneumothorax†	
Pulmonary embolism (PE)†: Prolonged immobilization, fracture of hip or femur, surgery, stroke, congestive heart failure, obesity, childbirth, hypercoagulability, oral contraceptives, malignancy protein C deficiency, protein S deficiency, antithrombin III deficiency, presence of Factor V Leiden	
Viral pleuritis†	
Gastroesophageal or Intestinal	
GERD (erosive reflux esophagitis)	Esophageal dysmotility: Achalasia (hypertensive lower sphincter), spasm (diffuse or nutcracker), nonspecific; radiation esophagitis; infectious esophagitis (cytomegalovirus, herpes, candida); cholelithiasis or cholecystitis; pancreatitis; peptic ulcer; non-ulcer dyspepsia; colitis; diverticulitis

*The chest pain is *sometimes* pleuritic. †The chest pain is *more commonly* pleuritic.
PE, Pulmonary embolism; *GERD,* gastroesophageal reflux disease.   *Continued*

Box 15-1
Differential Diagnosis of Chest Pain—cont'd

Common Causes	Less Common Causes
Chest Wall and Cervical or Thoracic Spine Disease	
Costochondritis (Tietze's syndrome)†	Degenerative or inflammatory lesion of shoulder†
Rib fracture or trauma to chest wall†	Thoracic outlet syndrome†; anterior chest wall syndrome†; intercostal neuritis (herpes zoster, diabetes mellitus)†
Psychological	
	Depression*
	Anxiety*
	Panic disorder*
Miscellaneous	
	Heightened visceral sensitivity

*The chest pain is *sometimes* pleuritic. †The chest pain is *more commonly* pleuritic.
PE, Pulmonary embolism; *GERD,* gastroesophageal reflux disease.

Clinical Features that Suggest a Specific Cause of Chest Pain

In the current case, the clinical features suggest that PE is a likely cause of this patient's chest pain. The specific characteristics of pain (i.e., sudden onset, worsening on deep inspiration, and onset after recent hip surgery and immobilization), combined with the associated symptoms of shortness of breath, cough, and hemoptysis and with the systemic symptoms of diaphoresis, dizziness, and anxiety, are highly suggestive of PE.

Notably, it is the occurrence of these findings in combination that suggests PE rather than any one finding alone. For example, considering all patients presenting with a symptom of pleuritic chest pain to the emergency room, only 21% of patients in an American series and 1.1% of patients in a British series were found to have PE. Although PE accounts for the minority of patients with pleuritic chest pain, most pulmonary emboli are *not* recognized based on the clinical features. Several series suggest that PE was not recognized before death in 50% to 92% of patients confirmed to have PE at post-mortem examination. This may be explained because only one-third of patients with PE present with the classic triad of chest pain, dyspnea, and hemoptysis, although 85% of patients may have pleuritic chest pain. Thus PE is a challenging diagnosis, and the clinical suspicion should always be high.

Since chest pain has many causes and atypical presentations are common, the clinician should recognize features that suggest specific causes of chest pain. Table 15-1 presents the characteristics of pain and associated clinical features that suggest specific causes.

TABLE 15-1
Interpreting Signs and Symptoms of Patients with Chest Pain

Possible Causes	Mechanisms	Suggestive Clinical Features
Myocardial ischemia or infarction	"Not "pain" but often "pressure" or "tightness," usually retrosternal or left precordial; commonly radiates to left shoulder, left arm, neck, lower jaw, or upper abdomen; precipitated by exertion, meals, and stress; relieved by rest; unrelated to posture or respiration.	Dyspnea, nausea, vomiting, diaphoresis, dizziness, palpitations, tachycardia, bradycardia, cardiac murmur, or gallop
Aortic dissection*	Sudden onset, severe tearing sensation, commonly radiates to back, maximum intensity at onset	Weak or absent pulses and reduced blood pressure on the left side and in the lower extremities; neurologic deficits causing weakness
Aortic stenosis	Angina pectoris	Syncope with exertion, congestive heart failure, systolic ejection murmur
Pericarditis†	Substernal pleuritic pain relieved by sitting	Dyspnea, pericardial friction rub, fever, leukocytosis, specific features based on the etiology
Pneumonia†	Localized to site of infiltrate	Fever, cough, expectoration, dyspnea
PE†	Sudden onset, crushing, shooting, or deep	Dyspnea, tachycardia, diaphoresis, and hemoptysis
Pleuritis†	Sharp, worsened by cough, sneezing, deep breathing, or movement; may be referred to shoulder	Dyspnea, pleural effusion causing reduced breath sounds and dullness
Spontaneous pneumothorax†	Sudden onset, may resemble angina or myocardial infarction	Dyspnea, emphysema, or other cystic lung disease such as eosinophilic granuloma predispose to pneumothorax
GERD	Pain located in lower central chest and upper abdomen, occurs after heavy meals or in recumbent position, relieved by antacids, sucralfate, or H_2 receptor antagonists	Sour regurgitation into the mouth, belching and flatulence

*The chest pain is *sometimes* pleuritic. †The chest pain is *more commonly* pleuritic.
PE, pulmonary embolism; *GERD,* gastroesophageal reflux disease.   *Continued*

TABLE 15-1
Interpreting Signs and Symptoms of Patients
with Chest Pain—cont'd

Possible Causes	Mechanisms	Suggestive Clinical Features
Esophageal spasm	Located retrosternally, relieved by nitrates and calcium channel blockers	
Anxiety	Sharp, stabbing pain not related to exertion, lasts for only seconds, but heaviness may persist for hours or days	Associated with dyspnea, nausea, vomiting, diarrhea, tremors, fatigue, palpitation, insomnia, and headache
Anterior chest wall syndrome†	Sharp, localized tenderness of intercostal muscles	
Costochondritis (Tietze's syndrome)†	Diffuse pain over chest	Warm, swollen, and red costochondral junctions; localized tenderness
Intercostal neuritis†	Localized to a dermatome	Herpes zoster rash follows, diabetes mellitus
Cervical or thoracic spine disease	Sudden sharp pain commonly located in neck or chest, radiates to outer aspect of the arm and the thumb and index fingers, related to specific movements of neck or spine, straining, or lifting	May be associated with tingling, numbness, or weakness of the extremities
Heightened visceral sensitivity	Pain effectively controlled with antidepressant	Sensitive to a variety of minor noxious visceral stimuli

*The chest pain is *sometimes* pleuritic. †The chest pain is *more commonly* pleuritic.
PE, pulmonary embolism; *GERD,* gastroesophageal reflux disease.

Diagnostic Tests in the Evaluation of a Patient with Chest Pain

The choice of diagnostic tests for the patient with chest pain is dictated by the desire to exclude serious acute causes (e.g., PE, MI, and aortic dissection) and to concentrate on the most likely causes, which are assessed by a careful history and physical examination. This distinction, although difficult, determines the initial choice of diagnostic tests (e.g., chest x-ray, lung scan, computed tomography [CT] of chest, and so forth).

Table 15-2 presents the commonly used diagnostic tests and specific comments helpful in evaluating a patient with chest pain. A chest x-ray and ECG should be obtained in every patient with pleuritic chest pain. Sometimes, a therapeutic trial without specific diagnostic tests may help in the differential diagnosis (e.g., omeprazole therapy for suspected GERD).

TABLE 15-2
Diagnostic Tests Commonly Used in the Evaluation
of a Patient with Chest Pain

Diagnostic Test	Comment
Pulmonary	
Sputum Gram's stain and culture sensitivity	Helps in etiologic diagnosis of pneumonia, does not differentiate infection from colonization
Chest x-ray	Useful in diagnosis of pneumonia and pleural effusion, nonspecific abnormalities in PE (wedge-shaped density, atelectasis, oligemia, or prominence of pulmonary arteries)
ABG	Not helpful in diagnosis of PE, helps manage hypoxemia due to associated conditions
Serum D-dimer level	High sensitivity but poor specificity due to false-positive results in liver disease, disseminated intravascular coagulation, etc
Ventilation-perfusion ($\dot{V}/\dot{Q}$) scanning	Useful in diagnosis of PE, normal result rules out (no further testing required), high-probability result is very specific for diagnosis (no angiography required), low or intermediate probability results need further testing
Spiral (helical) CT of chest	Recently used promising but unproven technology; high sensitivity (63%-98%) and specificity (80%-95%), especially for emboli in proximal pulmonary arteries
MRA	Recently used, promising but unproven technology; high sensitivity and specificity (similar to spiral CT)
Duplex ultrasonography of deep veins	High sensitivity and specificity (up to 95%); if a patient with suspected PE has DVT, then pulmonary angiography is not needed
Venography	Gold standard for definitive diagnosis of DVT but invasive and expensive, thus replaced by invasive tests
Pulmonary angiography	Gold standard for definitive diagnosis of PE but invasive and expensive, thus performed only when invasive tests are inconclusive; intraluminal defect or an arterial cutoff is diagnostic
Thoracentesis, pleural fluid examination, and pleural biopsy	Differentiates various etiologies of pleural effusion and empyema
Cardiopulmonary exercise test	Differentiates cardiac, pulmonary, and other causes of symptoms
Cardiovascular	
Serum cardiac enzymes and isoenzymes	Elevated in MI
Chest radiography	Detects ventricular hypertrophy, pericardial effusion
ECG	ST depression and T-wave inversion in myocardial ischemia; ST elevation and T-wave inversion in myocardial infarction; low QRS voltage in pericardial effusion; electrical alternans, if present, is pathognomonic of pericardial effusion

ABG, Arterial blood gases; *PE,* pulmonary embolism; *CT,* computed tomography; *DVT,* deep venous thrombosis; *MI,* myocardial infarction; *EGD,* esophagogastroduodenoscopy; *MRI,* Magnetic resonance imaging; *ECG,* electrocardiography; *MRA;* magnetic resonance angiography.   *Continued*

TABLE 15-2
Diagnostic Tests Commonly Used in the Evaluation of a Patient with Chest Pain—cont'd

Diagnostic Test	Comment
Cardiovascular—cont'd	
Exercise ECG	Most useful invasive test for myocardial ischemia
Echocardiography (transthoracic or transesophageal with exercise or dobutamine stress)	Detects regional wall motion abnormality and its reversibility, valvular abnormality
	Detects pericardial effusion and its hemodynamic effects (tamponade)
Myocardial perfusion scintigraphy (thallium or technetium-99m with exercise, dipyridamole or adenosine)	Useful when resting ECG is abnormal, localizes ischemia and differentiates it from infarction
Radionuclide thallium scanning	Images left ventricle, measures ejection fraction and wall motion
Coronary angiography and left ventriculogram	Definitive diagnostic test for coronary artery disease, localizes and identifies severity of stenoses, assesses global and regional left ventricular function
Aortic angiography	Diagnostic for aortic dissection
Dynamic CT scanning	Useful in aortic dissection
MRI	Diagnostic of aortic dissection
Cardiopulmonary exercise test	Differentiates cardiac, pulmonary, and other causes of symptoms
Pericardiocentesis, pericardial fluid examination, and pericardial biopsy	Differentiates various etiologies of pericarditis and pericardial effusion
Gastroesophageal or Intestinal	
EGD	Reflux esophagitis demonstrated by endoscopy (erythema, friability, and erosions of mucosa) and biopsy in 50% with proven acid reflux
Barium esophagography	Limited role in identifying reflux, mucosal abnormality, or esophageal stricture
Ambulatory esophageal pH monitoring	Best study for acid reflux demonstration, but unnecessary in most patients; indicated (1) before surgery if patient has no reflux esophagitis on endoscopy, (2) for symptoms unresponsive to therapy, (3) to document association between atypical symptoms and reflux episodes
Esophageal manometry	Indicated before esophageal pH probe placement to locate lower sphincter and for preoperative assessment for antireflux surgery

ABG, Arterial blood gases; *PE*, pulmonary embolism; *CT*, computed tomography; *DVT*, deep venous thrombosis; *MI*, myocardial infarction; *EGD*, esophagogastroduodenoscopy; *MRI*, Magnetic resonance imaging; *ECG*, electrocardiography; *MRA*; magnetic resonance angiography.

In PE, the chest x-ray is usually abnormal, but the abnormality is non-specific and often related to chronic pulmonary or cardiac disease. The presence of a pulmonary infiltrate and elevation of a hemidiaphragm are the most common abnormalities. Atelectasis, regional oligemia, prominence of the pulmonary arteries, and a small unilateral pleural effusion are sometimes seen. A homogenous, wedge-shaped, pleural-based infiltrate pointing toward the hilum is highly suggestive of pulmonary infarction (called *Hampton's hump*) but is uncommon. The most common abnormality in ECG is sinus tachycardia, whereas the specific changes of S1, Q3, and T3 (presence of S wave in lead I, and a Q wave and inverted T wave in lead III) are present in a small percentage of patients with large emboli. Other features suggesting PE are arterial hypoxemia in a patient with shortness of breath without preexisting lung disease and with a normal chest x-ray. If the perfusion pattern on a ventilation/perfusion ($\dot{V}/\dot{Q}$) scan is "normal," then PE is ruled out. On the other hand, a "high probability" pattern on the $\dot{V}/\dot{Q}$ scan almost confirms the diagnosis and often obviates the need for pulmonary angiogram. However, "low probability" and "intermediate probability" perfusion scans are more common, and patients with these patterns require further testing, including tests to detect deep venous thrombosis and possibly pulmonary angiography. Pulmonary angiography remains the definitive test for the diagnosis of PE because of its high sensitivity and specificity. However, because the angiogram is invasive and expensive, its use is reserved for circumstances when invasive tests are inconclusive or inadequate.

Approximately 30% of patients with chest pain who undergo cardiac evaluation do not have an apparent cardiac cause. However, because coronary artery disease is common, serious, and may have atypical presentations, it should be excluded before evaluation for other non-cardiac causes. Finally, esophageal manometry is not routinely recommended in evaluating patients suspected of esophageal dysmotility because of its low specificity.

Treatment of Chest Pain

Treatment of acute chest pain depends on its severity and the underlying cause. Serious causes of chest pain, such as PE, MI, and aortic dissection, should be diagnosed immediately and treated aggressively with specific therapy to prevent ominous consequences.

Specific therapy for PE includes anticoagulation with intravenous heparin, inferior vena caval filter (if intravenous heparin is contraindicated or ineffective), and thrombolytic agents such as tissue plasminogen activator (t-PA) or streptokinase (in acute right heart failure due to PE). Long-term management includes anticoagulation with oral agents such as warfarin for 3 to 6 months.

Acute MI should be treated with intravenous heparin (if not contraindicated), aspirin, beta-blockers, angiotensin-converting enzyme (ACE) inhibitors, and anti-arrhythmic medications (if required), along with supportive treatment and vascular interventions such as coronary angioplasty and stent placement, or coronary artery bypass graft surgery, if indicated.

Acute aortic dissection needs immediate diagnosis and surgical management, if surgery is an option, along with aggressive blood pressure control with antihypertensives.

Supportive symptomatic pharmacotherapy may be used to relieve pleuritis (analgesics and anti-inflammatory drugs, e.g., indomethacin), cough (antitussives such as codeine), GERD (omeprazole for 4 weeks), etc. "Heightened visceral sensitivity" may be effectively treated with low doses of antidepressants.

Pitfalls and Common Mistakes in the Assessment and Treatment of the Patient with Chest Pain

Common pitfalls in the assessment of a patient with pleuritic chest pain include inadequate attention to historical features that might suggest a specific underlying cause, such as features of cardiovascular, pulmonary, gastroesophageal, or musculoskeletal disease. A specific diagnosis should not be excluded because of the absence of a classic symptom or sign. Also, a specific diagnosis should not be based solely on the presence of a classic symptom or sign. Several of the underlying causes of chest pain may present with similar symptoms or signs (e.g., chest pain caused by PE and empyema may get worse on deep inspiration due to increased irritation of the parietal pleura). Thorough and definitive pursuit of serious causes of chest pain (e.g., PE, MI, and aortic dissection) is needed.

▼ BIBLIOGRAPHY

Branch WT Jr, McNeil BJ: Analysis of the differential diagnosis and assessment of pleuritic chest pain in young adults, *Am J Med* 75:671-679, 1983.

Chauhan A: Esophageal abnormalities and "linked-angina" in syndrome X. In Kaski JC (editor): *Chest pain with normal coronary angiograms: pathogenesis, diagnosis, and management*, Boston, 1999, Kluwer Academic Publishers, pp 39-60.

Chesnutt MS, Prendergast TJ: Lung. In Tierney LM Jr, McPhee SJ, Papadakis MA (editors): *Current medical diagnosis and treatment*, Stamford, Conn, 1999, Appleton and Lange, pp 255-338.

Chest pain. In Holmes HN, Foley M, Johnson PH (editors): *Professional guide to signs and symptoms*, ed 2, Springhouse, Penn., 1997, Springhouse Corporation, pp 153-162.

De Caestecker JS: Esophageal chest pain. In Kaski JC (editor): *Chest pain with normal coronary angiograms: pathogenesis, diagnosis, and management*, Boston, 1999, Kluwer Academic Publishers, pp 33-47.

Jones K, Raghuram A: Investigation and management of patients with pleuritic chest pain presenting to the accident and emergency department, *J Accid Emerg Med* 16:55-59, 1999.

Massie BM, Amidon TM: Heart. In Tierney LM Jr, McPhee SJ, Papadakis MA (editors): *Current medical diagnosis and treatment*, Stamford, Conn, 1999, Appleton and Lange, pp 339-431.

McQuaid KR: Alimentary tract. In Tierney LM Jr, McPhee SJ, Papadakis MA (editors): *Current medical diagnosis and treatment*, Stamford, Conn., 1999, Appleton and Lange, pp 538-637.

Potts SG, Bass C: Chest pain with normal coronary arteries: psychological aspects. In Kaski JC (editor): *Chest pain with normal coronary angiograms: pathogenesis, diagnosis, and management*, Boston, 1999, Kluwer Academic Publishers, pp 13-32.

Ryu JH, Olson EJ, Pellikka PA: Clinical recognition of pulmonary embolism: problem of unrecognized and asymptomatic cases, *Mayo Clin Proc* 73:873-879, 1998.

Thomas L, Reichl M: Pulmonary embolism in patients attending the accident and emergency department with pleuritic chest pain, *Arch Emerg Med* 8:48-51, 1990.

Tierney LM Jr, Messina LM: Blood vessels and lymphatics. In Tierney LM Jr, McPhee SJ, Papadakis MA (editors): *Current medical diagnosis and treatment*, Stamford, Conn, 1999, Appleton and Lange, pp 453-484.

CHAPTER 16

NON-PLEURITIC CHEST PAIN

Gary W. Falk

Key Terms

▼ Unexplained chest pain
▼ Gastroesophageal reflux disease (GERD)

▼ Non-pleuritic chest pain
▼ Gallbladder

▼ Neuromuscular disease
▼ Peptic ulcer disease

▼ THE CLINICAL PROBLEM

A 55-year-old man presents with recurring bouts of substernal chest pain. He describes the pain as a sense of substernal pressure lasting for up to 2 to 3 hours at a time. The episodes do not have any predictable precipitating factors and occur in a variety of scenarios. He has experienced pain while exercising on a treadmill at home and after a heavy meal. Sometimes the pain wakes the patient from sleep. The pain is not positional in nature. Lately, the frequency of the pain has increased, and the patient is very worried about this because his father died at age 65 from a massive myocardial infarction (MI).

The last episode occurred 48 hours before this visit; the patient's wife drove him to a local emergency room. He was held overnight and told his electrocardiogram was normal and blood tests for an MI were negative. There is no history of heartburn, dysphagia, or regurgitation. He does eat late meals because of his busy work schedule. There are no other symptoms at the time of his visit. His past medical history is significant for hypertension and hypercholesterolemia. He smokes 1 pack/day. Medications include enalapril and lovastatin. Physical examination is normal. In particular, there is no tenderness on palpation of the sternum or the xyphoid.

The patient brought a copy of his emergency room evaluation. The chest x-ray was normal, and the electrocardiogram revealed normal sinus rhythm with no ST or T wave abnormalities. A complete blood count and metabolic profile were normal.

What is the differential diagnosis for this patient's chest pain, and what is the most likely cause?

Differential Diagnosis of Non-Pleuritic Chest Pain

Recurring substernal chest pain is a common clinical dilemma. The most common causes of non-pleuritic chest pain are shown in Box 16-1. Typically, the etiology of non-pleuritic chest pain is cardiac, gastrointestinal, musculoskeletal, or psychological. The most important task for the physician is to exclude a cardiac source of chest pain because of the potential life-threatening nature of cardiac ischemia. Once cardiac disease has been excluded, attention may be directed to other causes of chest pain.

Some patients with chest pain and normal coronary arteries may have cardiac ischemia from microvascular angina. These patients have normal epicardial arteries by angiography, but an abnormal coronary vasodilator reserve in response to atrial pacing and ergonovine, as well as reduced left ventricular ejection fractions during exercise. Under these conditions, coronary artery resistance increases instead of decreases, causing chest pain. The physiologic significance of microvascular angina is uncertain because similar studies have not been performed in age-matched, normal individuals.

Chest pain is commonly reported by patients with mitral valve prolapse. Symptoms may be exertional or non-exertional. The duration of pain is highly variable, lasting from minutes to hours. The cause of chest pain in these patients is unknown, although many different mechanisms have been postulated. Many patients with

---

Box 16-1
Differential Diagnosis
of Non-Pleuritic Chest Pain

Common Causes	Less Common Causes
Coronary artery disease	Microvascular angina
GERD	Mitral valve prolapse
Musculoskeletal disorders	Esophageal motility disorders
	Peptic ulcer disease
Psychological	Gallstones
Brain-gut dysfunction	
Panic attacks	

GERD, Gastroesophageal reflux disease.

mitral valve prolapse have concurrent panic disorders, but a cause and effect relationship between the two disorders has not been proven. The diagnosis of mitral valve prolapse is made by the characteristic auscultatory findings of a mid-systolic click accompanied by a late or holosystolic murmur. The diagnosis is confirmed by echocardiography. Beta-blocker therapy decreases chest pain in some patients.

Once cardiac causes of chest pain are excluded, attention is directed toward the esophagus. The cause of chest pain in patients with esophageal diseases remains poorly understood. Whereas the term *esophageal spasm* was once synonymous with non-cardiac chest pain, it is now clear that the most common cause of esophageal chest pain is gastroesophageal reflux disease (GERD). GERD may present with chest pain as the major and sometimes sole symptom. However, most patients report heartburn, regurgitation, or both, if closely questioned. It is important to remember that acid reflux may coexist and cause chest pain in patients with known coronary artery disease. Furthermore, drugs commonly used to treat coronary artery disease, such as nitrates and calcium channel antagonists, can decrease lower esophageal sphincter pressure and distal esophageal contraction amplitudes, thereby predisposing these patients to gastroesophageal reflux. Some studies report that up to two thirds of patients with known coronary artery disease with recurrent episodes of atypical chest pain and the maximum medical and surgical therapy have chest pain related to gastroesophageal reflux events.

Chest pain is a common presenting symptom in patients with esophageal motility disorders, especially the spastic variety. However, it is now apparent that the majority of patients with unexplained chest pain have normal esophageal motility studies and the remainder have a variety of generally non-specific abnormalities of questionable significance. In large studies of patients with unexplained chest pain, no more than approximately one third have an esophageal motility disorder. Nutcracker esophagus is the most common motility disorder, followed by non-specific disorders, diffuse esophageal spasm, hypertensive lower esophageal sphincter, and achalasia.

Nutcracker esophagus is a manometric diagnosis characterized by high-amplitude peristaltic contractions greater than 180 mm Hg. The cause of nutcracker esophagus is unknown. Structural and esophageal transit tests are normal. However, patients with nutcracker esophagus frequently have abnormal psychological profiles (depression, somatization, anxiety) similar to that reported in patients with the irritable bowel syndrome. Furthermore, many patients with nutcracker esophagus have gastroesophageal reflux disease. As such, nutcracker esophagus may simply be a marker of abnormal brain-gut interactions or GERD in patients with non-cardiac chest pain.

Diffuse esophageal spasm is an uncommon motility abnormality in patients with non-cardiac chest pain. The primary manometric criterion for diagnosing diffuse esophageal spasm is the presence of frequent simultaneous contractions (greater than 10%) associated intermittently with normal peristalsis. A variety of other manometric findings may be encountered in diffuse esophageal spasm, but they are not required for the diagnosis. The hypertensive lower esophageal sphincter is observed in a small number of patients with non-cardiac chest pain. The cause of this disorder is also unknown. It is a manometric diagnosis defined as a mean lower esophageal sphincter pressure greater than 45 mm Hg with normal sphincter relaxation. Radiographic studies are usually normal, although sometimes a solid bolus travels slowly through the sphincter. A number of other esophageal motility patterns are clearly not normal but do not neatly fit into the criteria for either of these disorders or for achalasia. These non-specific esophageal motility disorders are of questionable significance.

The causal relationship between these esophageal motility disorders and chest pain is difficult to prove. Patients rarely have chest pain at the time of manometry, even if a motility abnormality is present. Furthermore, provocation of pain with pharmacologic agents is often not accompanied by motility abnormalities. Studies with 24-hour ambulatory esophageal manometry reveal that chest pain is associated with motility abnormalities in only 10% to 20% of cases.

Psychological abnormalities may also contribute to unexplained chest pain. Recent studies suggest that abnormal visceral pain perception (visceral hypersensitivity) may contribute to non-cardiac chest pain. Intra-esophageal balloon distension reproduces chest pain in these patients at a lower distension volume compared with control subjects who infrequently develop pain. This lower visceral pain threshold is similar to the response to rectal balloon distension studies by patients with the irritable bowel syndrome. The etiology of visceral hypersensitivity is unknown, but this abnormality of pain perception may be due to abnormal processing of information in the central nervous system.

Other similarities with the irritable bowel syndrome include the high frequency of psychiatric diagnosis, especially depression, anxiety, and somatization disorders, described in patients with unexplained chest pain. Panic attacks are encountered in approximately one third of chest pain patients with normal coronary arteries. Panic attacks consist of a generalized anxiety state characterized by chest pain associated with intense fear, palpitations, diaphoresis, paresthesias, dizziness, or breathlessness. Chest pain symptoms, psychiatric diagnoses, and motility disturbances observed in a subset of these patients can be linked by the observation that experimental stressors can increase esophageal contraction amplitude and produce simultaneous contractions in patients with the nutcracker esophagus more so than in healthy subjects. Thus alterations in sensory afferent input, central nervous system processing, and efferent muscle responses may all play a role in disturbed brain-gut interactions in some patients with unexplained chest pain.

Chest wall muscles, ribs, and cartilage may all cause unexplained chest pain. These patients have pain and tenderness in the anterior chest wall that may radiate across the chest and increase with inspiration. Pressure applied to the anterior chest on physical examination may reproduce the pain, but it is important to remember that some of these patients may also have underlying cardiac disease. The cause of musculoskeletal chest pain is uncertain, with radiographic studies typically demonstrating no abnormalities. Symptoms may decrease with non-steroidal anti-inflammatory drug (NSAID) therapy, steroid injections into costosternal or costoclavicular joints, or with trigger point injections.

On occasion, patients with peptic ulcer disease present with unexplained chest pain. Classic dyspepsia may be absent in these patients. Biliary colic is typically described as severe right upper quadrant pain occurring post-prandially. Pain may radiate to the chest or back, and substernal pain may sometimes be the only manifestation of biliary disease. An ultrasound of the gallbladder is the simplest way to confirm the diagnosis.

Clinical Features that Suggest a Specific Cause of Non-Pleuritic Chest Pain

Esophageal and cardiac disorders are common conditions that may occur together. Chest pain related to myocardial ischemia typically is related to exertion, whereas esophageal chest pain typically occurs at rest. However, chest pain of cardiac etiology may be impossible to distinguish clinically from chest pain of esophageal etiology. Both types of pain may be induced by exercise because exercise can induce gastro-esophageal reflux. Furthermore, both types of pain may also occur at rest.

Some features of pain, however, may help to distinguish esophageal from cardiac chest pain (Table 16-1). Esophageal causes are more likely to be associated with background esophageal symptoms such as classic heartburn, regurgitation, dysphagia, or odynophagia, and respond to antacids or over-the-counter histamine H_2-receptor antagonists. However, these features of esophageal pain are also found in some patients with ischemia-induced chest pain. Similarly, panic attacks, which may include symptoms such as chest pain, dyspnea, and diaphoresis, may be difficult to distinguish from angina-induced chest pain.

In the current case, clinical features that increase the possibility of coronary artery disease are the patient's age as well as risk factors for coronary artery disease, including the family history, hypertension, and tobacco use. However, as outlined above, coronary artery disease and GERD can have similar presentations.

TABLE 16-1
Interpreting Signs and Symptoms in the Patient with Non-Pleuritic Chest Pain

Possible Causes	Mechanisms	Suggestive Clinical Features
Coronary artery disease	Myocardial oxygen demand unable to be met by coronary blood flow	Exertional chest pain that decreases with rest; pain may also be precipitated by stress; risk factors for coronary artery disease
Microvascular angina	Myocardial ischemia due to inadequate vasodilator reserve of the coronary microcirculation	Typical anginal symptoms with normal coronary arteries on angiography
Mitral valve prolapse	Disordered autonomic nervous system function and increased sensitivity to pain	Most common in women of child-bearing age; unpredictable onset unrelated to exertion; mid-systolic click accompanied by a late or holosystolic murmur heard best at the apex
GERD	Stimulation of acid-sensitive nociceptors in the esophagus	Substernal burning after meals that may also be related to bending or the supine position; often accompanied by acid regurgitation; symptoms decrease with antacids or over-the-counter histamine-H_2 receptor antagonists

GERD, Gastroesophageal reflux disease.

Continued

TABLE 16-1
Interpreting Signs and Symptoms in the Patient
with Non-Pleuritic Chest Pain—cont'd

Possible Causes	Mechanisms	Suggestive Clinical Features
Esophageal motility disorders	Stimulation of mechanoreceptors in the esophagus during abnormal motility, which may be accompanied by visceral hypersensitivity	Associated with symptoms of dysphagia or regurgitation
Peptic ulcer disease	Sensitization of gastroduodenal afferent nerves to hydrogen ions	Burning epigastric pain or discomfort that may be relieved by antacids or over-the-counter histamine-H_2 receptor antagonists
Gallstones	Intermittent obstruction of the cystic duct, causing smooth muscle spasm	Sudden onset of severe unremitting pain in the epigastrium or right upper quadrant that may or may not be related to large meals
Musculoskeletal pain	Joint inflammation	Pain reproduced by palpation of the sternum, costochondral junction, or xyphoid; pain often positional
Visceral hypersensitivity	Abnormal sensory perception of normal events caused by either a decrease in the threshold of esophageal sensory nerve endings or abnormalities of sensory pathways in the central nervous system	Accompanying history of psychiatric disorders such as panic attacks, depression, or anxiety; all diagnostic testing will be negative

GERD, Gastroesophageal reflux disease.

Furthermore, both diseases are common in older patients and frequently coexist. The physical examination reveals no findings of costochondral tenderness, which essentially excludes a musculoskeletal cause of pain. Panic attacks remain a possibility. However, neither panic attacks nor visceral hypersensitivity related to brain-gut dysfunction should be considered until the life-threatening problem of coronary artery disease and the easy-to-treat GERD have been excluded. Peptic ulcer disease is a rare cause of chest pain, as are gallstones. Furthermore, the patient's symptoms are atypical for biliary colic.

Therefore, while the patient's symptoms are non-specific, coronary artery disease and GERD need to be dealt with before considering another less likely diagnosis.

Diagnostic Testing in the Evaluation of the Patient with Non-Pleuritic Chest Pain

A strategy for evaluating chest pain is shown in Figure 16-1. Diagnostic testing in this patient should first focus on excluding a cardiac cause of chest pain. The intensity of the evaluation depends on factors such as patient age and risk factors for

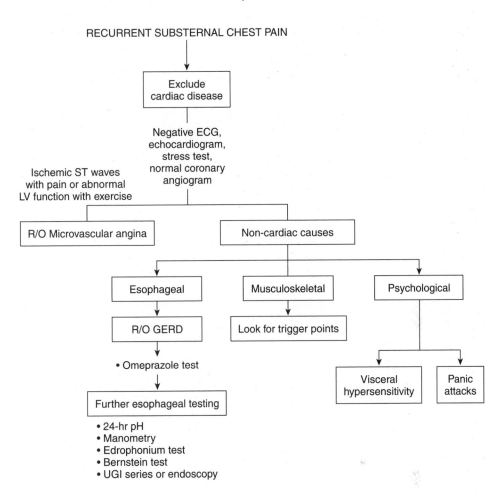

RECURRENT SUBSTERNAL CHEST PAIN

Exclude cardiac disease

Negative ECG, echocardiogram, stress test, normal coronary angiogram

Ischemic ST waves with pain or abnormal LV function with exercise

R/O Microvascular angina

Non-cardiac causes

Esophageal

R/O GERD

• Omeprazole test

Further esophageal testing

• 24-hr pH
• Manometry
• Edrophonium test
• Bernstein test
• UGI series or endoscopy

Musculoskeletal

Look for trigger points

Psychological

Visceral hypersensitivity

Panic attacks

▼ **Figure 16-1**   Diagnostic algorithm for the approach to the patient with unexplained chest pain. *LV,* Left ventricular; *R/O,* rule out; *GERD,* gastroesophageal reflux disease.

coronary artery disease. This evaluation should be done under the supervision of a cardiologist who can then choose the best diagnostic study, whether it is immediate catheterization, echocardiography, or nuclear perfusion imaging.

Once a cardiac cause of chest pain is excluded, the patient's evaluation should shift to possible esophageal causes of chest pain. There are a number of diagnostic studies that can evaluate the structure and function of the esophagus, including barium radiography, esophagogastroduodenoscopy, esophageal manometry, 24-hour pH testing, 24-hour esophageal manometry, and esophageal provocative tests such as edrophonium infusion. However, the yield of each of these tests is low, and current guidelines of the American Gastroenterological Association suggest deferring esophageal diagnostic testing until an adequate trial of proton pump inhibitor therapy. Upper endoscopy has a yield of only 10% to 15% in these patients and should likewise not be considered early in the evaluation of unexplained chest pain. A recent study suggests that the "omeprazole test" is both sensitive and specific for diagnosing GERD in patients with unexplained chest pain. Furthermore, it results in significant cost savings by decreasing the use of diagnostic tests in these patients. This test consists of omeprazole given as 40 mg in the morning and 20 mg in the evening for 7 days. If the patient responds, anti-secretory therapy is continued. If the patient fails to respond, further esophageal diagnostic studies are indicated, although it may be reasonable to extend the empirical trial up to 4 weeks.

If the omeprazole test is negative, 24-hour pH monitoring can be considered. In this type of monitoring, a transnasal pH probe is placed 5 cm above the manometrically determined lower esophageal sphincter. Data are collected in a small box worn on the belt and then analyzed on a computer after completion of the test. Data collection assesses esophageal acid exposure in the supine, upright, and combined positions, and the relationship between reflux events and chest pain can be determined. If the 24-hour pH study is non-contributory, esophageal manometry can be done to determine if an esophageal motility disorder is present. However, most patients will have normal manometric studies.

Other gastrointestinal causes of chest pain are best evaluated by a careful history and upper endoscopy. The latter study may identify an unsuspected peptic ulcer, esophageal ulcer, or other evidence of GERD that can be appropriately treated. A gallbladder ultrasound is the best way to evaluate the patient for gallstones. Despite this exhaustive evaluation, many patients will still not have a diagnosis. In these patients, formal psychological testing or an empiric trial of antidepressants should be considered.

Assessment of Therapy for Non-Pleuritic Chest Pain

It is estimated that up to one third of the patients undergoing first-time cardiac catheterization will have no evidence of coronary artery disease. The prognosis for these patients is uniformly excellent. However, many of these patients continue to have chest pain, which they believe is cardiac in origin. This misunderstanding results in continued health care costs related to emergency room visits, office visits, hospital admissions to exclude MI, more diagnostic tests, therapeutic trials, as well as functional impairment in the ability to work and quality of life.

Reassuring the patient that cardiac disease is absent is the first step in managing non-cardiac chest pain. Musculoskeletal causes of chest pain may be treated by injecting a local anesthetic into painful trigger points. If GERD is present, therapy with the proton pump inhibitors (omeprazole 20 mg twice daily, lansoprazole 30 mg twice daily, or rabeprazole 20 mg twice daily) should be given for 8 to 12 weeks. In patients with a good response, treatment can be titrated downward in the ensuing months to the lowest dose necessary to control symptoms.

Should these measures fail, supportive reassurance based on the results of additional esophageal testing that demonstrates an esophageal etiology for pain may alleviate some of the patient's worries, may enable the patient to work, and may decrease the need for prescription drugs, physician and emergency room visits, and further hospitalizations.

A variety of smooth muscle relaxants, including hydralazine, anticholinergics, nitrates, and calcium channel blockers have been studied in patients with esophageal motility disorders and non-cardiac chest pain. None of these smooth muscle relaxants is reliably effective. It is important to exclude GERD before a trial of these agents, since they all promote acid reflux.

Psychotropic medications may be very helpful in patients with lower pain thresholds or psychiatric diagnoses contributing to their chest pain syndrome. In clinical trials, trazodone (100 to 150 mg daily) and imipramine (50 mg at bedtime) improve global esophageal symptoms when compared with placebo. Other effective agents include amitriptyline, desipramine, and nortriptyline. Often these drugs improve symptoms at lower doses than required for treating psychiatric diseases, suggesting that they are working by improving pain thresholds. The selective serotonin reuptake inhibitors have not been extensively studied but may also play a role in treatment, since this class of drugs may be better tolerated than tricyclic antidepressants. Patients with panic attacks can improve with alprazolam or imipramine.

More aggressive therapy of esophageal motility disorders with botulinum toxin injection, pneumatic dilatation, or surgical myotomy should be avoided except in selected patients with diffuse esophageal spasm accompanied by intractable symptoms.

Pitfalls and Common Mistakes in the Assessment and Treatment of Non-Pleuritic Chest Pain

The key thing to remember in the approach to unexplained chest pain is to always exclude a cardiac cause first. Coronary artery disease is a potentially life-threatening problem that should be entertained first in all such patients. Of course, this is much less likely in young otherwise healthy patients without apparent risk factors and more common in older patients with risk factors for coronary artery disease. Unfortunately, the history is not always reliable. The physical examination should entail an assessment of tenderness or pain in the vicinity of the sternum and xyphoid, since costochondral causes of chest pain are easily treatable and often missed. Diagnosing GERD first is important because it can be treated and some cardiac medications (nitrates, calcium channel blockers) have the potential to make reflux worse.

Attention is appropriately directed early in the evaluation of unexplained chest pain to the esophagus. However, it should be remembered that comprehensive diagnostic testing, including upper endoscopy, esophageal manometry, and 24-hour pH testing, has a low yield in the evaluation of these patients and should only be reserved for patients who fail the omeprazole test.

Finally, it is important to remember the less common causes of chest pain in patients with persistent intractable symptoms. Additional diagnostic possibilities, such as peptic ulcer disease, gallstones, and mitral valve prolapse, should be considered in these patients as well.

▼ BIBLIOGRAPHY

Achem SR, DeVault KR: Unexplained chest pain at the turn of the century, *Am J Gastroenterol* 94:5-8, 1999.
Beitman BD, Mukerji V, Lamberti JW, et al: Panic disorder in patients with chest pain and angiographically normal coronary arteries, *Am J Cardiol* 63:1399-1403, 1989.
Cannon RO, Bonow RO, Bacharach SL, et al: Left ventricular dysfunction in patients with angina pectoris, normal epicardial coronary arteries, and abnormal vasodilator reserve, *Circulation* 71:218-226, 1985.

Cannon RO, Quyyumi AA, Mincemoyer R, et al: Imipramine in patients with chest pain despite normal coronary angiograms, *N Engl J Med* 330:1411-1417, 1994.

Clouse RE, Lustman PJ: Psychiatric illness and contraction abnormalities of the esophagus, *N Engl J Med* 309:1337-1342, 1983.

Fass R, Fennerty MB, Ofman JJ, et al: The clinical and economic value of a short course of omeprazole in patients with noncardiac chest pain, *Gastroenterology* 115:42-49, 1998.

Frobert O, Funch-Jensen P, Bagger JP: Diagnostic value of esophageal studies in patients with angina-like chest pain and normal coronary angiograms, *Ann Intern Med* 124:959-969, 1996.

Kahrilas PJ, Clouse RE, Hogan WJ: An American Gastroenterological Association medical position statement on the clinical use of esophageal manometry, *Gastroenterology* 107:1865-1884, 1994.

Kahrilas PJ, Quigley EM: American Gastroenterological Association medical position statement: guidelines on the use of esophageal pH recording, *Gastroenterology* 110:1981-1996, 1996.

Prakash C, Clouse RE: Long-term outcome from tricyclic antidepressant treatment of functional chest pain, *Dig Dis Sci* 44:2373-2379, 1999.

Richter JE, Barish CF, Castell DO: Abnormal sensory perception in patients with esophageal chest pain, *Gastroenterology* 91:845-852, 1986.

Singh S, Richter JE, Hewson EG, et al: The contribution of gastroesophageal reflux to chest pain in patients with coronary artery disease, *Ann Intern Med* 117:824-830, 1992.

CHAPTER 17

UPPER LOBE PULMONARY INFILTRATE

Laurence A. Smolley

Key Terms

▼ Pulmonary infiltrates
▼ Nodules
▼ Upper and lower lobes
▼ Bacterial pneumonia
▼ Primary tuberculosis
▼ Atypical mycobacterial infection
▼ Fungal infection
▼ Histoplasmosis

▼ Blastomycosis
▼ Coccidioidomycosis
▼ Aspergillus
▼ Centriacinar emphysematous bullae
▼ *Pneumocystis carinii*
▼ Silicosis
▼ Coal worker's pneumoconiosis

▼ Sarcoidosis
▼ Bronchogenic carcinoma
▼ Metastatic cancer
▼ Langerhans' cell histiocytosis
▼ Ankylosing spondylitis
▼ Histiocytosis x

▼ THE CLINICAL PROBLEM

A 49-year-old man who has not seen a doctor in 3 years establishes himself as a new patient. He complains of a cough productive of small amounts of pale yellow sputum and slight dyspnea on exertion. He is found to have a nodular infiltrate in the apical and posterior segments of the right upper lobe. There has been no fever, night sweats, or weight loss, but he had minimal hemoptysis twice during

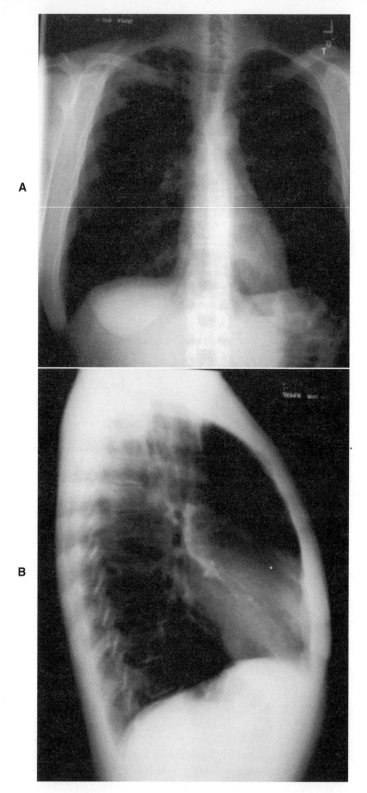

▼ **Figure 17-1** **A,** Anteroposterior (AP) chest x-ray showing right upper lobe disease. **B,** Lateral chest x-ray showing apical and posterior disease.

the previous 3 years. He has had intermittent lower back pain over the last 15 years and had a spontaneous pneumothorax on the right side about 5 years ago.

He smoked 1 to 2 packs/day for 10 years until about 7 years ago when he quit. He drinks one glass of wine with dinner on Friday and Saturday nights. He works as a computer software designer, which he has done since he finished graduate school 12 years ago. He has been married for 10 years and has two healthy children. He has not traveled out of the New England area except to visit Florida.

His past medical history is remarkable for an appendectomy 30 years ago. His skin tests for tuberculosis were negative when he was in elementary and high school. He takes no medications except for an occasional acetaminophen or ibuprofen tablet for headache or backache.

On physical examination, his vital signs are normal except for a temperature (oral) of 100° F. Salient findings include slightly decreased breath sounds and a few coarse rales in the region of the upper right lobe.

Laboratory tests were remarkable only for 12,000 white blood cells (WBCs) with 40% lymphocytes and 12% monocytes and a minimally elevated calcium and alkaline phosphatase.

His chest radiographs are shown in Figure 17-1, and representative cuts from the thoracic computed tomography (CT) are shown in Figure 17-2.

What is the differential diagnosis for this patient's cough, dyspnea and pulmonary infiltrate? What is the most likely cause?

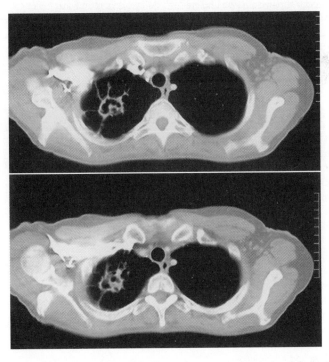

▼ **Figure 17-2**   CT of right upper lobe disease. There is cavitation or bronchiectasis.

Differential Diagnosis of Upper Lobe Infiltrates

Pulmonary infiltrates of the upper lobes may be caused by acute or chronic infectious diseases or benign or malignant non-infectious diseases. Diseases that predominantly involve the upper lobes may be distinguished from those that tend to affect mainly the lower lobes.

Bacterial pneumonia or other infections should be suspected in patients with lower respiratory symptoms such as cough, sputum production, and dyspnea associated with signs such as fever, altered breath sounds, and rales. The presence of fever with rigors and shaking chills and purulent sputum increases the likelihood that the pulmonary infiltrates are due to a bacterial infection.

The differential diagnosis of lower respiratory tract symptoms and signs can be quite extensive, as shown in Boxes 17-1 and 17-2. The chest radiograph is some-

---

Box 17-1
Differential Diagnosis of Upper Lobe Pulmonary Infiltrates

Infectious Causes	Non-Infectious Causes
Klebsiella-Enterobacter-Acinetobacter-Serratia pneumonia	Sarcoidosis (especially when cavitated, may have fungus ball)
Mycobacterium tuberculosis: primary and post-primary atypical mycobacteria	Bronchogenic carcinoma (especially when cavitated)
Fungal infections (histoplasmosis, blastomycosis, coccidioidomycosis, aspergillosis)	Silicosis
Infected centriacinar emphysematous bullae	Coal worker's pneumoconiosis
Pneumocystis carinii (cystic or cavitary)	Ankylosing spondylitis
	Langerhans' cell histiocytosis (formerly known as eosinophilic granuloma)

Box 17-2
Differential Diagnosis of Lower Lobe Pulmonary Infiltrates

Infectious Causes	Non-Infectious Causes
Streptococcus pneumoniae	Idiopathic pulmonary fibrosis
Legionella species	Desquamative interstitial pneumonitis
Mycoplasma pneumoniae	Collagen-vascular disease (systemic lupus erythematosus, scleroderma, rheumatoid arthritis)
Escherichia coli	
Pseudomonas aeruginosa	
Actinomyces species	Asbestosis
Nocardia species	Hematogenous metastasis
Cryptococcus neoformans	Lymphangitic carcinomatosis
Echinococcus granulosus	Intra-lobar sequestration
Entamoeba histolytica	Hydrostatic pulmonary edema
Chlamydia psittaci and *C. pneumoniae*	
Coxiella burnetti (Q fever)	
Septic thromboemboli	
Viruses (influenza and adenovirus)	

times helpful for determining the diagnosis, particularly if the distribution of lesions and the specific characteristics of the opacities are typical of one disease process or another. An appropriate, detailed medical history including associated symptoms, other illnesses, and occupational or other exposures is indispensable in narrowing the list of differential diagnoses. The clinician should prioritize the additional tests needed to confirm the specific diagnosis so that effective treatment may be applied. It must be emphasized that respiratory symptoms such as cough, dyspnea and hemoptysis are non-specific.

In primary tuberculosis, a lobar or segmental, well-defined airspace consolidation may be present in any lobe but is more likely in an upper lobe. Associated pleural effusion and hilar or mediastinal adenopathy is quite common. Reactivation tuberculosis most commonly involves the apical and posterior segments of the upper lobes. These infiltrates tend to be bilateral, asymmetric, less well defined and tend to cavitate. Pleural effusion and enlarged lymph nodes are rare. On plain chest radiographs, atypical mycobacterial infections are usually very similar in appearance to primary tuberculosis. Pleural effusion and hilar adenopathy are much less common, and there is a tendency to produce thin-walled cavities with little surrounding infiltrate.

The radiographic presentation of fungal infections is as diversified as the fungi themselves. Chronic pulmonary histoplasmosis may produce unilateral or bilateral fibronodular apical infiltrates that may simulate tuberculosis. Blastomycosis may present as a chronic pulmonary infiltrate that resembles a mass in an upper lobe, whereas coccidioidomycosis may begin as a patchy infiltrate and develop into a thin-walled cavity.

Apergillus may materialize as evanescent infiltrates in the upper lung regions or may appear as branching homogenous fingerlike shadows of mucoid impaction that extend up from the hila. Upper lobe fibrosis or honeycombing may develop in chronic disease. This fungus often becomes a secondary infection or colonizer in a damaged bronchial tree or in an old cavity as noted in the discussions of sarcoidosis and ankylosing spondylitis.

In people over age 50, especially if they smoked cigarettes, there is a propensity to develop centriacinar emphysematous bullae involving the upper lobes. These bullous lesions can become infected with bacteria, such as anaerobes, or the usual pathogens that cause community-acquired pneumonias.

Pneumocystis carinii pneumonia produces abnormal chest radiographs in 80% to 90% of the cases, with the classic findings of diffuse interstitial or reticulonodular infiltrates. Nodular disease, which may evolve into cystic or cavitary lesions (especially if located in the upper lobes), has been reported.

Patients with upper lobe opacifications that are nodular may have silicosis, coal worker's pneumoconiosis, sarcoidosis, or neoplasm (primary or metastatic) of the lung. In silicosis, there are three main patterns of radiographic abnormalities. In simple silicosis, reticular and nodular patterns are frequent. The nodules range in size from 1 mm to less than 10 mm in diameter, predominate in the upper lobes, and usually have very distinct margins. Hilar lymph node enlargement is common, and about 5% of those nodes have the classic "egg-shell" calcification, once considered pathognomonic for silicosis, which has been reported in cases of sarcoidosis and tuberculosis. Progressive massive fibrosis is characterized by densities that are 10 mm or larger in diameter and often conglomerated into larger masses. In chronic silicosis, the masses in the upper lobes may cavitate and become colonized with mycobacteria. Simple coal worker's pneumoconiosis shows a profusion of small, rounded densities. Complicated coal worker's pneumoconiosis or progressive massive fibrosis is associated with opacities greater than 1 cm in diameter (some experts require lesions bigger than 2 cm for the diagnosis to be established).

Sarcoidosis of the upper lobes may be nodular and may cavitate. There may or may not be associated hilar adenopathy. A cavity may become colonized with aspergillus. The radiographic sign is a mycetoma or fungus ball, which is a solid homogenous rounded mass separated from the cavity wall by a crescentic clear space. Other cavitated nodular lesions, particularly if large, may be due to bronchogenic carcinoma. Metastatic cancer may present as singular or multiple nodules. Primary lung cancer in the upper lobes predominates, whereas metastases are more common in lower lung fields. Cystic changes or micronodular shadows are characteristic of Langerhans' cell histiocytosis.

In ankylosing spondylitis, the chest radiograph initially shows a nodular or reticular pattern in the apical or sub-apical areas. This pattern may coarsen, become confluent, and eventually densely consolidate. The pulmonary hilar structures may be pulled upward as volume is lost in the upper lobes. Involvement initially may be unilateral, but eventually both sides are affected in most cases. The apical lesions usually cavitate and are surrounded by fibrosis. Aspergillomas and atypical mycobacteria may colonize the cavities and cause hemoptysis.

Clinical Features that Suggest a Specific Cause of Upper Lobe Infiltrates

In the current case, clinical features such as intermittent lower backache and a history of spontaneous pneumothorax suggest ankylosing spondylitis. His negative PPD skin tests in the past do not preclude tuberculosis. The absence of a history of exposure to silica dust goes against silicosis. Travel to Florida, particularly to the northern counties, raises suspicion of blastomycosis and histoplasmosis, especially if he explored any caves where bats may have been living. Coccidioidomycosis is much less likely, since he has not been to the southwestern United States where this organism is endemic. Sarcoidosis remains a possibility given the history because sarcoidosis may be associated with arthralgias. He has no predisposing risk factors to suggest *P. carinii* infection, and the mode of presentation is not consistent with an acute bacterial process. Bronchogenic carcinoma is possible, since he did smoke.

Diagnostic Testing in the Evaluation of Upper Lobe Infiltrates

Since there is nothing pathognomonic about the radiographic appearance of the nodular infiltrates in this case, additional testing is required. A diagnosis can be made by isolating a pathogen, such as a fungus or mycobacteria, in the expectorated sputum or by finding malignant cells. Various blood tests and serologies are not that helpful in this case for determining a specific infectious agent. If the sputum specimens do not provide adequate information, then an invasive biopsy technique would be necessary.

Before an invasive procedure is done, the patient's pulmonary function should be assessed with spirometry and oxygenation by pulse oximetry to be sure that he can safely undergo a procedure that potentially could be complicated by pneumothorax. The ideal biopsy would be chosen by an experienced pulmonologist after review of a CT scan of the patient's chest. If a lesion in question is of sufficient size and is close or contiguous to the pleura, a needle biopsy would be an appropriate approach. If the lesion or lesions are more diffuse or ill-defined or large enough and deeper in the lung parenchyma, fiberoptic bronchoscopy for bronchial brushings and washing with transbronchial biopsy would be advisable. Occasionally, a surgeon would be required to perform a biopsy by thoracoscopic or other means. The specimens must be examined by a pathologist with experience in pulmonary disease.

Sometimes, as in the present patient, the histologic manifestations may be nonspecific. Tissue from the nodular lesions of ankylosing spondylitis may show a nondescript interstitial mononuclear cell infiltrate with variable degrees of fibroblastic proliferation and fibrosis. There may be thin-walled bullae and cavities or bronchiectasis. In these situations, a blood test for the histocompatibility antigen HLA-B27 may be positive, and radiographic signs of inflammation in the sacroiliac joints may be supportive in establishing the diagnosis.

Assessment of Therapy

There is no definitive treatment for ankylosing spondylitis. No medication has been shown to actually modify the course of the disease, particularly in the lung, but non-steroidal anti-inflammatory drugs (NSAIDs) and drugs, such as methotrexate, sulfsalazine, and others, have been used to palliate the arthritis.

Pitfalls and Common Mistakes in the Assessment and Treatment of Upper Lobe Infiltrates

One of the main challenges in finding the etiology of an upper lobe pulmonary infiltrate is choosing the safest biopsy procedure that can afford the highest chance of defining the disease process. The risk of an invasive procedure in an elderly patient with poor pulmonary function reserve always has to be weighed against the therapeutic implications. Invasive procedures are associated with a finite risk of pneumothorax, which sometimes requires tube thoracostomy. Bleeding and cardiac dysrhythmias are other potential complications.

A common mistake is applying an empiric therapy, such as prescribing an antibiotic, and then failing to follow-up the clinical symptoms for improvement and not ordering radiographs for resolution of the lesions.

▼ BIBLIOGRAPHY

Eisenberg RL: *Clinical imaging: an atlas of differential diagnosis*, ed 3, Philadelphia, 1996, Lippincott-Raven.

Fraser RS, Muller NL, Colman N, Pare PD: *Diagnosis of diseases of the chest*, ed 4, Philadelphia, 1999, WB Saunders.

Putman CE, Ravin CE: *Textbook of diagnostic imaging*, ed 2, Philadelphia, 1994, WB Saunders.

Rosenow EC, Strimlan CV, Muhm JR, Ferguson RH: Pleuroparenchymal manifestations of ankylosing spondylitis, *Mayo Clin Proc* 52:641-649, 1977.

CHAPTER 18

WHEEZING

Mani S. Kavuru

Key Words

▼ Wheezing
▼ Stridor
▼ Asthma

▼ Chronic obstructive pulmonary disease (COPD)

▼ Cardiac asthma
▼ Airflow obstruction

▼ THE CLINICAL PROBLEM

A 55-year-old man presents with episodic wheezing and shortness of breath. He describes the wheezing as worse at night, as well as with exertion. The wheezing is often accompanied by a dry cough. His wife and co-workers have commented that the wheezing is audible several feet away. He denies exertional chest pain, orthopnea, or hemoptysis. He is a former smoker (one pack/day for 25 years, quit 10 years ago). His past medical history is remarkable for childhood asthma, allergic rhinitis, and hypertension (for which he is on therapy with a beta-blocker).

On physical examination, his blood pressure is 142/78, and he is mildly dyspneic with a respiratory rate of 20. He is awake and conversant and he does not have "drooling." Neck examination revealed mild wheezes during expiration only. There were no palpable masses in the neck. Cardiac examination was unremarkable. Auscultation of the chest revealed loud wheezes throughout the expiratory phase, which was prolonged. Inspiratory phase was fairly clear. The intensity of the wheezes in the chest was much louder than in the neck. The remainder of the examination was unremarkable.

Chest x-ray showed a normal size heart and the lung fields were somewhat hyperinflated but clear.

What is the differential diagnosis for this patient's wheezing and what is the most likely cause?

Differential Diagnosis of Wheezing

The term *wheezing* may be used to describe both a respiratory symptom that a patient complains about and a finding during a physical examination (a sign). Wheezing is generally considered an abnormal or adventitious lung sound and is typically a continuous sound that is high-pitched (as opposed to a low-pitched continuous sound, which is referred to as a rhonchus). The presence of wheezing generally indicates partial obstruction of an airway lumen.

Common causes of wheezing include bronchial asthma with a largely reversible component, chronic obstructive pulmonary disease (COPD) with a largely fixed component, congestive heart failure (CHF) ("cardiac asthma"), and an obstructing lesion at any level of the airway (Box 18-1). Although wheezing usually is not present in normal individuals during quiet breathing, it may be brought on by a forced expiratory maneuver in otherwise normal individuals.

Infrequent causes of wheezing include other parenchymal lung disease (i.e., pneumonia), pulmonary embolism, psychogenic or functional ("factitious") causes, or a reaction to a medication (i.e., beta-blocker). Table 18-1 summarizes signs and symptoms as well as mechanisms for wheezing in a variety of disease states.

Wheezing is a hallmark of most patients with bronchial asthma. In asthmatics, wheezing is loudest in the chest (as opposed to over the neck) and is typically present throughout the expiratory phase. When the airflow obstruction is more severe, it may be present both during inspiration as well as expiration. In general,

---

**Box 18-1
Differential Diagnosis of Wheezing**

Common Causes	Less Common Causes
Asthma	Endobronchial lesions (both benign and malignant)
COPD	
CHF ("cardiac asthma")	Pneumonia
Upper airway disease	Pulmonary embolism
	Bronchiectasis
	Drug reaction (i.e., beta-blocker)
	Factitious or psychogenic

COPD, Chronic obstructive pulmonary disease; *CHF,* congestive heart failure.

TABLE 18-1
Interpreting Signs and Symptoms in the Patient with Wheezing

Possible Causes	Mechanisms	Suggestive Clinical Features
Asthma	Partial narrowing of small and medium size airways, bronchospasm, airway inflammation with mucosal edema	Episodic symptoms; wheezing is generalized (both sides); strong family history, atopic state with associated seasonal allergies, rhinitis; definite and/or dramatic improvement with therapy (including inhaled and oral corticosteroids)
COPD	Partial narrowing of small airways, bronchospasm, airway inflammation with mucosal edema and secretions, loss of elastic recoil with dynamic airway collapse	Symptoms are present on most days with only partial improvement with therapy; decreased intensity of background lung sounds
CHF ("cardiac asthma")	Partial narrowing of small airways, reflex bronchospasm due to local release of mediators, submucosal edema due to venous engorgement	Presence of other features of heart disease including exertional chest pain, orthopnea, palpitations, dizziness; examination may indicate jugular venous distension, crackles (in addition to wheezes), edema; abnormal chest x-ray, electrocardiogram, etc
Upper airway obstruction	Narrowing of the large airway by any process (paralyzed vocal cords, foreign body, tumor, infection)	Stridor, hoarseness, difficulty with secretions or swallowing, wheezing loudest over the neck, usually worse with inspiration
PE	Reflex bronchospasm due to release of mediators (serotonin, histamine)	Acute onset of symptoms including dyspnea, chest pain, hemoptysis (in addition to wheezing); underlying risk factors for venous thromboembolism (i.e., stasis, obesity, etc)
Localized airway tumors	Bronchogenic carcinoma with localized narrowing, obstruction of large or medium size airways with post-obstructive atelectasis and/or pneumonitis	Smoking history, hemoptysis, localized or focal wheeze on examination, chest x-ray usually shows a mass

COPD, Chronic obstructive pulmonary disease; CHF, congestive heart failure; PE, pulmonary embolism.

bi-phasic wheezing is associated with lower peak expiratory flow than only expiratory wheezing, and loudness and high-pitched wheezing are associated with more severe obstruction. Occasionally, with very severe airflow obstruction, wheezing may actually decrease or disappear (the so-called *silent chest*).

An objective assessment of airflow obstruction by a handheld peak flow meter or spirometer should be obtained in most patients with asthma to assess the severity of airflow obstruction. It is postulated that the mechanism for a wheeze is that of a narrowed airway with opposing walls that oscillate or flutter between a nearly occluded position and a fully occluded position to produce the characteristic wheezing sound.

Wheezing may be present in patients with COPD in a manner similar in patients with bronchial asthma. Wheezing in this setting is also due to partial narrowing of the small airways as a result of bronchospasm, mucosal edema, and airway secretions. In patients with COPD, the presence of a wheeze on examination may suggest a more likely response to bronchodilators.

Wheezing may be a common symptom and physical finding in patients with cardiac decompensation and CHF. The term *cardiac asthma* describes patients with CHF who have wheezing; the mechanism is felt to be on the basis of airflow obstruction. Causes of airflow obstruction in cardiac asthma include airway mucosal and submucosal edema due to venous engorgement, and reflex bronchospasm due to release of local mediators.

Upper airway obstruction of any cause can produce a loud musical sound similar to wheezing in the neck and the chest. The adventitious sound known as *stridor* is generally loudest over the neck and may be transmitted to the lower airways and can occasionally be confused with asthma. When this noise is loudest on inspiration, then it is due to an upper airway obstruction (e.g., narrowing at the level of the glottis or vocal cords as in croup or epiglottitis).

Clinical Features that Suggest a Specific Cause of Wheezing

In the current case, clinical features suggest the cough is caused by either asthma or COPD. The wheezing is described as being episodic and is worse at nighttime, so CHF is in the differential diagnosis. However, the patient does not have a history of heart disease, known coronary artery risk factors, exertional chest pain, or orthopnea. Absence of these features along with a clear chest x-ray would make cardiac disease much less likely. The fact that he has a history of childhood asthma and allergic rhinitis increases the likelihood that wheezing is due to asthma. The fact that he is an ex-smoker raises the possibility of COPD.

Physical examination indicates that the wheezing is loudest in the chest rather than the neck, which strongly argues against upper airway obstruction as an important factor.

A spirogram showing a normal flow-volume loop would be very useful in further excluding upper airway obstruction. Clearly, the spirometry would show significant airflow obstruction (i.e., a reduced FEV_1 and FEV_1/FVC ratio), with or without a significant acute response to a bronchodilator to be most consistent with asthma or COPD.

This patient is on a beta-blocker, which is known to exacerbate airflow obstruction in patients with asthma and COPD. Therefore further history would need to be obtained to see if there is any temporal correlation between the start of beta-blocker therapy and the patient's symptoms. A normal chest x-ray would generally exclude other parenchymal causes for wheezing such as pneumonia and bronchiectasis. There is nothing acute in this patient's history to suggest an entity such as pulmonary embolism as a cause of wheezing.

Diagnostic Testing in the Evaluation of the Patient with Wheezing

Several simple diagnostic studies are useful in evaluating patients with wheezing. These include spirometry with special attention to both limbs of the flow-volume loop, as well as an anteroposterior (AP) and lateral chest radiograph. In general, a combination of a good history and physical examination with attention to the neck and chest examination, as well as a spirogram and a chest x-ray, are generally adequate to establish the likely cause of wheezing in an adult.

A typical scenario, as in the patient described, would be a normal configuration of the flow-volume loop and a normal chest x-ray, along with airflow obstruction, which would support a diagnosis of obstructive airway disease. In this setting, objectively assessing the severity of airflow obstruction and optimizing bronchodilator and anti-inflammatory therapy (including a systemic corticosteroid for several weeks) should improve the patient's symptoms. If the flow-volume loop is abnormal and there is history to suggest stridor, this would require additional evaluation, perhaps including laryngoscopy, bronchoscopy or CT scan of the neck and/or chest.

If the history suggests features of heart disease (i.e., orthopnea, exertional chest discomfort, paroxysmal nocturnal dyspnea, wheezing as well as crackles and edema on examination) this would require further evaluation with electrocardiograms, two dimensional echocardiogram, and perhaps a stress study as well as a heart catheterization. If the spirogram and chest x-rays are normal, then wheezing may still be on the basis of occult or atypical asthma.

A reasonable way to establish the presence of airway reactivity in this setting is to perform bronchoprovocation testing with methacholine or histamine. These studies are highly sensitive to detect airway hyperreactivity by demonstrating a 20% decrease in the FEV_1 by an incremental challenge procedure. Most patients with a history of wheezing or wheezing documented by physical examination can have the etiology established by this approach.

Pitfalls and Common Mistakes in the Assessment and Treatment of a Patient with Wheezing

When a patient presents with wheezing, the clinician must ensure there are no historical features to suggest CHF (e.g., orthopnea or exertional chest discomfort) or upper airway obstruction (hoarseness, drooling, difficulty swallowing, or stridor). Special emphasis on physical examination should be placed on auscultating the neck and making sure that the wheezing is originating in the chest rather than in the neck. By special attention to these issues, the cause of wheezing usually can be established.

▼ BIBLIOGRAPHY

Baughman RP, Loudon RG: Quantitation of wheezing in acute asthma, *Chest* 86:718-722, 1984.

Bettencourt PE, Del Bono EA, Spiegelman D, et al: Clinical utility of chest auscultation in common pulmonary diseases, *Am J Respir Crit Care Med* 150:1291-1297, 1994.

Forgacs P: The functional basis of pulmonary sounds. Chest 73:399-405, 1978.

Fraser RS, Müller NL, Colman N, Pare PD (editors): *Fraser and Pare's diagnosis of diseases of the chest*, ed 4, Philadelphia, 1999, WB Saunders, pp 394-395.

King DK, Thompson BT, Johnson DC: Wheezing on maximal forced exhalation in the diagnosis of atypical asthma, *Ann Intern Med* 110:451-455, 1987.

Marini JJ, Pierson DJ, Hudson LD, Lakshminarayan S: The significance of wheezing in chronic airflow obstruction, *Am Rev Respir Dis* 120:1069-1072, 1979.

Shim CS, Williams MH: Relationship of wheezing to the severity of obstruction in asthma, *Arch Intern Med* 413:890-892, 1983.

CHAPTER 19

STRIDOR

Tareq Jamil
Loutfi S. Aboussouan

Key Terms

▼ Stridor
▼ Hoarseness
▼ Trachea
▼ Dyspnea
▼ Epiglottitis

▼ Croup
▼ Angioedema
▼ Tracheotomy
▼ Tracheal stenosis

▼ Laryngospasm
▼ Goiter
▼ Flow-volume loop
▼ Spirometry

▼ THE CLINICAL PROBLEM

A 20-year-old male presents with progressively worsening dyspnea on exertion over the past 1 month. He also complains of a "hissing" sound during breathing that he first noticed 2 weeks earlier. He does report some shortness of breath at rest but denies any wheezing, hoarseness, cough, nasal congestion, runny nose, sore throat, or throat pain. There is no history of fever, chills, night sweats, weight loss, or episodic facial or lip swelling. He denies any history of asthma or lung problems in the past.

He is not on any medication and has no known drug allergy. His medical history is significant for head trauma that occurred 2 months ago when he fell off the back of a pick-up truck with resulting epidural hematoma. He was admitted to the intensive care unit and underwent surgery for hematoma evacuation. His hospital stay was complicated by a nosocomial pneumonia that required 12 days of orotracheal intubation.

He is currently back in college. He denies smoking or drug use but admits to occasional alcoholic beverages.

On physical examination, he is 5-foot tall and weighs 120 lbs. He is afebrile and has a blood pressure of 110/75 in the sitting position, respiratory rate of 14, and oxygen saturation of 95% on room air by pulse oximetry. He is in no acute distress and is not using accessory muscles of respiration. His voice is of normal male pitch and characteristics. Examination of head, eyes, ears, nose and throat reveals evidence of previous head surgery, and a harsh inspiratory sound is heard loudest at the base of the neck anteriorly. His chest is clear to percussion and auscultation. Cardiac examination is unremarkable, as is the rest of the physical examination.

Laboratory data available at this initial visit include a normal plain 2-view chest x-ray.

What is the differential diagnosis for this patient's symptoms, and what is the most likely cause?

Differential Diagnosis of Stridor

Stridor is a harsh blowing noise of constant pitch with a characteristic crowing or musical sound caused by obstruction in the upper airways, usually at the level of larynx or upper trachea. Significant anatomic narrowing precedes overt symptoms. For instance, dyspnea on exertion only starts when the airway is narrowed to about

---

Box 19-1
Differential Diagnosis of Stridor

Common Causes	Less Common Causes
Infectious Causes	**Infectious Causes**
Acute epiglottitis	Tonsillitis
Laryngotracheobronchitis	Pharyngitis
Ludwig's angina	Retropharyngeal abscess
Foreign body aspiration: Dental appliances in adults, bolus of food	Acute uvulitis
	Acute lingular cellulitis
Angioedema	Acute suppurative parotitis
Tumors and masses: Bronchogenic carcinoma, goiter or thyroid malignancy, Hodgkin's lymphoma, sarcoidosis	Neuromuscular causes: Shy-Drager syndrome, Parkinson's disease, laryngeal-pharyngeal dystonia, vocal cord paralysis
	Relapsing polychondritis
Trauma to upper airway: Functional vocal cord dysfunction	Tracheobronchomegaly
Intubation related: Glottic edema, tracheal stenosis, paralyzed vocal cords, tracheotomy scar, tracheomalacia	Miscellaneous: Vascular causes, hypoplastic trachea, tracheobronchopathia

8 mm, and dyspnea at rest and stridor develop when the diameter of airway is reduced to 5 mm. However, when upper airway obstruction is severe and alveolar hypoventilation occurs, stridor may be absent. Causes of upper airway obstruction associated with stridor are numerous, with the most common etiologies summarized in Box 19-1 and Table 19-1.

TABLE 19-1
Interpreting Signs and Symptoms in the Patient with Stridor

Possible Causes	Mechanisms	Suggestive Clinical Features
Acute epiglottitis	Bacterial infection and swelling of epiglottis and supraglottic structures	Rapid onset of symptoms of dysphagia, dysphonia, drooling, fever; absent cough; less fulminant onset in adults
Laryngotracheo-bronchitis	Viral infection and edematous narrowing of the subglottic area	Stridor, barking cough, and hoarseness after several days of cold symptoms
Ludwig's angina	Cellulitis of the floor of the mouth with posterior displacement of the tongue	Poor dental hygiene, dental extraction, toothache, pain, dysphagia, drooling, neck swelling (bull neck), "hot-potato" voice
Foreign body aspiration	Aspiration of food bolus, or iatrogenic aspiration of medical or dental appliances	Sudden choking and inability to breathe, advanced age, altered mental status
Angioedema	Laryngeal swelling as part of a generalized process of facial and mucous membranes edema	Non-pitting asymmetric facial edema; identified trigger, family history, or recent ACE inhibitor initiation
Tumors and masses	Airway compromise by tumor progression or benign masses (i.e., goiter)	Progressive onset of symptoms, history of malignancy, superior vena cava syndrome
Vocal cord causes	Recurrent laryngeal nerve dysfunction or cord paralysis with narrowed glottic aperture	Horseness, breathy voice; normal voice in bilateral cord paralysis; inspiratory and expiratory stridor may be present
Functional vocal cord dysfunction	Paradoxic inspiratory apposition of the vocal cords	Wheezing, stridor, shortness of breath, depression, histrionic personality disorder
Prolonged intubation	Vocal cord ulceration, granulomas, or paralysis; stenosis of trachea or posterior glottic commissure; pressure necrosis	Intubation for more than 10 days, increased tube caliber, severe respiratory failure, history of diabetes, female gender
Tracheotomy	Stomal or tracheal stenosis, bacterial contamination of larynx, tracheomalacia	History of tracheotomy, high placement of tracheal stoma

ACE, Angiotensin-converting enzyme.

Infectious Causes

Acute epiglottitis is a life-threatening condition requiring immediate securing of the airway. The most common causative agent is *Haemophilus influenzae.* The prevalence of this infection in children has declined dramatically in recent years due to widespread use of the anti-*Haemophilus influenzae* type B vaccine and it is therefore now more commonly observed in adults. Presenting features are dysphagia, dysphonia, drooling, and respiratory distress accompanied by stridor, fever, and generalized toxicity. Cough is typically absent. In adults, the symptoms are less fulminant in nature, with fever, sore throat, and pain on swallowing as usual symptoms, and occasional stridor and respiratory distress. Treatment consists of second- and third-generation cephalosporins.

Laryngotracheobronchitis (croup) is a common acute viral respiratory infection of children under the age of 4 and is due to edematous narrowing of the subglottic area. It presents with inspiratory stridor, barking cough, and hoarseness after several days of cold symptoms. The most common causative agents are para-influenza virus, respiratory syncytial virus, adenovirus, and influenza A and B viruses. Treatment consists of corticosteroids, mist therapy, and nebulized racemic epinephrine.

Other reported infectious causes of upper airway obstruction include Ludwig's angina (a potentially lethal cellulitis of the floor of the mouth and submandibular space), acute tonsillitis and pharyngitis with or without retropharyngeal abscess, acute suppurative parotitis with glottic obstruction, bacterial tracheitis, and rarely tuberculosis.

Foreign Body

Foreign body aspiration is much more common in children but can also occur in adults. The usual presentation in adults is sudden aspiration of a food bolus into the upper larynx or hypopharynx causing sudden respiratory distress, choking and inability to breathe (the *café coronary* syndrome). Emergency intervention, such as the Heimlich maneuver, can be lifesaving. Iatrogenic aspiration of medical and dental appliances accounts for 32% of cases of foreign body obstruction. Risk factors include advanced age, altered mental status due to alcohol or drugs, poor dentition, and neurologic conditions such as stroke and Parkinson's disease. Large esophageal foreign bodies can also compress the upper airway. Treatment is endoscopic removal, usually by rigid bronchoscopy.

Angioedema

Angioedema is characterized by transient episodes of painless, well-demarcated, non-pitting, asymmetric edema that affects the face, eyelids, lips, tongue, and mucous membranes. Laryngeal edema occurs in about 20% of cases and may lead to severe life-threatening upper airway obstruction. Allergic IgE-mediated reactions are characterized by rapid onset of upper airway edema and possible associated urticaria. Hereditary angioneurotic edema is due to a deficiency of C1 esterase inhibitor and is characterized by upper airway edema progressing over several hours and typically no urticaria. Acquired C1 esterase inhibitor deficiency usually presents after the fourth decade and is often associated with hematologic malignancies. Non-IgE mediated angioedema can also be caused by narcotics, radiocontrast material, non-steroidal anti-inflammatory drugs including aspirin, and angiotensin-converting enzyme (ACE) inhibitors. It can also be idiopathic, caused by physical stimuli, such as cold, heat, and stress, or related to connective tissue diseases associated with circulating immune complexes. Recent initiation of ACE inhibitors has been implicated in up to 35% of cases of angioedema. The mechanism is unclear but patients with history of idiopathic angioedema are at increased risk. Treatment includes securing the airway, epinephrine, antihistamines, or corticosteroids.

Tumors and Masses

Benign or malignant tumors of the pharynx, larynx, and trachea may produce slow and progressive upper airway obstruction. Bronchogenic carcinoma is the most common tumor affecting the trachea. Secondary tracheal involvement occurs with local spread of laryngeal, esophageal, bronchogenic, thyroid carcinomas or Hodgkin's lymphoma, and sarcoidosis. Endotracheal metastasis can also cause upper airway obstruction. Enlargement of the thyroid gland (goiter) surrounding the anterolateral wall of the extra-thoracic trachea may result in airway obstruction.

Trauma

Acute obstruction of the airway may be caused by blunt trauma to the face, neck, and chest, commonly after motor vehicle accidents or assault with penetrating injuries caused by knife or gunshot wounds. Oropharyngeal or hypopharyngeal edema, hematomas, subcutaneous emphysema, fractures, and laceration of laryngeal cartilage cause airway compromise. Inhalation of noxious fumes and heated gases can also cause severe tracheobronchitis and sloughing of the mucosa, leading to airway obstruction. Subsequent intubation injury may delay healing and result in formation of granulation tissue, scarring and stenosis. Treatment options include stenting with silastic tubes, subglottic reconstruction, and tracheal reconstruction.

Vocal Cord Causes

Unilateral vocal cord paralysis resulting from recurrent laryngeal nerve dysfunction or injury (commonly from thyroid surgery) usually presents with hoarseness with a breathy voice character. Bilateral vocal cord paralysis usually causes inspiratory and expiratory stridor. If insidious in onset, the patient may be asymptomatic at rest and the voice may be quite normal, since the vocal cords are symmetrically apposed in midline. Thyroid surgery, neck trauma, and tumor invasion from anaplastic thyroid or esophageal carcinoma are common causes. Immobility of the vocal cords can also occur from cricoarytenoid arthritis caused by severe advanced rheumatoid arthritis.

Several reports describe a syndrome called *functional vocal cord dysfunction* that is characterized by paradoxic apposition of the vocal cords intermittently during inspiration in the absence of organic disease. The signs and symptoms of functional stridor resemble those of laryngeal edema, laryngospasm, vocal cord paralysis, or asthma. A typical presentation includes dramatic onset of wheezing, stridor and shortness of breath, and hypoxemia without respiratory acidosis in an individual with a psychiatric history. Direct laryngoscopy may be normal or show adduction of vocal cords on expiration, inspiration, or both. The underlying problem is depression and histrionic personality disorder. Although some patients are unaware of the self-induced nature, others appear to have secondary gain. Treatment includes psychiatric counseling, speech therapy, and relaxation techniques.

Iatrogenic Causes

Most common iatrogenic complications affecting the larynx and trachea result from prolonged endotracheal intubation. Tracheotomy may also cause upper airway obstruction immediately after the procedure, as well as months to years later.

Vocal cord ulceration, edema, and granulomas are the most common complications of prolonged intubation and usually resolve spontaneously within 8 to 12 weeks. More serious stenosis occurs at the posterior glottic commissure in 6% to 12% of cases and is thought to be caused by movement of the tube and pressure necrosis of the mucosa. Predisposing factors include prolonged translaryngeal intubation (<6 days prevalence 2%, 6-10 days prevalence 5%, >10 days prevalence 12%), increased tube caliber, oral versus nasal intubation, severe respiratory failure, diabetes mellitus, and female gender.

Vocal cord paralysis is also a cause of post-extubation airway obstruction and can result from trauma, surgery, recurrent laryngeal nerve injury, or cricoarytenoid joint ankylosis.

Tracheal stenosis may also occur as late sequelae of intubation caused by ischemic injury and pressure necrosis to the mucosa caused by the tube cuff. The use of low pressure, high volume cuffs has reduced this complication.

Glottic edema as a post-extubation complication is more commonly seen in children, especially with burns and trauma, and may necessitate reintubation in about 1% of cases. In adults, the prevalence varies from 2% to 22% and the risk factors are intubation for more than 36 hours and female gender.

Laryngospasm is an exaggerated glottic closure reflex that can be elicited by stimulating the superior laryngeal nerve and by various stimuli, including intubation. Glottic closure may persist long after the initiating stimulus. Laryngospasm appears to be a rare cause of post-extubation stridor.

Tracheotomy frequently is associated with stomal stenosis from scarring. Stenosis can occur at the subglottic area from a highly placed stoma. Tracheotomy itself may also exacerbate laryngeal injury after prolonged intubation by retrograde bacterial contamination of the larynx and impairment of vocal cord abduction. Tracheomalacia due to the thinning of the tracheal cartilage may occur and can cause upper airway obstruction by itself or with development of tracheal stricture.

Nebulized racemic epinephrine and corticosteroids are used in the empiric treatment of post-extubation laryngeal edema. Racemic epinephrine treatments may need to be repeated frequently to prevent reintubation. There is no proven benefit of routine steroid use in preventing post-extubation laryngeal edema in children or adults.

Laryngotracheal resection and reconstruction can treat tracheal stenosis and tumors, an experienced surgeon is believed to be an important predictor of successful outcome.

Clinical Features that Suggest a Specific Cause of Stridor

In the case presented, the history is suggestive of gradual onset of upper airway obstruction (worsening dyspnea on exertion) and development of stridor as evidenced by dyspnea at rest and a harsh inspiratory sound that is loudest at the neck. The history and physical examination permit exclusion of infectious etiologies, foreign body, angioedema, inhalation injury, or neuromuscular disorder.

The history of recent and prolonged endotracheal intubation in the wake of head trauma with subsequent nosocomial pneumonia should focus our attention on the possibility of vocal cord pathology or tracheal stenosis. Important additional factors include his relatively small body frame and weight. Although a suggestive history is not available, it is conceivable that intubation with a conventionally sized endotracheal tube for his gender may have exceeded the recommended size, and increased the possibility of upper airway injury. This includes vocal cord paralysis, excessive granulation tissue on the cords or upper trachea, or tracheal stenosis.

Voice characteristics may be helpful in the diagnosis. For instance, hoarseness is often a sign of laryngeal pathology, and muffling of the voice without hoarseness may represent a supraglottic process. Our patient's normal voice does not completely exclude vocal cord pathology since bilateral paralysis can be associated with a normal voice due to symmetric apposition of the cords.

In our case, computed tomographic (CT) scanning and bronchoscopy revealed a 2.5 cm segment of tracheal stenosis at the thoracic inlet with narrowing of the lumen to a diameter of 6 mm. The patient was treated surgically with sternal split tracheal resection and end-to-end anastomosis with resolution of symptoms and correction of the stricture.

Diagnostic Testing in the Evaluation of Patient with Stridor

Plain Chest X-Rays and Neck Films

Plain chest x-ray may be helpful as a screening test by identifying tracheal deviation, compression, foreign body, or vascular abnormality. Neck films with the head in extension during inspiration can be used in differentiating croup and epiglottitis. The "steeple" sign, found in 40% to 50% of cases, is the classic sign of croup with narrowing of the subglottic space on anteroposterior (AP) neck films. However, this sign is non-specific and may also be seen in 5% of cases of epiglottitis. The lateral neck film may also show a swollen epiglottis or hypopharyngeal dilatation in epiglottitis. However, the false positive rate is about 24% to 30%. Some authors believe the test is unwarranted because of the inaccuracy with lateral neck films and potential delay in securing the airway.

Spirometry and Flow-Volume Loops

The flow-volume loop is a graphic representation of inspiratory and expiratory airflow on the Y-axis versus volume of air moved on the X-axis during maximal inspiratory and expiratory efforts. Substantial information is readily available from this simple test, including diagnosis and localization of airflow obstruction. The inspiratory curve of the loop is a relatively symmetric saddle-shaped curve. The expiratory part of the curve is characterized by a rapid rise to the peak expiratory flow rate and then followed by an almost linear decline in flow toward residual volume. The flow rate at the midpoint of both the expiratory and inspiratory flow loop is approximately equal. The location and nature of upper airway obstruction determines whether inspiratory, expiratory, or both flows are limited (Figure 19-1).

In variable extra-thoracic obstruction, also known as *dynamic* or *non-fixed extra-thoracic obstruction*, the inspiratory maneuver causes further narrowing of the extra-thoracic airway, appearing as a flattening in the inspiratory loop due to flow

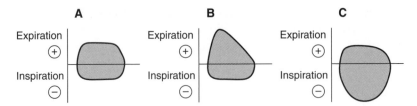

▼ **Figure 19-1** Flow-volume loops in upper airway obstruction. **A,** Fixed upper airway obstruction with flow limitation and flattening of both the inspiratory and expiratory limbs of the loop. **B,** Dynamic or variable, non-fixed extra-thoracic obstruction with flow limitation and flattening of the inspiratory limb of the loop. **C,** Dynamic or variable, non-fixed intra-thoracic obstruction with flow limitation and flattening of the expiratory limb of the loop. From Kryger M, Bode F, Antic R, et al: *Am J Med* 61(1): 85-93, 1976.

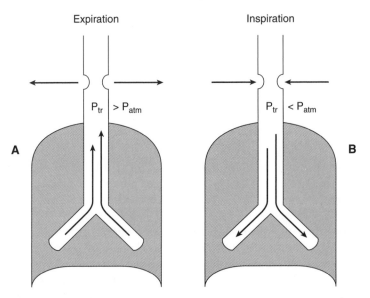

▼ **Figure 19-2** Effect of dynamic extra-thoracic airway obstruction. **A,** During forced expiration, intra-tracheal pressure (P_{tr}) exceeds the pressure around the airway (P_{atm}), lessening the obstruction. **B,** During forced inspiration, intra-tracheal pressure falls below the atmospheric pressure causing the obstruction to worsen with flow limitation. From Kryger M, Bode F, Antic R, et al: *Am J Med* 61(1): 85-93, 1976.

limitation (Figures 19-1, *B,* and 19-2). This pattern is usually associated with benign etiologies such as tracheomalacia and vocal cord processes.

In variable intra-thoracic obstruction, also known as *dynamic* or *non-fixed intra-thoracic obstruction,* the relative negative pleural pressure surrounding the intra-thoracic airway during inspiration does not cause any inspiratory flow impairment. However, during forced expiration, as the pleural pressure becomes positive relative to the trachea, narrowing of the intra-thoracic airway can occur with flattening of the expiratory loop due to worsening of any obstructing lesion in this region (Figures 19-1, *C,* and 19-3). This pattern can be associated with intra-thoracic tracheomalacia or malignant tracheal lesions.

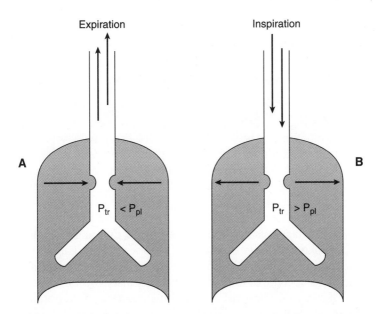

Expiration   Inspiration

A   B

$P_{tr} < P_{pl}$ $P_{tr} > P_{pl}$

▼ **Figure 19-3**   Effects of dynamic intra-thoracic airway obstruction. **A,** During forced expiration, the intra-thoracic intra-tracheal pressure (P_{tr}) is less than the pleural pressure (P_{pl}), worsening the obstruction. **B,** During forced inspiration, intra-tracheal pressure exceeds the pleural pressure, lessening the degree of obstruction. From Kryger M, Bode F, Antic R, et al: *Am J Med* 61(1): 85-93, 1976.

In fixed upper airway obstruction, a firm obstructing lesion prevents the modulating or narrowing effect of transmural pressures across the wall, resulting in flow limitation in both inspiration and expiration with flattening of both limbs of the loop (Figure 19-1, *A*).

Spirometry with flow-volume loops is not a sensitive test for the diagnosis of stridor and upper airway obstruction because it reflects the functional rather than the anatomic severity of the obstruction. Despite this limitation, it is a simple and available test and should be ordered in the appropriate clinical setting. However, because of its poor sensitivity, a normal flow-volume loop should be followed up with further evaluation when clinical suspicion is high.

Tomography

Conventional tomography has largely been replaced by CT for imaging airway lesions. Present indications for conventional tomography are (1) post-intubation tracheal stenosis where mediastinal abnormalities are not expected, (2) pre-operative assessment of the length of the lesion (better appreciated with tomography), and (3) post-operative assessment of the bronchial anastomoses. CT scanning is useful for the evaluation of mediastinal masses and compressive airway lesions but is limited by its inability to image the trachea along its long axis.

Magnetic Resonance Imaging

Magnetic resonance imaging (MRI) is the preferred imaging technique in infants and young children. Its advantages include lack of ionizing radiation, multiplanar imaging, good resolution without contrast, estimation of the length and degree of occlusion, and evaluation of the mediastinum.

Pitfalls and Common Mistakes in the Assessment and Treatment of Stridor

It is essential to distinguish between stridor and lower airway sounds, but errors can be made since asthmatic wheezes and stridor can have similar pitch and frequency. To facilitate this distinction, stridor is usually heard in inspiration and is loudest in the neck, with maneuvers increasing flow, such as voluntary hyperventilation, accentuating it. Tumors of the trachea and carina usually cause a gradual decrease in airway diameter. Patients often present with signs and symptoms of chronic airflow obstruction and wheezing for months, and some cases mislead the physician toward a diagnosis of asthma. Therefore a diagnosis of asthma of recent onset should provoke a closer evaluation of the upper airway. Failure to elicit a good history or inadequate attention to historical features, such as hoarseness or a muffled voice, that suggest a specific underlying cause may also result in missed or delayed diagnosis. The absence of a particular suggestive feature should not prevent further evaluation by other methods when the clinical index of suspicion is very high for a particular etiology, such as in the case of a near-normal flow-volume loop.

Another common pitfall is the confusion of functional vocal cord dysfunction with asthma. Pulsus paradoxus can be present in functional vocal cord dysfunction, and the dramatic presentation can lead to intubation, tracheotomy, and prolonged steroid therapy. A high degree of suspicion should be present if the patient has little difficulty completing full sentences, can hold his or her breath, can abolish the laryngeal-induced sounds during a panting maneuver or cough and with sedation and anesthesia despite the severe respiratory distress. Laryngeal sounds may also decrease with switching from mouth to nose breathing and during talking.

▼ BIBLIOGRAPHY

Aboussouan LS, Stoller JK: Diagnosis and management of upper airway obstruction, *Clin Chest Med* 15(1):35-53, 1994.

Baughman RP, Loudon RG: Stridor: differentiation from asthma or upper airway noise, *Am Rev Respir Dis* 139(6):1407-1409, 1989.

Colice GL, Stukel TA, Dain B: Laryngeal complication of prolonged intubation, *Chest* 96(4): 877-884, 1989.

Kryger M, Bode F, Antic R, et al: Diagnosis of obstruction of the upper and central airways, *Am J Med* 61(1):85-93, 1976.

Megerian CA, Arnold JE, Berger M: Angioedema: 5 years' experience with a review of the disorder's presentation and treatment, *Laryngoscope* 102(3):256-260, 1992.

Morton NS, Barr GW: Stridor in an adult: an unusual presentation of functional origin, *Anaesthesia* 44(3):232-234, 1989.

CHAPTER 20

CAVITARY PULMONARY INFILTRATE

David L. Longworth

▼ Cavitary pulmonary
  infiltrate
▼ Tuberculosis

▼ Histoplasmosis
▼ Lung abscess
▼ Aspiration

▼ Pneumonia
▼ Lung cancer

▼ THE CLINICAL PROBLEM

A 45-year-old man presents in the emergency room with a 4-week history of low-grade fever, cough productive of yellow sputum, anorexia, night sweats, and a 15-pound weight loss. Today, he has coughed up approximately 1 teaspoon of blood, prompting his visit to the emergency room.

Past medical history is notable for a seizure disorder that developed after head trauma 15 years ago. He is poorly compliant with his phenytoin, and his last seizure was 6 weeks ago. He says that on several occasions over the past 10 years he has been hospitalized for an infection of the heart valves, but he cannot provide further details. On additional questioning, he says he uses intravenous heroin several times a week and occasionally shares needles. His last drug use was yesterday. His only medication is phenytoin 300 mg daily.

His family history is notable for an uncle who died of pulmonary tuberculosis; the patient was exposed to him as a child when growing up in rural Kentucky but was never skin tested. Social history is notable for the fact that he smoked 1 pack/day for the past 30 years, but he denies alcohol use. He came to Cleveland 4 months ago after hitchhiking cross-country from Los Angeles, where he lived for the past 5 years. He says he spent several weeks in Las Vegas visiting a friend and that they traveled out into the desert to several nearby national parks. He has done odd jobs over the years and for the past 3 months has worked as a construction worker in downtown Cleveland, where he is involved in excavation for a new office tower. Performing his job has become increasingly difficult with this illness. He lives alone and has no pets. He is heterosexual but has not been sexually active in recent years.

On physical examination, he is a thin, chronically ill man in no apparent distress. His temperature is 100° F, blood pressure 125/70 mm Hg, heart rate 82 and regular, and respiratory rate 14 and unlabored. His skin is notable only for track marks on his arms. The examination of the head, eyes, ears, nose, and throat discloses normal conjunctiva and sclera and poor dentition with multiple carious teeth. There is no adenopathy. His chest is clear to auscultation and percussion. On cardiac examination, the rate is regular and there is a grade 2/6 systolic murmur at the lower left sternal border radiating to the apex, increased with forced expiration. There are no gallops. The abdomen is soft, non-tender, and without organ enlargement. The extremities are unremarkable, the joints are normal, and the neurologic examination is intact.

Several routine diagnostic studies are obtained. His leucocyte count is 12,100 cells/mm^3 with a differential that includes 80% granulocytes, 12% monocytes, 5% lymphocytes, and 3% eosinophils. The hemoglobin is 10.2 g/dL, and platelet count 125,000 cells/mm^3. The electrolytes, liver function studies, and urinalysis are normal. A chest x-ray discloses a 2 × 2-cm cavity with surrounding infiltrate in the right upper lobe (Figure 20-1, A). Computed tomography (CT) of the chest confirms these findings (Figure 20-1, B). Pulse oximetry discloses an oxygen saturation of 96% on room air.

What is the differential diagnosis for this patient's problem? What further tests are indicated? How should the patient be managed?

Differential Diagnosis of the Cavitary Pulmonary Infiltrate

The differential diagnosis of a cavitary pulmonary infiltrate includes both infectious and non-infectious etiologies. Common and less common causes are summarized in Box 20-1 and are further classified by the type of organism. The pace of the illness is also helpful in assessing the likely cause of a cavitary pulmonary infiltrate. Classifying the illness as acute versus subacute or chronic can further narrow the differential diagnosis as shown in Box 20-2.

In the developed world, the most common causes of cavitary pulmonary infiltrates are tuberculosis, pyogenic lung abscess, histoplasmosis, blastomycosis, coccidioidomycosis, and pulmonary aspergillosis in selected patient populations. *Mycobacterium tuberculosis* has undergone a resurgence in the United States in the past 15 years, owing in part to the acquired immunodeficiency syndrome (AIDS) epidemic. Pulmonary tuberculosis can present as a primary pneumonia (usually

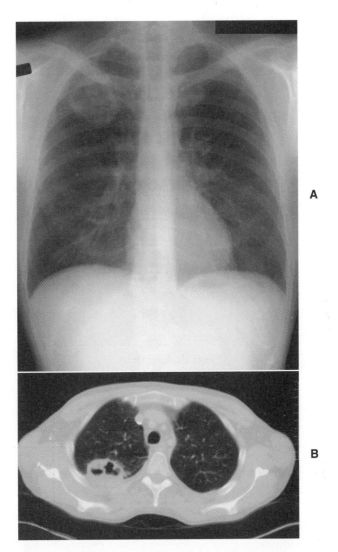

▼ **Figure 20-1**   **A,** Right upper lobe cavity is present on the plain film of the chest. **B,** Small surrounding infiltrate is seen on the CT scan.

involving a lower lobe) when infection is initially acquired, or as a subacute pulmonary process, often with an upper lobe cavitary infiltrate, when the disease reactivates.

Reactivation pulmonary tuberculosis occurs most commonly in the first 5 to 10 years following primary infection, but can occur decades later. Reactivation pulmonary tuberculosis may occur in the setting of immunosuppression, including in patients with recognized or unrecognized human immunodeficiency virus (HIV) infection or in those receiving immunosuppressive medications for malignancy, transplantation, or other medical illnesses. Patients with reactivation pulmonary tuberculosis typically present with a subacute or chronic illness over weeks to several months characterized by fever, productive cough (occasionally with hemoptysis),

Box 20-1
Differential Diagnosis of a Cavitary Pulmonary Infiltrate

Common Causes	Less Common Causes
Bacterial Infections	**Bacterial Infections**
Tuberculosis	Non-tuberculous mycobacterial infections
Pyogenic lung abscess	Nocardiosis
	Staphylococcus aureus pneumonia
	Gram-negative pneumonia
	Legionellosis
	Septic pulmonary infarct
	Melioidosis
	Corynebacterium equi
	Cysts or bullae with fluid collections
	Bronchiectasis
	Empyema with air fluid level
Fungal Infections	**Fungal Infections**
Histoplasmosis	Pulmonary zygomycosis
Blastomycosis	Paracoccidioidomycosis
Coccidioidomycosis	Cryptococcosis
Aspergillosis	
	Parasitic Infections
	Echinococcosis
	Pragonimiasis
	Amebiasis
	Non-Infectious Causes
	Malignancy
	Pulmonary infarct
	Wegener's granulomatosis
	Polyarteritis nodosa
	Pulmonary sequestration

PCP, Pneumocystis carinii pneumonia.

night sweats, anorexia, and weight loss. Pulmonary tuberculosis occurs with higher frequency in HIV-infected individuals, especially in selected urban areas, and may be the presenting manifestation of HIV infection. In individuals with suspected or proven tuberculosis, a risk history for HIV infection should be obtained.

Pyogenic lung abscess is usually a polymicrobial infection involving mouth organisms and arises following an aspiration event. This may be recognized or unrecognized, but the diagnosis should be entertained in those with underlying illnesses likely to result in aspiration, such as seizure disorder, syncope, substance abuse complicated by obtundation, and neurologic disorders characterized by loss of the gag reflex. Although occasionally the clinical illness may be acute, patients with pyogenic lung abscess more typically present with a subacute or chronic illness over weeks or even a few months characterized by fever, cough productive

Box 20-2
Causes Associated with an Acute Versus Subacute
or Chronic Presentation*

Acute Presentation	Subacute or Chronic Presentation
Staphylococcus aureus pneumonia	Tuberculosis
Gram-negative pneumonia	Pyogenic lung abscess
Legionellosis	Histoplasmosis
Septic or bland pulmonary infarct	Coccidioidomycosis
Pyogenic lung abscess	Blastomycosis
Aspergillosis	Aspergillosis
	Nocardiosis
	Non-tuberculous mycobacterial infections
	PCP
	Zygomycosis
	Paracoccidioidomycosis
	Melioidosis
	Echinococcosis
	Malignancy

PCP, Pneumocystis carinii pneumonia.
*An *acute* process is defined as a duration of illness of less than 1 week. A *subacute* or *chronic* process is defined as a duration of illness of several weeks to a few months.

of foul sputum, weight loss, and constitutional symptoms. An episode of loss of consciousness may have preceded the onset of the illness by several weeks.

Histoplasmosis is endemic in the upper midwestern United States, especially in the Ohio and Mississippi river valleys. It is produced by the dimorphic fungus, *Histoplasma capsulatum*. Infection is acquired by inhalation of dust or dirt containing the organism. Like tuberculosis, it may produce a primary pneumonia, although this is usually self-limited and may not come to medical attention unless the inhalational exposure is significant. More often, histoplasmosis presents as a subacute or chronic cavitary pneumonia, which may mimic cavitary pulmonary tuberculosis, characterized by fever, cough, or sputum that may be blood-tinged and constitutional symptoms.

Blastomycosis is produced by the fungus *Blastomyces dermatitidis* and produces an illness and cavitary pneumonia that may mimic reactivation pulmonary tuberculosis or chronic cavitary histoplasmosis. Blastomycosis is endemic throughout the Southeastern United States and the upper Midwest. The organism is found along waterways, and a history of such exposure should be carefully sought, especially to beaver dams. Infection may also be acquired at construction or excavation sites. Subcutaneous nodules occur in up to 10% of patients with blastomycosis, and the finding of such nodules on physical examination may provide a helpful clinical clue to the diagnosis.

Coccidioides immitis is the causative fungal agent of coccidioidomycosis and is acquired by inhalation of the organism, which is endemic in the southwestern

United States and in the San Joaquin Valley of central California. The diagnosis should be considered in patients with recent travel or residence in those areas, especially if they recall inhalational exposure to dust, sand, or dirt. Like histoplasmosis, pulmonary coccidioidomycosis may present as a self-limited acute pneumonia without cavitation, often accompanied by eosinophilia and occasionally by erythema nodosum, and as a subacute or chronic illness with a cavitary pulmonary infiltrate and constitutional symptoms.

Aspergillosis can produce five clinical syndromes involving the lung. These include allergic bronchopulmonary aspergillosis, acute aspergillus pneumonia, semi-invasive pulmonary aspergillosis, invasive pulmonary aspergillosis, and an isolated non-invasive fungus ball in a pre-existing cavity. The latter three are associated with the presence of cavitary pulmonary infiltrates.

Semi-invasive pulmonary aspergillosis and fungus balls in pre-existing cavities are most often seen in patients with underlying chronic lung disease. Patients usually present with a subacute illness characterized by cough and constitutional symptoms. Fever is often absent. Hemoptysis is common and may be the symptom that prompts the patient to seek medical attention. The cavity may or may not have a significant surrounding infiltrate and often has a "fungus ball" within the cavity; biopsy of the wall of the cavity may be necessary to distinguish semi-invasive disease from an isolated fungus ball. In semi-invasive disease, the cavity wall may contain organisms, but they generally do not invade the lung parenchyma.

Invasive pulmonary aspergillosis is almost always a disease of immunocompromised individuals, and is most often seen in bone marrow transplant recipients, patients with leukemia, or lymphoreticular malignancies receiving chemotherapy, and, less often, other patients receiving chronic immunosuppression for a variety of conditions. The infiltrate may or may not be cavitating. Rare cases have been reported in immunocompetent individuals following significant inhalational exposure to dust or dirt containing *Aspergillus* species; most such cases have occurred in those with underlying lung disease.

The clinical presentation in immunocompromised hosts can be acute, subacute, chronic, or even asymptomatic. When acute, the initial presentation is often one of new onset hemoptysis; fever may or may not be present. Patients with subacute or chronic presentations may complain of fever, cough, hemoptysis, and constitutional symptoms. Pulmonary aspergillosis is occasionally recognized in at-risk asymptomatic individuals, such as bone marrow transplant recipients, in whom a routine chest x-ray or computed tomographic scan of the chest is performed for another reason. In such patients, the finding of a cavitary pulmonary infiltrate necessitates a diagnostic evaluation, even in the absence of symptoms. Because of the propensity of *Aspergillus* species to invade blood vessels when present in the lung, hemoptysis is frequent and is often the sentinel complaint in patients with invasive pulmonary aspergillosis. A history of hemoptysis in such an individual should suggest the diagnosis.

There are many less common causes of cavitary pulmonary infiltrates as summarized in Box 20-1. Patients with acute bacterial pneumonia due to *Staphylococcus aureus*, gram-negative bacilli, and *Legionella* species may occasionally have infiltrates accompanied by cavities. In general, cavities are small and occur within sizeable surrounding infiltrates. In the case of *S. aureus* and gram-negative bacilli, these typically thin-walled cavities are termed "pneumatoceles." Non-tuberculous mycobacteria such as *Mycobacterium kansasii* can produce a cavitary infiltrate and a clinical illness resembling pulmonary tuberculosis. *M. kansasii* has been described in HIV-infected individuals in the Southern United States.

Nocardiosis, produced by one of several *Nocardia* species, occurs predominantly in immunocompromised individuals receiving chronic medications that suppress cell-mediated immunity. At-risk individuals include transplant recipients and those receiving chronic corticosteroid therapy, usually in excess of 20 mg of prednisone per day. Nocardiosis is rare in HIV-infected individuals but has been described. Trimethoprim-sulfamethoxazole prophylaxis given for prevention of *Pneumocystis carinii* pneumonia (PCP) is effective in preventing nocardiosis. In individuals at risk for nocardiosis who are not receiving such prophylaxis, the diagnosis should be considered.

Corynebacterium equi may produce cavitary infiltrates in HIV-infected individuals and in transplant recipients receiving chronic immunosuppressive therapy. A history of exposure to horses, which carry the organism and shed it in their stool, should suggest the diagnosis. Infection is acquired by inhalation of the organism. Melioidosis is produced by the gram-negative bacillus *Pseudomonas pseudomallei*, which is endemic in Southeast Asia. Melioidosis may present as an acute and fulminant gram-negative pneumonia, as bacteremia producing sepsis syndrome, or as a subacute or chronic illness mimicking pulmonary tuberculosis accompanied by a cavitary pulmonary infiltrate.

Pulmonary emboli may occasionally produce cavitary pulmonary infiltrates, which tend to be peripheral and pleural-based on the chest x-ray. These most often represent septic (or infected) pulmonary infarcts seen in the setting of right-sided infective endocarditis (most often seen in intravenous drug users) or in patients with chronic indwelling central venous catheters who develop infected lines and/or surrounding venous thrombi that embolize to the lung. The clinical presentation is usually acute.

Less common fungal causes of cavitary infiltrates include the zygomycoses (produced by *Mucor, Absidia,* and *Rhizopus* species), paracoccidioidomycosis, and cryptococcosis. The zygomycoses usually produce cavitary pneumonias in patients who are immunosuppressed by virtue of underlying leukemia or organ transplantation. In organ transplant recipients, zygomycosis is most often seen months to years following transplantation. *Paracoccidioides brasiliensis* is endemic in Central and South America and may mimic tuberculosis in its presentation. Pulmonary cryptococcosis occurs predominantly in chronically immunosuppressed individuals who are receiving corticosteroids or who are HIV-infected, but occasionally can produce clinical illness in immunocompetent hosts. The illness is usually subacute in presentation and accompanied by a patchy or nodular lung infiltrate; cavitation is uncommon, but occurs.

PCP is seen in HIV-infected individuals with CD4 counts less than 200 cells/μL who are not receiving appropriate prophylaxis, and in patients receiving medications that chronically suppress cell-mediated immunity, especially solid organ transplant recipients not receiving PCP prophylaxis. Pneumonia usually presents as a subacute illness with dry cough and progressive dyspnea on exertion. The chest x-ray typically discloses diffuse interstitial infiltrates, although it may be normal in patients with early infection. A small percentage of patients will also have small thin-walled cavities accompanying the infiltrates; cavities without infiltrates should not be ascribed to PCP.

The helminthic parasite *Echinococcus granulosus* can produce cystic lesions of the lung that mimic cavitary pulmonary infiltrates; however, the lesions are cysts rather than true cavities. The liver is the most common organ involved in echinococcosis, but pulmonary involvement occurs in 25% of infected individuals. Echinococcosis, also termed *cystic hydatid disease,* is endemic in the Mediterranean and throughout the developing world and is acquired through the ingestion of food contaminated with eggs of the parasite, most often shed in stool of infected sheepdogs. Patients usually present with cough and occasionally hemoptysis. Travel to or residence in an endemic area, even in the remote past, should prompt consideration of the diagnosis, which is also often suggested by the radiographic appearance of the cyst.

Paragonimiasis is another helminthic infection that may produce lung cysts that resemble small cavities in the chronic phase of the illness. Paragonimiasis is most often produced by *Paragonimus westermani,* which is endemic in Southeast Asia. Infection is acquired by ingesting raw or undercooked freshwater crustaceans, such as crabs and crayfish. Rare cases produced by other *Paragonimus* species and acquired in this fashion have been described in the Southern United States in the Mississippi River basin.

Amebiasis is produced by the protozoan parasite *Entamoeba histolytica,* which is endemic throughout the developing world and which may produce dysentery and occasionally liver abscess. On rare occasion, amebic liver abscesses may rupture through the diaphragm and produce a parasitic empyema and cavitary pulmonary infiltrate; this most often involves the right lower or right middle lobes.

Other rare causes of cavitary pulmonary infiltrates include Wegener's granulomatosis (a granulomatous vasculitis with a propensity to involve lung, kidney, and the paranasal sinuses), pulmonary cysts that become secondarily infected, pulmonary sequestration, bronchiectasis, and malignancies (such as lymphomas or primary or metastatic carcinomas).

Clinical Features that Suggest a Specific Cause of a Cavitary Pulmonary Infiltrate

A number of features of a patient's illness may help to elucidate the cause of a cavitary pulmonary infiltrate. As outlined in Box 20-2, the pace of the illness may be very helpful. A sudden and acute respiratory illness of less than a week's duration accompanied by fever and a cavitary infiltrate is most likely to be bacterial in origin. In profoundly immunosuppressed individuals, such as bone marrow transplant recipients, the sudden onset of hemoptysis and a cavity on the chest x-ray should suggest invasive pulmonary aspergillosis. Mycobacterial, fungal, parasitic, and malignant causes of cavitary infiltrates usually produce more indolent and subacute illnesses in which patients present either with less severe symptoms at the outset or a history of escalating symptoms over several weeks or even months. Occasionally, however, hemoptysis may be the sentinel symptom that prompts evaluation.

Box 20-3 summarizes aspects of the history that should be explored in every patient with a cavitary pulmonary infiltrate, as they may provide clues to the etiology. These include an assessment concerning prior exposure to and skin test-

Box 20-3
Essential History Considerations
in a Cavitary Pulmonary Infiltrate

Prior exposure to tuberculosis
Prior skin tests for tuberculosis
Recent contacts with sick individuals
Recent loss of consciousness
Travel and residence history
Risk factors for human immunodeficiency virus infection
Underlying illnesses and past history
Medications
Occupation
Hobbies and unusual exposures
Associated symptoms such as pleuritic chest pain, headache,
   or the presence of subcutaneous masses

ing for tuberculosis. In patients who have such a history, further information should be obtained regarding the results of prior chest x-rays and whether isoniazid prophylaxis was administered. In many instances, it is helpful to obtain old chest x-rays for comparison. Recent contact with individuals with active respiratory illnesses should also be assessed.

A careful travel and residence history should be elicited to explore potential recent or remote exposure to histoplasmosis, blastomycosis, coccidioidomycosis, paracoccidioidomycosis, echinococcosis, paragonimiasis, and tuberculosis. In individuals who have resided in or traveled to parts of the world where these diseases are endemic, further questioning should explore activities while in these areas that might heighten the risk of acquiring these pathogens. As an example, someone who recently traveled to California and spent the entire time in Los Angeles would be at very low risk of having acquired coccidioidomycosis. On the other hand, travel to the San Joaquin Valley where a dust storm was encountered would significantly heighten the risk of acquiring the disease.

Risk factors for HIV infection should be obtained in all individuals with a cavitary infiltrate, as should a careful medical history regarding underlying illnesses and medication use, especially corticosteroid and immunosuppressive medications. The issue of recreational marijuana use should be explored, as this has been associated with the development of invasive aspergillosis in immunocompromised individuals. A careful history regarding occupation, hobbies, and unusual recent activities or exposures should be obtained. Finally, a careful review of systems should be performed, as the presence of certain associated symptoms may help to narrow the differential diagnosis. This should specifically explore whether the patient has lost consciousness in recent weeks and whether specific aspiration events are recalled. In selected individuals, a dietary history may be very relevant, as discussed below.

Table 20-1 outlines specific features of the history that should suggest specific causes for a cavitary infiltrate. The presence of one of these historical features by no means assures that the infiltrate is caused by the associated organism(s), but it should heighten one's concern and prompt aggressive diagnostic evaluation.

A prior history of exposure to tuberculosis, especially if in the recent past, should suggest the diagnosis. Patients with even a remote exposure history, however, may develop reactivation cavitary tuberculosis, especially if they are immunosuppressed and if they have never received isoniazid prophylaxis. Pulmonary tuberculosis may be the presenting illness in patients with underlying HIV infection, and risk factors for HIV should be elicited in every patient with an unexplained cavity on chest x-ray. Other causes of cavitary disease in HIV-infected individuals include histoplasmosis, coccidioidomycosis, *M. kansasii*, and, rarely, nocardiosis or *Corynebacterium equi*.

In addition to the risk of acquiring HIV infection, intravenous drug use is also associated with the development of infective endocarditis, most often due to *Staphylococcus aureus*, gram-negative bacilli such as *Pseudomonas aeruginosa*, and, rarely, *Candida albicans*. Intravenous drug users may infect valves on the left or right sides of the heart but have a higher incidence of right-sided endocarditis involving the tricuspid valve, compared with otherwise healthy individuals who develop endocarditis. Right-sided endocarditis may result in vegetations on the tricuspid valve, which break off and embolize to the lungs, producing septic pulmonary infarcts. Such events typically present with the sudden onset of pleuritic chest pain and shortness of breath. Chest x-rays classically reveal peripheral wedge-shaped pleural-based infiltrates that go on to cavitate. Occasionally, however, such cavities are more central. The presence of chronic indwelling central venous catheters in a patient with a cavity on chest film should also suggest pulmonary infarct as the most likely cause, as such individuals may develop bland or septic thrombi involving the line and surrounding vein, which may occasionally embolize.

Residence in urban shelters for the homeless or nursing homes should suggest tuberculosis, which occurs with higher frequency in such settings. Residence in or travel to selected parts of the United States and abroad should prompt consideration of certain organisms endemic in these specific locales, as summarized in Table 20-1. Bone marrow transplant recipients and patients with acute leukemia who have received multiple cycles of intensive chemotherapy and who present with a cavitary pulmonary infiltrate have fungal disease, such as aspergillosis or zygomycosis, until proven otherwise. In other individuals receiving chronic immunosuppression with corticosteroids, such as solid organ transplant recipients, the differential diagnosis may include aspergillosis, tuberculosis, nocardiosis, cryptococcosis, *Corynebacterium equi*, and cavitary pneumocystosis. Health care workers with a cavitary infiltrate should have the diagnosis of tuberculosis pursued aggressively, especially if a contact history can be elicited. Construction workers and other individuals exposed to construction or excavation sites are at special risk for blastomycosis and histoplasmosis in parts of the country where these diseases are endemic, as well as to legionellosis.

Exposure to rivers and beaver dams in the upper midwestern and southeastern United States should suggest blastomycosis; a history of exposure to fresh or standing water should also suggest legionellosis, especially if the patient has inhaled

TABLE 20-1
Historical Clues to the Cause of a Cavitary Pulmonary

History	Potential Causes
General	
Prior exposure to or positive skin test for tuberculosis, especially if immunocompromised and not on prophylaxis	Tuberculosis
Residence in homeless shelters, nursing home	Tuberculosis
Travel or residence in upper midwestern US or Ohio or Mississippi river valleys	Histoplasmosis, blastomycosis
Southeastern US, Kentucky, Tennessee	Blastomycosis
Southwestern US or central California	Coccidioidomycosis
Southeast Asia	Tuberculosis, melioidosis, paragonimiasis
Central or South America	Paracoccidioidomycosis, tuberculosis
Risk factor for HIV infection	Tuberculosis, histoplasmosis, coccidioidomycosis, non-tuberculous mycobacteria, nocardiosis, *Corynebacterium equi*
Intravenous drug use	Septic pulmonary infarct due to right-sided infective endocarditis, tuberculosis (HIV positive)
Recent loss of consciousness	Pyogenic lung abscess
Bone marrow transplant recipient	Aspergillosis
Acute leukemia on intensive therapy	Zygomycosis
Chronic indwelling central venous catheter	Septic pulmonary embolus
Chronic corticosteroids, immunosuppression	Aspergillosis, tuberculosis, nocardiosis, cryptococcosis, *Corynebacterium equi*
Occupation	
Health care worker	Tuberculosis
Construction worker (in appropriate locale)	Histoplasmosis, blastomycosis, legionellosis
Farmer (chickens)	Histoplasmosis
Hobbies and Exposures	
Rivers, beaver dams	Blastomycosis
Spelunker, clean gutters, exposure to bird or chicken feces	Histoplasmosis
Horses	*Corynebacterium equi*
Construction or excavation sites (in appropriate locale)	Legionellosis, histoplasmosis, blastomycosis
Fresh or standing water (lake, etc)	Legionellosis
Associated Symptoms	
Sudden pleuritic chest pain	Septic pulmonary embolus
Subcutaneous masses or nodules	Nocardiosis, blastomycosis, cryptococcosis
Erythema nodosum	Tuberculosis, histoplasmosis, coccidioidomycosis
Headache, seizures, or neurologic symptoms	Tuberculosis, histoplasmosis, cryptococcosis, nocardiosis, aspergillosis, legionellosis, echinococcosis
Sinus symptoms	

HIV, Human immunodeficiency virus.

aerosolized sprays. The presence of headache, seizures, or neurologic symptoms should suggest tuberculosis with meningitis or tuberculoma, cryptococcosis with meningitis or cryptococcoma, histoplasmosis with meningitis, coccidioidomycosis with meningitis, nocardiosis with brain abscess, or legionellosis. The rash of erythema nodosum consists of tender erythematous nodules involving the shins and is associated with tuberculosis, histoplasmosis, and coccidioidomycosis. Subcutaneous nodules are associated with nocardiosis and blastomycosis in about 10% of cases and rarely with cryptococcosis; in the latter instance, the nodules may ulcerate and drain. Sinusitis or glomerulonephritis should suggest the possibility of a systemic vasculitis such as Wegener's granulomatosis.

The physical examination is often unhelpful in patients with a cavitary pulmonary infiltrate, although certain physical findings may help to narrow the differential diagnosis if present, as summarized in Table 20-2; these are rarely diagnostic, however. Findings that should suggest the diagnosis of pyogenic lung abscess include fetid breath, poor dentition, an absent gag reflex, clubbing (in the setting of congenital heart disease), and a succussion splash. The latter finding is elicited by listening over the chest with a stethoscope, rocking the patient back and forth, and listening for the presence of a splash, which is produced by the presence of shifting fluid in a large cavity that communicates with the endobronchial tree (and thus contains air). Tracks from intravenous drug use or stigmata of infective endocarditis involving the skin, nailbeds, or mucous membranes should suggest the diagnosis of right-sided endocarditis with septic pulmonary infarct.

TABLE 20-2
Findings on Physical Examination Suggestive of the Cause of a Cavitary Pulmonary Infiltrate

Physical Finding	Likely Causes
Fetid breath, gingivitis, poor dentition, absent gag reflex	Pyogenic lung abscess
Tracks from intravenous drug use	Septic pulmonary embolus from right-sided infective endocarditis; causes of cavitary infiltrates associated with underlying HIV infection
Cutaneous stigmata of infective endocarditis (Osler's nodes, Janeway lesions, conjunctival petechiae)	Septic pulmonary embolus from right-sided infective endocarditis (although these suggest concomitant left-sided disease)
Erythema nodosum	Tuberculosis, histoplasmosis, coccidioidomycosis
Subcutaneous nodules	Nocardiosis, blastomycosis; cryptococcosis
Tricuspid regurgitation	Septic pulmonary infarct from right-sided infective endocarditis
Succussion splash	Pyogenic lung abscess
Cranial neuropathies	Tuberculosis; histoplasmosis, coccidioidomycosis, cryptococcosis
Clubbing	Pyogenic lung abscess

HIV, Human imunodeficiency virus.

Diagnostic Testing in the Evaluation of the Patient with a Cavitary Pulmonary Infiltrate

Diagnostic testing in patients with a cavitary pulmonary infiltrate is driven by the pace and severity of the illness, clues in the history that suggest a specific pathogen, host factors, the presence of associated findings that suggest other sites of involvement, and the location of the cavity. General guidelines are presented in Table 20-3.

As outlined in Box 20-2, immunocompetent patients with an acute presentation who are symptomatic for less than a week usually have a bacterial infection. Thus the diagnostic evaluation should include a sputum Gram's stain and culture and

TABLE 20-3
Diagnostic Testing in the Evaluation of Cavitary Pulmonary Infiltrate

Clinical Setting	Diagnostic Tests
Acute Presentation	
Immunocompetent host	Blood cultures, sputum Gram's stain and culture, sputum DFA for *Legionella*, *Legionella* urinary antigen, acute and convalescent *Legionella* serologies, bronchoscopy occasionally indicated
Immunocompromised host	As above, bronchoscopy usually indicated
Suggestive Clues	
Pyogenic lung abscess	Sputum Gram's stain, blood cultures, bronchoscopy, transthoracic needle aspiration sometimes indicated
Fungal pathogens	Sputum for KOH, fungal culture, fungal serologies, serum cryptococcal antigen, histoplasma urinary antigen, bronchoscopy indicated if above work-up negative
Tuberculosis or MOTT infection	Sputum AFB smears and cultures, PPD with controls, HIV EIA, bronchoscopy indicated if smears negative
Nocardiosis	Sputum for modified AFB smears and cultures, bronchoscopy often indicated if smears negative
PCP	Sputum for PCP, bronchoscopy indicated if sputum unavailable or smears negative
Septic pulmonary infarct	Blood cultures, echocardiogram, duplex ultrasound or venography in those with indwelling central lines and suspected thrombi
Paragonimiasis, echinococcosis, amebiasis	Serology, sputum for ova and parasites, bronchoscopy indicated if above non-diagnostic
Malignancy	Sputum cytology, bronchoscopy, thoracotomy, mediastinoscopy
Wegener's granulomatosis	C-ANCA, sinus endoscopy and biopsy, bronchoscopy and biopsy or surgical lung biopsy

DFA, Direct fluorescent antibody; *AFB,* acid-fast bacilli; *PPD,* purified protein derivative (tuberculin); *HIV EIA,* human immunodeficiency virus electroimmunoassay; *PCP, Pneumocystis carinii* pneumonia; *C-ANCA,* cytoplasmic anti-neutrophilic cytoplasmic antibody.   *Continued*

TABLE 20-3
Diagnostic Testing in the Evaluation of Cavitary
Pulmonary Infiltrate—cont'd

Clinical Setting	Diagnostic Tests
Immunocompromised Host	Bronchoscopy almost always indicated
Neurologic findings	CT brain, lumbar puncture
Subcutaneous nodules	Biopsy and culture of nodules
Sinusitis	Sinus endoscopy and biopsy
Glomerulonephritis	C-ANCA; renal biopsy
Peripheral cavity	Transthoracic needle aspiration sometimes indicated
Subacute or chronic presentation, no clues	PPD with controls; sputum smears and cultures for AFB, fungi; fungal serologies; sputum cytology, urinalysis; serum creatinine; C-ANCA; bronchoscopy indicated if above non-diagnostic; transthoracic or open lung biopsy if bronchoscopy non-diagnostic

CT, Computed tomography; C-ANCA, cytoplasmic anti-neutrophilic cytoplasmic antibody. PPD, purified protein derivative (tuberculin); AFB, acid-fast bacilli.

cultures of the blood. In those individuals in whom legionellosis is a possibility, a legionella urinary antigen should be obtained. This test is usually positive within 3 days of the onset of the illness in patients infected with *Legionella pneumophila* serogroup 1, which accounts for 80% of cases of legionellosis in the United States. The test is negative in the remaining 20% who have legionellosis due to another species or serogroup, and thus a negative test does not exclude the diagnosis of Legionnaire's disease. If legionellosis is suspected, direct fluorescent antibody testing of sputum for *Legionella* species should also be performed; it has a sensitivity of 40%. Serologies are often negative early in the illness, but an acute specimen should be collected so as to permit follow-up testing of a convalescent specimen 4 to 6 weeks later, which may be helpful in retrospectively establishing the diagnosis of Legionnaire's disease.

Bronchoscopy is occasionally indicated in immunocompetent hosts with an acute illness and a cavitary infiltrate, especially in those who are quite ill, unable to produce sputum, or in whom the routine studies outlined above are unrevealing. By contrast, immunocompromised hosts with an acute presentation and a cavity in the lung are almost always candidates for early diagnostic fiberoptic bronchoscopy, since the microbial differential diagnosis is broader, and, in selected individuals, such as bone marrow transplant recipients and leukemics, includes invasive aspergillosis.

In those with clues to the diagnosis in the history or on physical examination, diagnostic testing may be more focused. In patients with suspected pyogenic lung abscess, blood cultures should be collected, but are positive in only a small minority of cases. A sputum Gram's stain of an adequately collected specimen typically shows many polymorphonuclear leukocytes, few squamous epithelial cells, and mixed flora. In patients in whom the diagnosis is still uncertain, fiberoptic bronchoscopy or transthoracic aspiration of the cavity, if accessible, may help to confirm the diagnosis. In patients with suspected fungal pathogens such as *H. capsulatum*, *Blastomyces dermatitidis*, *Coccidioides immitis*, and *Cryptococcus neoformans*, sputum should be collected for microscopic examination and culture. Direct microscopy is positive for the organisms in fewer than 50% of cases and cultures require 4 to 6 weeks to grow; these studies may fail to establish the diagnosis at the time the patient presents.

Fungal serologies should also be obtained and are helpful if strongly positive, but may also be negative in the initial weeks of the illness, or in those who are immunocompromised. A serum cryptococcal antigen is positive in 25% to 30% of patients with pulmonary cryptococcosis. The urinary antigen test for *H. capsulatum* is positive in approximately 75% of patients with chronic pulmonary histoplasmosis. In those individuals in whom a fungal pathogen is suspected but who have negative stains of sputum and negative serologies, fiberoptic bronchoscopy is indicated if the cavity or surrounding infiltrate are accessible. Bronchoalveolar lavage and transbronchial biopsy should be performed for histopathology with appropriate staining for fungal organisms, as well as for culture. On occasion, when all studies are unrevealing, more invasive procedures such as lung biopsy may be indicated; convalescent fungal serologies performed 4 to 6 weeks later are also sometimes helpful in establishing a diagnosis.

In those with a history to suggest pulmonary tuberculosis or non-tuberculous mycobacterial infection (also termed *MOTT,* or Mycobacterium Other Than Tuberculosis), the first expectorated sputum of the morning should be collected, stained, and examined for acid-fast bacilli (AFB). Patients with cavitary disease usually have a high organism burden, and the sensitivity of direct microscopy on three sputum specimens is high in detecting mycobacteria. Cultures of sputum for mycobacteria should also be obtained but may take up to 6 weeks to grow. Molecular techniques have been developed to more rapidly identify mycobacteria isolated in culture based on recognition of a species' unique DNA sequence. Studies are underway to assess the utility of these techniques in detecting mycobacterial genetic material directly in expectorated sputum. All patients with suspected or confirmed tuberculosis should be questioned about risk factors for HIV infection, and HIV testing should be offered to those at risk. Finally, in those individuals in whom mycobacterial disease remains a diagnostic concern and in whom smears of sputum are unrevealing, fiberoptic bronchoscopy should be performed.

In patients with suspected nocardiosis, sputum specimens should be examined using a modified acid-fast stain, and cultures for *Nocardia* species should be performed. Direct microscopy is often unrewarding, however, and the organism may take several weeks to grow. Therefore bronchoscopy is frequently necessary to obtain fluid and tissue for additional smears and cultures.

P. carinii may be detected in expectorated sputum utilizing one of several stains; the sensitivity of direct microscopy in those able to produce sputum ranges from 40% to 80% in the literature. Most patients with PCP have a dry cough and are unable to produce sputum; bronchoscopy for smear is therefore usually indicated in those in whom the diagnosis is suspected. Cultures for *P. carinii* are not routinely performed.

In patients with suspected pulmonary infarcts from pulmonary emboli, diagnostic evaluation should focus on identifying the origin of the thromboembolus.

In those at risk for right-sided infective endocarditis, two-dimensional echocardiography should initially be performed in search of tricuspid or pulmonic valve vegetations. If this study is unrevealing, a transesophageal study is indicated and may detect vegetations not evident on surface echocardiography. In patients with chronic indwelling central venous catheters, pacemakers, or implantable cardiac defibrillators, duplex ultrasonography or venography of the upper extremity venous system should be performed to detect the presence of thrombi. Multiple cultures of blood collected over several hours should be obtained prior to the initiation of antimicrobial chemotherapy in patients with suspected endocarditis. In those with suspected infection of a chronic indwelling central venous catheter, quantitative blood cultures collected through each lumen of the catheter and peripherally may help prove that the line is infected and localize the involved lumen. The presence of a tenfold-higher concentration of organisms in blood drawn through the catheter compared with blood collected from a peripheral vein incriminates the line as the source of the bacteremia; negative peripheral blood cultures in the setting of positive blood cultures collected through the line also suggest the line as the source of infection.

In patients with a history to suggest potential exposure to paragonimiasis, amebiasis, or echinococcosis, serologic tests for the suspected organism are often helpful. Sputum specimens for ova and parasites may demonstrate the characteristic ova of *Paragonimus westermani* or the hooklets of *Echinococcus granulosus.*

In patients with suspected malignancy, sputum for cytology should be obtained, if possible. If non-diagnostic, further invasive studies such as bronchoscopy, mediastinoscopy, and open lung biopsy should be pursued. In patients with suspected lymphoma, such as those with lymphadenopathy or splenomegaly, biopsy of an enlarged lymph node or bone marrow examination may establish the diagnosis.

In patients with sinus or joint symptoms or findings to suggest glomerulonephritis, the diagnosis of Wegener's granulomatosis should be pursued in several ways. The C-ANCA blood test is positive in approximately 85% to 90% of individuals with Wegener's granulomatosis. Biopsy of sinus mucosa or the kidney may demonstrate the presence of granulomatous vasculitis, which is characteristic of the disease. If these tests are non-diagnostic, bronchoscopy or open lung biopsy may be necessary to obtain tissue for histopathologic examination for the presence of vasculitis.

The presence of localizing signs or symptoms may be helpful in further focusing the diagnostic evaluation. For example, the presence of focal neurologic findings should prompt a CT scan of the brain in search of a space-occupying mass lesion or abscess, which may be amenable to biopsy. The presence of meningeal signs or symptoms mandates a lumbar puncture and appropriate testing for tuberculous, fungal, and carcinomatous meningitis. Subcutaneous nodules should be biopsied, and specimens should be stained and cultured for mycobacteria, *Nocardia* species, and fungi. Patients with sinus symptoms should undergo a CT scan of the sinuses; if sinusitis is present, sinus endoscopy and biopsy should be performed in search of Wegener's granulomatosis. An active urinary sediment with red blood cell casts should prompt consideration of this diagnosis as well.

In immunocompetent patients with a subacute presentation who lack clues in the history and physical examination as to the cause of the infiltrate, initial diagnostic testing should include a skin test for tuberculosis with appropriate controls, sputum smears and cultures for mycobacteria and fungi, fungal serologies, sputum for cytology, a serum creatinine and urinalysis, and a C-ANCA. If these are unrevealing, fiberoptic bronchoscopy should be pursued if the lesion is accessible. If this is non-diagnostic or the lesion is inaccessible, open lung biopsy or resection is indicated. In immunocompromised hosts without clues in the history or physical examination, invasive tests such as bronchoscopy, mediastinoscopy, and lung biopsy are almost always indicated early in the diagnostic evaluation. In patients with peripheral cavities, transthoracic needle aspiration and biopsy is occasionally helpful.

Assessment of Therapy in a Cavitary Pulmonary Infiltrate

The tempo of the clinical response to therapy in the patient with the cavitary pulmonary infiltrate is determined by the underlying disease process, the size of the cavity, and host factors such as immunocompetence and the presence of comorbid illnesses. A detailed discussion of the appropriate therapy of the many illnesses that may produce cavitary pulmonary infiltrates is beyond the scope of this chapter. Nevertheless, several generalizations regarding response to therapy can be made.

Patients with bacterial pneumonias accompanied by cavitary infiltrates usually begin to improve clinically within several days to a week of initiation of appropriate therapy, although improvement in the cavitary infiltrate may lag behind and take longer. In those with septic pulmonary infarcts produced by right-sided infective endocarditis or infected chronic indwelling central venous catheters, clinical response is similarly fairly prompt.

Patients with pyogenic lung abscess generally defervesce and begin to improve clinically within 7 to 10 days of the initiation of appropriate antimicrobial chemotherapy. Radiographic resolution of the abscess may take several months, however, and some patients are left with a residual small cavity. Patients with cavitary tuberculosis, non-tuberculous mycobacterial infections, or fungal infections may require several weeks of therapy before a clinical response is evident; radiographic improvement typically takes weeks to months, and prolonged therapy is required. Depending on the specific infection, this may range from 6 to 18 months. In patients with cavitary pulmonary tuberculosis, sputum smears may remain positive for acid-fast bacilli (AFB) for several weeks. Persistently positive smears beyond this may be seen in those with extensive cavitary disease, but should raise concerns about poor compliance with therapy or drug resistance.

Patients with invasive pulmonary aspergillosis should begin to improve within 1 to 2 weeks of initiation of antifungal therapy, although the infection may be fatal despite aggressive treatment. Every effort should be made to withdraw immunosuppression to the extent possible. Radiographic resolution of the cavity may take weeks to months, and the duration of antifungal therapy is dictated by clinical and radiographic progress, as well as the degree of ongoing immunosuppression of the host. At a minimum, 1.5 g of amphotericin B (usually 4 to 6 weeks of therapy) are required.

Patients with nocardiosis usually respond clinically with 1 to 2 weeks of initiation of antibacterial therapy. Radiographic improvement takes longer, and 4 to 6 months of therapy is typically necessary. Patients with paragonimiasis usually improve within weeks of initiating antihelminthic therapy, and those with pulmonary hydatid disease usually require resection for cure. The response to therapy in patients with cavitary pulmonary malignancies depends on the histology of the tumor and the type of therapy chosen. Lymphomas are treated with multidrug chemotherapy, and radiographic and clinical improvement typically takes several weeks. Patients with primary lung cancers should undergo curative resection if possible; in those with unresectable disease, the clinical and radiographic response to radiation or chemotherapy typically takes weeks or even months.

Pitfalls and Common Mistakes in the Assessment and Treatment of Patients with a Cavitary Pulmonary Infiltrate

There are several common pitfalls and mistakes in the assessment and management of patients with a cavitary pulmonary infiltrate. First is the failure to take a detailed history, especially with regard to potential exposures to tuberculosis and to fungal pathogens. Asking the right question may unlock the case. Patients often fail to volunteer information that is vital and relevant, such as remote exposure to a relative with tuberculosis or travel within recent months to geographic locales that they perceive to be irrelevant to their current illness. In many instances, very specific questions must be asked to identify a relevant exposure, especially to fungal pathogens such as *H. capsulatum* or *Blastomyces dermatitidis.*

Another common mistake is the failure to nevertheless consider tuberculosis when it seems unlikely. Tuberculosis is undergoing a resurgence in the United States and should be considered in every patient with a cavity in the lung. In those admitted to hospital, respiratory isolation is mandatory until the diagnosis is excluded. Failure to take such appropriate infection control precautions is a common mistake that may lead to the unnecessary exposure of health care workers and hospitalized patients to *M. tuberculosis.*

Another common mistake is to fail to consider the presence of underlying HIV infection in patients with tuberculosis. Not all patients will admit to an HIV risk behavior, and HIV testing should be offered to all individuals with tuberculosis, even if the risk of HIV infection appears by history to be low. An additional pitfall is failure to perform appropriate contact tracing in patients with tuberculosis. Tuberculosis is a reportable disease, and state and local public health departments should be notified of newly diagnosed cases. In most instances, they will assist with contact tracing and testing, but the respiratory clinician also bears responsibility to ensure that these activities are performed appropriately.

Several pitfalls in management merit comment. In patients with pulmonary tuberculosis, compliance with therapy is essential to avoid the emergence of drug resistance. Respiratory clinicians must have a very low threshold for employing directly observed therapy (DOT) in those with newly diagnosed tuberculosis. Failure to improve within several weeks of initiating therapy should raise the specter of drug resistance, but should also prompt concern about compliance in those not receiving DOT.

Another pitfall in management relates to duration of therapy for selected diseases, such as pyogenic lung abscess, invasive pulmonary aspergillosis, nocardiosis, and cavitary fungal infections. The optimal duration of antimicrobial therapy for these respective infections has not been defined through well-controlled comparative clinical trials. A common mistake is to discontinue therapy prematurely. As a general rule, treatment of these respective infections should continue until clinical symptoms have resolved and until radiographic resolution of the process is demonstrated. In some instances, patients may be left with residual pulmonary parenchymal scarring and small cavities; however, before therapy is discontinued, the stability of these processes should be documented through serial chest x-rays and CT scans.

In this era of declining reimbursement for health care services and increased emphasis on shortening hospital length of stay and shifting care to the outpatient setting, patients with infective endocarditis rarely complete their parenteral antimicrobial therapy in hospital. In most instances, therapy is completed at home or in a subacute setting. This generally requires placement of a chronic indwelling central venous device. In patients with right-sided infective endocarditis in the setting of intravenous drug use, such devices provide a portal for ongoing intravenous drug use. Such patients may require these types of venous access, but should complete their therapy in observed settings such as extended care facilities with skilled nursing. In addition, these devices should be removed promptly following completion of therapy and negative follow-up test of cure blood cultures.

Evaluation and Management of the Patient with a Cavitary Pulmonary Infiltrate

The current patient presents with a subacute febrile illness, cough with hemoptysis, and a cavitary right upper lobe infiltrate. The history and physical examination are notable for several important clues. He has a history of active intravenous drug use along with findings on examination of track marks, raising the possibility of underlying HIV infection and right-sided bacterial endocarditis. He has a murmur, but it is more suggestive of mitral regurgitation rather than tricuspid regurgitation, since it increases in intensity with forced expiration (rather than inspiration, as occurs with tricuspid regurgitation) and radiates to the cardiac apex. He has a remote exposure to an uncle with tuberculosis, grew up in rural Kentucky where histoplasmosis is endemic, recently traveled through rural Nevada where coccidioidomycosis is present, and has worked on a construction site where he could have been exposed to histoplasmosis, blastomycosis, or legionellosis. In addition, he has a seizure disorder and last had a seizure 6 weeks ago, at which time he could have aspirated, raising the possibility of a pyogenic lung abscess.

The patient's lack of fetid breath on physical examination speaks against this diagnosis, but he has poor dentition with multiple carious teeth, making this a concern. On laboratory examination, he has anemia and mild thrombocytopenia. The anemia is non-specific and could be seen with multiple causes of a cavitary infiltrate. The thrombocytopenia raises several possibilities, however, including occult HIV infection and disseminated tuberculosis or fungal infection with marrow involvement. The differential diagnosis in this patient therefore includes tuberculosis, bacterial endocarditis, histoplasmosis, coccidioidomycosis, blastomycosis, legionellosis, and pyogenic lung abscess. In addition, underlying HIV infection must also be considered.

The appropriate diagnostic tests include sputum specimens for Gram's stain, routine culture for bacteria and *Legionella* species, direct fluorescent antibody (DFA) testing for *Legionella* species, and AFB and fungal smears and cultures. In addition, fungal serologies, a skin test for tuberculosis with controls, and HIV testing (after informed consent) should be performed. Several sets of blood cultures should be collected over several hours. Given the uncertainty regarding the diagnosis and the clinical stability of the patient, antibiotics should be withheld, pending establishing a diagnosis. An echocardiogram should be considered in the next 24 to 48 hours, especially if blood cultures are positive. If sputum smears are negative, a urine specimen should be sent for *Legionella* and *Histoplasma* urinary antigen testing, and an acute serum specimen should be sent for *Legionella* serology. The patient should be placed in respiratory isolation because of the concern about pulmonary tuberculosis.

The patient's initial sputum specimen is positive for AFB, and an HIV test is positive. Blood cultures and fungal serologies are negative. Four-drug antituberculous chemotherapy is commenced, and the patient is reported to the local and state public health departments, who contact his co-workers for screening. The sputum ultimately grows drug-susceptible *M. tuberculosis*. Serial sputum specimens are obtained over the next 10 days, which become smear negative. He is dismissed from hospital to receive daily, observed antituberculous therapy at home. His CD4 count is found to be 250 cells/mm^3, and he begins antiretroviral therapy.

▼ BIBLIOGRAPHY

Bradsher RW: Histoplasmosis and blastomycosis, *Clin Infect Dis* 22:5102-5111, 1996.

Finegold SM: Lung abscess. In Mandell G, Bennett J, Dolin R, (editors): *Principles and practice of infectious diseases*, ed 5, Philadelphia, 2000, Churchill Livingstone, pp 751-755.

Griffith DE: Mycobacteria as pathogens of respiratory infection, *Infect Dis Clin N Am* 12:593-612, 1998.

Kirkland TN, Fierer J: Coccidioidomycosis: a reemerging infectious disease, *Emerg Infect Dis* 2:192-199, 1996.

Lerner PI: Nocardiosis, *Clin Infect Dis* 22:891-905, 1996.

Patterson TF, Kirkpatrick WR, White M, et al: Invasive aspergillosis: disease spectrum, treatment practices, and outcomes, *Medicine (Baltimore)* 79:250-260, 2000.

Wheat LJ, Wass J, Norton J, et al: Cavitary histoplasmosis occurring during two large urban outbreaks: analysis of clinical, epidemiologic, roentgenographic, and laboratory features, *Medicine (Baltimore)* 63:201-209, 1984.

CHAPTER 21

BILATERAL HILAR ADENOPATHY

John E. Heffner

▼ Sarcoidosis
▼ Lymphoma
▼ Potato nodes
▼ Erythema nodosum

▼ Tuberculosis
▼ Human immunodeficiency virus (HIV)

▼ Adenopathy
▼ Berylliosis
▼ Interstitial lung disease

▼ THE CLINICAL PROBLEM

A 22-year-old white man presents with a 2-week history of painful lesions over both shins and aching knees and ankles. He denies cough, shortness of breath, weight loss, abdominal pain, or exposure to tuberculosis. He was born in South Carolina and has not traveled out of the state. His family physician performed a general health screen, which demonstrated normal results for his complete blood count, serum electrolytes, renal indices, and urinalysis. A chest x-ray was described as "abnormal," showing "hilar fullness."

He smokes 1 pack/day and has for the last 5 years. He has not had any previous health problems, and his only medications are non-prescription analgesics used occasionally for headaches.

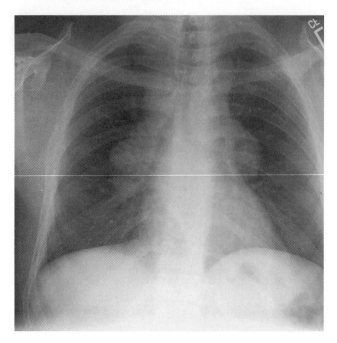

▼ **Figure 21-1** Anteroposterior (AP) chest x-ray showing bilateral hilar adenopathy (BHA). Notice the fullness in the hilum (where the pulmonary arteries emerge from the mediastinum).

On physical examination, his vital signs are normal. Examination of the skin shows raised, red, and tender placques scattered across both regions. His eye examination is normal. His chest is clear to auscultation and percussion. Cardiac examination demonstrates a grade I/VI systolic ejection murmur. The remainder of his examination is normal.

The previously performed blood studies were reviewed and confirmed to be normal. His chest x-ray is shown in Figure 21-1.

What is the differential diagnosis for this patient's clinical presentation? How would you manage his condition?

Differential Diagnosis of Bilateral Hilar Adenopathy

The term *hilum* refers to the region where the pulmonary vessels and bronchi emerge from the center of the chest (mediastinum). *Hilar adenopathy* refers to enlargement of the lymph nodes in this area.

The differential diagnosis of bilateral hilar adenopathy (BHA) with a normal pulmonary parenchyma includes malignant tumors in addition to infectious, congenital, immunologic, inhalational, and idiopathic disorders (Box 21-1). The likelihood of any of the conditions associated with hilar adenopathy depends on the patient's clinical presentation, age, associated underlying conditions, geographic residence, and radiographic appearance of the hilum. The major differential diagnosis usually

Box 21-1
Differential Diagnosis of Bilateral
Hilar Adenopathy*

Common Causes	Less Common Causes
Sarcoidosis	Tuberculosis
Hodgkin's and non-	Extra-thoracic neoplasms
Hodgkin's lymphoma	Lung cancer
Endemic fungi	Leukemia
H. capsulatum	Amyloidosis
C. immitis	Silicosis
	Angioimmunoblastic
	lymphadenopathy

*In the absence of parenchymal findings.

settles on lymphoma, sarcoidosis, and infections, such as tuberculosis, *Histoplasma capsulatum*, and *Coccidioides immitis*.

Sarcoidosis, an idiopathic systemic granulomatous disorder, is the most common cause of symmetric BHA. Enlarged lymph nodes usually have a lobular appearance. Bronchopulmonary amyloidosis can also cause bilar adenopathy in the absence of pulmonary involvement, although most patients have associated lung radiographic findings.

Both primary intra-thoracic and extra-thoracic malignancies cause hilar adenopathy. Lung cancer usually causes unilateral hilar adenopathy after regional spread occurs to hilar lymph nodes but can rarely (1% of patients) produce bilateral hilar enlargement in an asymmetric pattern. BHA with evidence of parenchymal disease occurs most commonly with small cell carcinoma. Metastases from extra-thoracic malignancies that spread to hilar lymph nodes include renal cell carcinoma and melanoma.

Hodgkin's and non-Hodgkin's lymphomas commonly produce mediastinal lymph node enlargement. BHA, however, is unusual and occurs in only 4% of patients with lymphoma at clinical presentation. Most patients with hilar lymph node enlargement have an asymmetric nodal distribution with associated enlargement of mediastinal lymph nodes, which most commonly involve the anterosuperior mediastinum. Angioimmunoblastic lymphadenopathy, a type of lymphoma, can produce a radiographic appearance identical to Hodgkin's disease. Leukemias, especially chronic lymphocytic, are less common causes of BHA.

Primary tuberculosis with hilar node enlargement almost always presents with associated parenchymal findings in non-immunocompromised hosts. Patients with tuberculosis and underlying human immunodeficiency virus (HIV) infection are more likely to present with BHA and normal lung parenchyma. Other infections include the endemic fungi, *H. capsulatum* and *C. immitis*.

Silicosis is the only inhalational disorder that can cause BHA without associated parenchymal findings, although this radiographic presentation is rare.

TABLE 21-1
Interpreting Signs and Symptoms in the Patient
with Bilateral Hilar Adenopathy

Possible Causes	Suggestive Clinical Features
Sarcoidosis	Absence of systemic symptoms such as fever, weight loss, sweats; presence of erythema nodosum and arthralgias (Löfgren's syndrome) in a patient who has not traveled to areas endemic for *C. immitis*
Lymphoma	Systemic symptoms of fever, weight loss, dyspnea, or sweating; associated peripheral lymphadenopathy
Endemic fungi	Travel to areas endemic for *H. capsulatum* or *C. immitis,* presence of symptoms of cough or fever
Tuberculosis	Symptoms of weight loss, fever, and cough; risk factors for HIV infection
Lung cancer	Airway symptoms of cough or hemoptysis
Metastatic cancer	Manifestations of the underlying neoplasm such as abdominal pain, jaundice, hematuria, abnormal eye grounds
Leukemia	Spontaneous mucosal hemorrhage and abnormal blood counts

Clinical Features that Suggest a Specific Cause of Bilateral Hilar Adenopathy

The clinical manifestations of the major conditions in the differential diagnosis for BHA are listed in Table 21-1.

In the present patient, several features of the clinical presentation suggest sarcoidosis as the cause of the BHA. Sarcoidosis presents most commonly in previously healthy patients under the age of 40. Symmetric BHA in a young patient without any associated symptoms, normal blood counts, and no evidence of HIV infection is due to sarcoidosis in 95% of patients. This patient, however, had arthralgias and raised, red, and tender pretibial lesions, which are typical of erythema nodosum. This cutaneous disorder commonly affects patients with an acute onset of sarcoidosis associated with BHA. The triad of acute polyarthritis, BHA, and erythema nodosum defines Löfgren's syndrome. Most experts believe that this characteristic presentation of sarcoidosis allows a presumptive diagnosis to be made in the appropriate clinical setting without tissue confirmation.

A "rheumatologic" presentation similar to Löfgren's syndrome can affect patients with coccidoidomycosis. The current patient, however, had not traveled to any area that would place him at risk for endemic fungi. Moreover, the symmetric and lobular appearance of the lymph nodes is characteristic of sarcoidosis.

Patients with lymphoma presenting with BHA almost always have systemic symptoms, such as fever or weight loss, or these patients experience non-specific chest pains or dyspnea. Most patients have associated mediastinal lymph node enlargement, and many have peripheral lymphadenopathy. Tuberculosis commonly presents with fever, cough, and other respiratory complaints. Erthema nodosum has not been described in patients with HIV disease with BHA due to tuberculosis or their underlying viral infection.

The patient's young age, short smoking history, and absence of chest symptoms lower the likelihood of lung cancer. The polyarthralgias, erythema nodosum, and normal urinalysis decrease the probability of metastatic renal cell cancer. Melanoma metastatic to the chest is a difficult diagnosis to exclude but appears unlikely in a patient presenting with the characteristic features of Löfgren's syndrome.

Diagnostic Testing in Evaluating the Patient with Bilateral Hilar Adenopathy

Because of the importance of distinguishing sarcoidosis from the various infectious and neoplastic disorders associated with BHA, a careful patient evaluation is required. Asymptomatic patients with symmetric BHA in a characteristic pattern of sarcoidosis probably do not need further confirmation of the diagnosis if the CBC, urinalysis, and physical examination are normal and HIV disease can be excluded. A negative PPD skin test and an elevated serum level of angiotension-converting enzyme (ACE) further support the diagnosis of sarcoidosis. Approximately 75% of patients with sarcoidosis have an elevated ACE level, and false positive results occur in less than 5% of patients evaluated for sarcoidosis. The presence of Löfgren's syndrome further supports a clinical diagnosis of sarcoidosis, if coccidioidomycosis appears unlikely. Patients with BHA diagnosed with sarcoidosis on clinical grounds should be reevaluated in 3 months with a repeat chest x-ray and further evaluated if lymph nodes continue to enlarge.

Patients suspected of having sarcoidosis who present with symptoms (except classic symptoms of Löfgren's syndrome) and patients with asymmetric hilar adenopathy regardless of symptoms require laboratory confirmation of their disease. When sarcoidosis remains a likely diagnosis, patients can undergo biopsy of palpable parotid glands to detect non-caseating granulomas. In the absence of accessible lesions, patients should undergo fiberoptic bronchoscopy with transbronchial lung biopsy with appropriate studies to exclude fungal and mycobacterial infections. The failure to detect non-caseating granulomas in lung parenchyma or evidence of an alternative diagnosis necessitates mediastinoscopy for lymph node biopsy or thoracoscopic lung biopsy. Cytologic evaluation of bronchoalveolar lavage fluid (BAL) obtained at bronchoscopy may suggest the presence of sarcoidosis or an alternative diagnosis, but is usually not diagnostic by itself. Gallium scans do not have diagnostic utility for sarcoidosis. Chest computed tomography (CT) scans are generally overutilized in examining patients undergoing evaluation for sarcoidosis.

Patients require a thoughtful selection of studies when sarcoidosis is not the leading differential diagnosis. Chest and abdominal CT scans are indicated for patients with suspected lymphoma to detect the characteristic anterosuperior mediastinal nodal distribution. Tissue confirmation of the diagnosis by biopsy of accessible or mediastinal nodal lymph nodes is mandatory. Endemic fungi are first evaluated with serologic studies. If results are non-diagnostic, sputum and urine should be examined for organisms. Some patients may require lymph node biopsy to confirm the presence of fungal disease. Sputum cultures and rarely lymph node biopsy are indicated in non-immunocompromised hosts. The presence of HIV disease requires an extensive evaluation of hilar lymph nodes with microbiologic studies of multiple tissue and fluid samples to establish a diagnosis; many patients require biopsy of enlarged lymph nodes. Patients with tuberculous lymphadenitis and HIV infection have a characteristic CT finding of hypodense central regions of involved lymph nodes, which have a contrast-enhancing rim.

Bronchogenic cancer is suspected by the typical clinical setting in which it occurs. Associated airway symptoms of cough and hemoptysis support the utility of bronchoscopy to detect an endobronchial lesion. Patients with normal airway examinations may have a diagnosis of lung cancer established by a bronchoscopic transbronchial needle biopsy or lymph node biopsy by thoracoscopy, mediastinoscopy, or a parasternal thoracotomy. Metastatic neoplasm as a cause of enlarged hilar lymph nodes is pursued by searching for evidence of the underlying tumor. An abnormal urinalysis should prompt an abdominal imaging study to exclude renal cell carcinoma. The skin and eye grounds should be carefully examined to detect a primary lesion of metastatic melanoma.

The present patient had the characteristic presentation of sarcoidosis described as Löfgren's syndrome. Because he had not traveled to a region endemic for coccidioidomycosis, a presumptive diagnosis of sarcoidosis was made. He improved rapidly with non-steroidal anti-inflammatory agents and did not experience a recurrence of his symptoms. The hilar lymph nodes resolved spontaneously over the next 3 months.

Pitfalls and Common Mistakes in the Assessment and Treatment of Patients with Bilateral Hilar Adenopathy

Common pitfalls in assessing patients with BHA include failure to examine patients closely for the presence of extrathoracic evidence of disease. Hematuria or a black retinal lesion may be immediate evidence that a metastatic tumor requires consideration. Physicians may also fail to recognize common presentations of sarcoidosis that could prevent an exhaustive diagnostic evaluation with multiple laboratory studies. Patients with BHA due to sarcoidosis often undergo bronchoscopy or mediastinoscopy to establish a diagnosis when a more accessible cutaneous lesion or peripheral lymph node is available for biopsy.

Another pitfall of diagnosis is the willingness of clinicians to attribute asymmetric BHA to sarcoidosis when this radiographic presentation is more typical of alternative diagnoses, such as lymphoma or tuberculosis in patients with HIV disease. HIV infection requires exclusion in any patient presenting with hilar adenopathy.

▼ BIBLIOGRAPHY

Carr JL et al: Noninvasive testing of asymptomatic bilateral hilar adenopathy, *J Gen Intern Med* 5:138-146, 1990.

Mana J et al: Excessive thoracic computed tomographic scanning in sarcoidosis, *Thorax* 50:1264-1266, 1995.

Newman LS, Rose CS, Maier LA: Sarcoidosis, *N Engl J Med* 333:1224, 1997.

North LB, Libshitz HI, Lorigan JG: Thoracic lymphoma, *Radiol Clin North Am* 28:745-762, 1990.

Patil SN, Levin DL: Distribution of thoracic lymphadenopathy in sarcoidosis using computed tomography, *J Thorac Imaging* 14:114-117, 1999.

Wilcke JT et al: Radiographic spectrum of adult pulmonary tuberculosis in a developed country, *Respir Med* 92:493-497, 1998.

PART III

COMMON PROBLEMS IN THE NON-ICU PATIENT

CHAPTER 22

PULMONARY INFILTRATE

David L. Longworth

▼ Fever
▼ Pulmonary infiltrate
▼ Hospitalized adult
▼ Inpatient
▼ Nosocomial pneumonia

▼ THE CLINICAL PROBLEM

A 64-year-old woman was admitted 4 days ago to the surgical service and underwent an elective open cholecystectomy for chronic cholecystitis and cholelithiasis. The post-operative course has been complicated by nausea and vomiting, ascribed to a post-operative ileus for which a nasogastric tube has been placed. Several hours ago she developed fever to 102.2° F and complained of dry cough and mild dyspnea. The clinician is called to evaluate the new-onset fever and a pulmonary infiltrate.

Her past medical history is notable for obesity, hypertension, a prior non-Q wave anteroseptal myocardial infarction (MI), chronic congestive heart failure (CHF), type 2 diabetes mellitus, and chronic venous stasis in her lower extremities. Her medications include digoxin, furosemide, verapamil CD, simvastatin, subcutaneous heparin post-operatively, and glyburide. She has smoked 1 pack/day for the past 40 years. Her immunizations are up to date.

On physical examination she is febrile to 101.5° F, her blood pressure is 120/70 mm Hg, her heart rate is 110 and regular, and her respiratory rate is 24. Her weight is 80 kg, 2 kg above her admission weight. Her skin is notable for ecchymoses on her abdomen at the sites of subcutaneous heparin injections. A right internal jugular central venous catheter is present, and the exit site is clean. There is no rash or jaundice. The head, eyes, ears, nose, and throat examination is notable for the absence of scleral icterus and for the presence of a nasogastric tube. Her chest has bibasilar rales, worse on the right compared with the left. Her cardiac examination discloses a regular rhythm, a grade 2/6 holosystolic murmur at the cardiac apex, and a soft summation gallop. Her abdomen is soft, and there is minimal tenderness at the surgical site, which is clean and healing nicely. Bowel sounds are absent. Her lower extremities are notable for chronic venous stasis changes and 1+ pretibial edema bilaterally, which are old. No cords are palpable.

Laboratory studies from earlier in the day disclose a WBC of 12,500 cells/mm^3 with 80% granulocytes, a hemoglobin of 14 g/dL, a platelet count of 225,000 cells/mm^3, a serum sodium of 131 mmol/L, a potassium of 3.3 mEq/dL, and a normal serum creatinine. A chest x-ray discloses bibasilar infiltrates (left worse than right), a poor inspiratory effort, slight elevation of the right hemidiaphragm, and borderline cardiomegaly. The upper lobe vasculature is prominent. A KUB and upright disclose dilated loops of small bowel with air fluid levels, air in the colon, and scant free air beneath the right hemidiaphragm. An electrocardiogram demonstrates sinus tachycardia and non-specific ST-T changes in the anterior leads, unchanged from prior tracings. A room air arterial blood gas discloses a pH 7.45, PaO_2 76, PCO_2 30, HCO_3^- 28.

What is the differential diagnosis of this clinical problem? What tests are indicated, and how should the patient be managed?

The Differential Diagnosis of Fever and a New Pulmonary Infiltrate

The differential diagnosis of fever and a new pulmonary infiltrate in hospitalized adults who are not in an intensive care unit (ICU) setting is broad and includes both infectious and non-infectious etiologies. These are summarized in Box 22-1.

Among the infectious causes of fever and a new lung infiltrate, pneumonia is the most likely differential diagnostic consideration and may include nosocomial pneumonia (defined as pneumonia developing beyond 48 hours of hospital admission), aspiration pneumonia (which implies a major aspiration event and may be infectious or chemical), and community-acquired pneumonia (which implies incubating infection at the time of admission and the development of symptoms within the first few days of hospitalization). This distinction has implications with regard to pathogenesis, microbiology, and empiric therapy. All three types of pneumonia may arise through aspiration of oropharyngeal contents, although the term *aspiration pneumonia* implies a large-volume aspiration of gastric or oropharyngeal secretions, which may lead to chemical or infectious pneumonitis, or both. In addition, some cases of pneumonia arise from inhalation of infectious agents, such as influenza or *Mycobacterium tuberculosis.*

The microbiology of these respective forms of pneumonia is summarized in Box 22-2. Different organisms are responsible for these different types of pneumonia, which has implications with regard to empiric and pathogen-specific therapy when these diagnoses are suspected. Aspiration pneumonia is usually a polymicrobial

Box 22-1
Differential Diagnosis of Fever and a New Pulmonary Infiltrate

Infectious Causes	Non-Infectious Causes
Common	PE/Infarction
Pneumonia	Chemical pneumonitis (aspiration)
Aspiration	CHF
Nosocomial	ARDS
Community-acquired	Drugs
Atelectasis	Alveolar hemorrhage
	Tracheoesophageal fistula
Uncommon	Radiation pneumonitis
Septic PE	
Intra-vascular device	
Right-sided endocarditis	
Contiguous spread of infection	
Sub-diaphragmatic abscess	

PE, Pulmonary embolism; CHF, congestive heart failure; ARDS, acute respiratory distress syndrome.

Box 22-2
Common Microorganisms Producing Community-Acquired, Aspiration, and Nosocomial Pneumonia

Community-Acquired	Aspiration	Nosocomial
Streptococcus pneumoniae	Mixed mouth aerobes	Gram-negative bacilli
Chlamydia pneumoniae	and anaerobes	Staphylococci
Legionella species		*Legionella* species
Mycoplasma pneumoniae		Influenza (winter)
Haemophilus influenzae		
Moraxella catarrhalis		

infection produced by aerobic and anaerobic organisms from the mouth. In residents of chronic care facilities or in recent recipients of antimicrobial therapy, aerobic gram-negative bacilli or staphylococci may colonize the oropharynx and contribute to lower respiratory tract infection when aspiration occurs. The microbiology of hospital-acquired (nosocomial) pneumonia varies from one hospital to another, and knowledge of local epidemiology and antimicrobial susceptibility profiles is essential in predicting the most likely cause and in choosing the most effective empiric antibiotic regimen. In most instances, hospital-acquired pneumonia is bacterial, but in winter months influenza may be transmitted within the hospital setting to patients from infected health care workers and must be considered in the differential diagnosis, especially in unimmunized hosts.

Uncommon infectious causes of fever and a new pulmonary infiltrate in hospitalized adults outside the ICU setting include septic pulmonary emboli from

TABLE 22-1
Historical Clues to Specific Causes of Fever and a New Pulmonary Infiltrate

Cause	Historical Clues
Aspiration pneumonia	Antecedent nausea and vomiting Loss of consciousness (seizure, syncope, etc) Obtundation Pre-existing conditions associated with an absent gag reflex Cough may be dry or productive
PE	Immobilization Central intra-vascular catheters Pre-existing conditions associated with hypercoagulable states Sudden onset dyspnea or pleuritic chest pain Hemoptysis Cough may be dry or absent; rarely productive Pain, swelling at central line site
Atelectasis	Presence of conditions that impair deep breathing Pain from surgical incision Sedation Immobilization Cough may be dry or absent
CHF	Pre-existing CHF or left-sided valvular heart disease New onset atrial fibrillation or supraventricular tachycardia Acute chest pain and dyspnea suggesting acute myocardial infarction
Contiguous spread of infection from the abdomen	Abdominal surgical procedure within the past 2 weeks Abdominal catastrophe
Tracheoesophageal fistula	Presence of esophageal or lung cancer Recent surgical procedure involving the airway or esophagus Recent dilation of esophageal stricture Fits of coughing precipitated by swallowing fluid or food
Alveolar hemorrhage	Antecedent radiation therapy to the lung or chemotherapy Thrombocytopenia or coagulopathy Cough may be dry or productive of blood-tinged secretions Recent bone marrow transplantation
Radiation pneumonitis	Recent radiation therapy to the lung

PE, Pulmonary embolism; *CHF,* congestive heart failure.

central venous catheters or right-sided endocarditis, or contiguous spread of infection from below the diaphragm in patients with intra-abdominal abscesses. In the former circumstance, staphylococci are the most common pathogens, whereas in the latter situation polymicrobial infections due to aerobic gram-negative bacilli and bowel anaerobes are most likely. When infection spreads to the lung from below the diaphragm, empyema also is almost always present.

Fever and a new pulmonary infiltrate are not synonymous with infection, and a number of non-infectious causes must be considered. Common and uncommon non-infectious causes are summarized in Box 22-1. Common causes include chemical pneumonitis from aspiration of acidic gastric contents, bland pulmonary embolism (PE) with or without pulmonary infarction, CHF in selected clinical settings (e.g., acute myocardial infarction or biventricular failure with hepatic congestion), the fibroproliferative phase of the adult respiratory distress syndrome and atelectasis. Uncommon causes include alveolar hemorrhage (most often seen in patients with thrombocytopenia and some form of lung injury), tracheoesophageal fistula (usually seen in patients with esophageal cancer or endobronchial lung malignancy with erosion of tumor), radiation pneumonitis (in patients receiving radiation therapy), and certain medications (such as amiodarone or bleomycin).

Clinical Features that Suggest a Specific Cause of Fever and a New Pulmonary Infiltrate

The history and physical examination may be very helpful in formulating the differential diagnosis of fever and a new pulmonary infiltrate in the hospitalized adult who is not in the intensive care unit. Some helpful clues are summarized in Tables 22-1 and 22-2.

TABLE 22-2
Clues on Physical Examination to Specific Causes of Fever and a New Pulmonary Infiltrate

Physical Finding	Cause of Pulmonary Infiltrate
Focal pulmonary rales	Pneumonia
Bibasilar pulmonary rales	Bibasilar pneumonia, CHF, atelectasis
Pleural friction rub	PE with infarct, pneumonia with pleural irritation or empyema
Venous cord	Deep venous thrombosis with PE
New unilateral limb swelling	Deep venous thrombosis with PE
Unilateral dilated chest wall veins	Subclavian deep venous thrombosis with PE
Cardiac S_3 or summation gallop	CHF
Increasing weight	CHF
Absent gag reflex	Aspiration pneumonia
Impaired mentation	Aspiration pneumonia

PE, Pulmonary embolism; CHF, congestive heart failure.

The presence or absence of cough and sputum production may be helpful in guiding the differential diagnosis. Cough is often absent in patients with CHF, atelectasis, and PE. It is frequently but not invariably present in patients with pneumonia. Purulent sputum production should suggest the presence of bacterial pneumonia. The presence of hemoptysis should suggest PE with infarct, but hemoptysis is present in a minority of patients with PE, and its absence does not exclude the diagnosis. Moreover, hemoptysis may also occur with bacterial pneumonia, significant acute CHF, and alveolar hemorrhage.

Historical clues to the diagnosis of aspiration pneumonia include recent vomiting, the presence of pre-existing conditions associated with an absent gag reflex (e.g., stroke), recent loss of consciousness (e.g., syncope, seizure, sedation for a procedure), and obtundation. The cough may be absent, dry, or productive in patients with aspiration pneumonia. On examination, specific clues to the diagnosis include an absent gag reflex and the presence of basilar rales. Patients who aspirate in the sitting or semi-recumbent position most frequently do so to the lower lobes (especially the right lower lobe), given the anatomy of the tracheobronchial tree. Aspiration to the upper lobes is distinctly uncommon, and the presence of upper lobe rales should suggest other causes of pneumonia.

PE should be considered in patients who have had prolonged bed rest and immobilization, in those with chronic indwelling central venous catheters (complicated by internal jugular or subclavian deep venous thrombosis with PE), and in those with hypercoagulable states. Cough is often absent and usually dry if present. Hemoptysis should prompt consideration of the diagnosis. The physical examination is rarely helpful in patients with PE, and health care professionals must have a high index of suspicion for the diagnosis in the appropriate clinical setting. Tachycardia is the most common physical finding but occurs in only about 70% of patients. A minority may have a pleural friction rub. In those with indwelling central venous catheters, the presence of a palpable venous cord, new unilateral limb swelling, inflammation or swelling at the catheter site, or unilateral dilation of chest wall veins, should suggest the diagnosis of PE in the presence of fever and a new pulmonary infiltrate. These findings occur in a small minority of patients with PE, however.

Atelectasis should be considered in patients with basilar pulmonary infiltrates who have conditions that may impair deep breathing. Examples include prolonged immobilization and bed rest, surgical procedures producing pain that impairs maximal inspiration, and sedation. Cough may be absent or dry in patients with atelectasis. On examination, rales are usually basilar and bilateral, but occasionally unilateral.

Congestive heart failure (CHF) should be considered as a cause of fever and new infiltrates in those with pre-existing or new-onset left ventricular dysfunction or valvular heart disease, especially if they become fluid overloaded. New-onset congestive failure may occur in the setting of acute myocardial infarction or infective endocarditis. The pattern of the infiltrates in CHF depends on the presence or absence of pre-existing chronic lung disease and the degree of congestive failure. In patients with healthy lungs, the infiltrates are usually interstitial and bilateral. Basilar involvement is typical in mild congestive failure; frank pulmonary edema may involve the upper lobes as well. Patients with pre-existing emphysema may have atypical radiographic patterns; if emphysema exists at the lung bases, congestive

TABLE 22-3
Classic Radiographic Patterns in Selected Causes of Pulmonary Infiltrates

Cause	Typical Radiographic Pattern
Aspiration pneumonia	Unilateral or bilateral basilar infiltrates
Bacterial pneumonia	Focal lobar or patchy infiltrates
Atelectasis	Linear plate-like infiltrates, usually basilar Basilar infiltrate or volume loss, often bilateral Focal lobar infiltrate (in the setting of mucous plugging)
CHF	Bilateral interstitial infiltrates with Kerley B lines Mild CHF involves lower lobes Bilateral bat-wing infiltrates in florid pulmonary edema Pleural effusions common
PE	Often no infiltrate Peripheral wedge-shaped infiltrate abutting pleura (Hampton's hump)
Alveolar hemorrhage	Patchy unilateral or bilateral infiltrates
Contiguous spread from below diaphragm	Unilateral basilar infiltrate with effusion
ARDS	Bilateral ground glass infiltrates Bilateral fibronodular infiltrates (chronic form)

CHF, Congestive heart failure; *PE,* pulmonary embolism; *ARDS,* acute respiratory distress syndrome.

failure may present with upper lobe interstitial infiltrates. Fever accompanies CHF in selected clinical settings, including acute myocardial infarction with pulmonary edema due to left ventricular dysfunction or ruptured papillary muscle, left-sided infective endocarditis resulting in valvular incompetency, and biventricular failure with hepatic congestion. The mechanism by which hepatic congestion produces fever is not known. Physical findings that should suggest the possibility of CHF include the presence of an S_3 or summation gallop, bibasilar rales, jugular venous distension, increased body weight compared to baseline, and new or worsening bilateral lower extremity edema.

Contiguous spread of infection to the lung from beneath the diaphragm is rare, and should be considered in patients with recent abdominal surgery or intra-abdominal catastrophe. Lung involvement is almost always basilar and unilateral with an accompanying pleural effusion.

The radiographic pattern of the infiltrate may also be helpful in narrowing the differential diagnosis as discussed above and summarized in Table 22-3. It is important to emphasize, however, that the classic radiographic patterns are not uniformly present in the various clinical entities and that a given entity may present with one of several radiographic findings (Figure 22-1).

In the present patient, the history is helpful in formulating a preliminary differential diagnosis. The clinician knows that she was admitted 4 days earlier for an elective cholecystectomy, complicated by nausea and vomiting ascribed to an ileus.

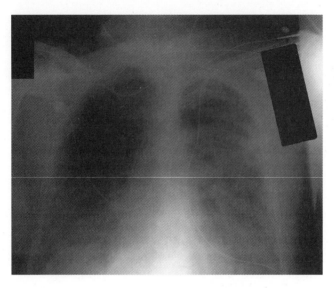

▼ **Figure 22-1**   Chest x-ray discloses right upper lobe and left upper lobe infiltrates.

During an episode of vomiting, she could easily have aspirated, leading to a chemical or bacterial pneumonitis. In a previously healthy individual without antecedent antibiotic therapy, an infectious aspiration pneumonia would most likely be caused by mouth aerobes and anaerobes; at post-operative day 4, staphylococcal or gram-negative pneumonia would be much less likely. She has a history of chronic CHF and is 2 kg above her admission weight at this time; this suggests the possibility of a component of worsening CHF. Although she has been receiving subcutaneous heparin post-operatively, she has at least two risk factors for PE, including her immobilization in bed and the presence of a right internal jugular central venous catheter. Atelectasis also should be a differential diagnostic concern given her bed rest and the fact that her incisional pain likely impairs her ability to take a maximal inspiration, thereby predisposing to basilar atelectasis. Finally, she has had an abdominal surgical procedure, raising the possibility of an occult subdiaphragmatic abscess with spread to the lung. This possibility is less likely in our patient for several reasons. First, it would be uncommon to have an abscess form by post-operative day 4. Post-operative intra-abdominal abscesses most often become manifest 1 to 2 weeks after surgery. Second, a right sub-diaphragmatic abscess would be more common following biliary surgery and if it traversed the diaphragm, it should produce a right pleural effusion and a right basilar pneumonia. This patient's chest x-ray discloses bibasilar infiltrates and no significant pleural effusion, which speaks against this diagnostic consideration.

This patient's physical examination is notable for increased weight, a summation gallop, and a murmur of mitral regurgitation. These findings should suggest a component of CHF. Bibasilar rales are present, consistent with congestive failure, bibasilar atelectasis, or bilateral lower lobe pneumonia. The chest x-ray discloses bibasilar infiltrates and mild upper zone redistribution. These findings suggest a component of CHF, but are also consistent with concomitant basilar atelectasis or pneumonia. The confusion regarding the correct diagnosis at this point in the eval-

**Box 22-3
Diagnostic Tests in Patients With
Fever and a New Pulmonary Infiltrate**

Indicated in All Patients
Complete blood count with differential
Blood cultures
Sputum Gram's stain and culture if feasible
Pulse oximetry or arterial blood gas measurement
   to assess oxygenation

Indicated in Selected Patients
Fiberoptic bronchoscopy
Venous duplex examination
Ventilation-perfusion scanning
Spiral CT of chest
Pulmonary angiography
CT of abdomen and chest
Gastrografin swallow study
Electrocardiography

CT, Computed tomography.

uation is not uncommon and illustrates two important points. First, the clinical distinction between pneumonia, atelectasis, and CHF may be difficult at the bedside. Second, patients may have more than one cause for fever and pulmonary infiltrates.

Diagnostic Testing in the Evaluation of the Patient with New Pulmonary Infiltrate

Diagnostic testing may be helpful in further elucidating the cause of a new pulmonary infiltrate in the hospitalized adult patient not in the ICU. Some general guidelines for testing are provided in Box 22-3; however, individual patient circumstances dictate whether some tests are indicated, as well as the order in which they should be performed. All patients should have a complete blood count with differential white cell count. The presence of leukocytosis and its magnitude may aid in diagnosis. Significant leukocytosis (e.g., exceeding 15,000 cells/mm^3) or a significantly left-shifted white blood cell differential should heighten concern about bacterial pneumonia. The absence of leukocytosis, however, does not exclude the diagnosis, and overwhelming and fulminant gram-negative or staphylococcal pneumonia may be accompanied by leukopenia, a poor prognostic sign. Oxygenation should be assessed in all patients by either pulse oximetry or arterial blood gas. This is essential for two reasons: first, to assure that the patient is adequately oxygenated, and, second, while hypoxemia can occur in all of the differential diagnostic concerns owing to ventilation-perfusion mismatch, an elevated alveolar-arterial gradient out of proportion to the pulmonary infiltrate if the latter is very small should suggest the possibility of PE.

Blood cultures should be obtained in all patients, recognizing that bacteremia occurs in only a minority of those with nosocomial, aspiration, or community-acquired pneumonia. Nevertheless, if bacteremia is documented, this is very useful in guiding the type and sometimes the duration of antimicrobial therapy.

The utility of sputum Gram's stain and culture in patients with pneumonia continues to be debated. If the sputum is purulent and can be obtained, a Gram's stain may be helpful in suggesting a pathogen and in guiding empiric antimicrobial therapy. If the specimen is adequate, which requires the presence of many leukocytes and few epithelial cells, detecting a predominant pathogen, or, alternatively, a mixture of different mouth flora (as would be seen in a polymicrobial aspiration), may be helpful in determining the cause of a pneumonia, as well as appropriate empiric therapy.

If the diagnosis of PE is suspected, several diagnostic strategies may be pursued, including venous duplex evaluation of the lower and upper extremity venous circulation, ventilation perfusion lung scanning, and pulmonary angiography. A detailed discussion of this issue is beyond the scope of this chapter, although some generalizations can be made. First, the presence of new unilateral limb edema or dilation of chest wall veins should prompt duplex examination of the involved venous system for the presence of thrombosis. If present, this would represent a source for PE. Thrombosis may nevertheless be present in venous systems without any overt clinical signs, and in patients with unexplained pulmonary infiltrates and fever, screening duplex examination may be indicated, especially in those with subtle infiltrates, focal infiltrates without sputum production, hypoxemia out of proportion to the infiltrate, hemoptysis or a pleural rub, hypercoagulable state, or prolonged immobilization.

Second, ventilation-perfusion lung scanning is less useful in patients with pulmonary infiltrates, as scans are frequently indeterminate in probability for pulmonary embolus. Ventilation-perfusion mismatch in an area of radiographically normal lung might nevertheless be helpful, although this happens infrequently. If screening duplex studies are negative and ventilation-perfusion scanning is indeterminate or unlikely to be helpful, pulmonary angiography or spiral computed tomography of the chest may be necessary to establish the diagnosis of PE.

Third, if contigious spread of infection from the abdomen to the chest is suspected by history, computed tomography of the abdomen and lower chest should be performed. Fourth, gastrografin swallow studies may be helpful to document the presence of recurrent aspiration or the presence of a tracheoesophageal fistula. Fifth, electrocardiography should be performed if cardiac ischemia with resultant CHF is suspected. Finally, fiberoptic bronchoscopy may be necessary in selected settings, including critically ill patients in whom the diagnosis is uncertain so as to establish a microbiologic diagnosis of pneumonia, in those with suspected alveolar hemorrhage, and in patients with suspected lobar collapse due to mucous plugging. In the latter circumstance, bronchoscopy may be therapeutic as well as diagnostic.

The present patient has a minimally elevated leukocyte count and no sputum production. She has mild hypoxemia. The most likely diagnoses are basilar atelectasis from splinting together with mild CHF. Because of the history of recurrent vomiting, aspiration pneumonia cannot absolutely be excluded. Blood cultures are collected, a program of vigorous pulmonary toilet with incentive spirometry is begun, and intravenous furosemide is administered. She is unable to provide sputum for Gram's stain and culture. Ampicillin-sulbactam is begun because of the concern about aspiration pneumonia and pending blood cultures.

Assessment of the Effect of Therapy

A detailed discussion of the appropriate therapy of the many entities that may produce fever and a new pulmonary infiltrate in the hospitalized adult is beyond the scope of this chapter, but a few comments are in order. Aspiration pneumonia should be treated with agents that adequately cover mouth anaerobes and aerobes. For those hospitalized for more than several days who aspirate, many authorities favor expanded coverage with agents active against nosocomial gram-negative bacilli and staphylococci, which may colonize the oropharynx of hospitalized individuals within 48 hours of admission. Knowledge of local hospital pathogens and their antimicrobial susceptibility profiles should guide empiric antibiotic selection. Agents such as ampicillin-sulbactam, ticarcillin-clavulanate, piperacillin-tazobactam, or even imipenem-cilastatin are sometimes employed in patients with suspected significant aspiration or nosocomial pneumonias. Patients with PE should be anticoagulated unless contraindications exist; in those with lower extremity deep venous thrombosis and a contraindication to anticoagulation, an inferior vena cava filter should be considered. CHF should be treated with diuresis and adjunctive cardiac medications to optimize left ventricular function. Atelectasis should be treated with aggressive pulmonary toilet.

Given the broad differential diagnosis of fever and a new pulmonary infiltrate in the hospitalized adult, it should not be surprising that the rapidity of response to therapy may be highly variable, depending on the diagnosis. For example, patients with aspiration pneumonitis may be febrile for several days, irrespective of whether the pneumonia is chemical or bacterial and despite appropriate antibiotic therapy. Patients with large pneumonias may defervesce more slowly than those with small pneumonias. Patients with nosocomial gram-negative or staphylococcal pneumonia may remain febrile for up to 7 to 10 days, even with appropriate therapy. As a general rule, radiographic improvement frequently lags days to weeks behind clinical response in patients with aspiration or nosocomial pneumonia.

Patients with fever due to PE and infarction may be febrile for up to 48 to 72 hours after anticoagulation; persistent fever beyond this should prompt consideration of alternative diagnoses. In patients with large myocardial infarctions and CHF, fever may persist for several days, even with effective therapy of the failure. In such circumstances, fever is likely due to ongoing myocardial necrosis. In those with biventricular failure and fever due to hepatic congestion, resolution of fever and pulmonary infiltrates usually correlates with adequate treatment of the congestive failure. Fever and radiographic abnormalities in those with atelectasis may take several days to remit; persistent signs and symptoms should suggest the possibility of inspissated secretions, for which bronchoscopy may be indicated. Following bronchoscopy, once atelectatic lung is reexpanded, fever and infiltrates generally resolve promptly.

Patients with tracheoesophageal fistulas may develop recurrent fever and infiltrates until the anatomic communication between the esophagus and tracheobronchial tree is corrected. In those with contiguous spread of infection from beneath the diaphragm, resolution of fever depends on adequate drainage of collections in the abdomen and pleural space, along with appropriate antimicrobial therapy. The duration of fever and radiographic pulmonary abnormalities may be highly variable in such individuals. Fever and infiltrates in the setting of alveolar hemorrhage may persist for several days, and even longer if bleeding is ongoing. With a self-limited event, most patients defervesce within a week, although radiographic improvement may lag.

Pitfalls and Common Mistakes in the Assessment and Treatment of the Patient with Fever and a New Pulmonary Infiltrate

Fever with a new pulmonary infiltrate is a common clinical problem in the hospitalized adult, yet, despite its frequency, pitfalls in evaluation and management await the unwitting clinician. A common mistake is to assume that all such patients possess respiratory tract infections and to fail to consider non-infectious etiologies. Such practice leads to overuse of antibiotics, and, more importantly, may lead to delayed consideration and diagnosis of potentially fatal illnesses such as PE.

PE is an insidious diagnosis, since a physical examination may be inconclusive and patients often lack physical findings to suggest the diagnosis. Deep venous thrombi in the lower extremities may be asymptomatic but may produce pulmonary emboli. Upper extremity venous thrombi involving the internal jugular and subclavian veins are increasingly common given the widespread use of central venous access devices. Such thrombi may eventuate in pulmonary emboli, yet are often asymptomatic before a sentinel pulmonary event. The respiratory clinician must be cognizant of the subtle physical signs that may belie the presence of such thrombi, which include a venous cord involving the internal jugular vein, subtle ipsilateral upper extremity swelling, and dilation of the veins on the ipsilateral chest wall. The latter two findings usually only occur in totally occlusive thrombi, yet non-occlusive thrombi can nevertheless produce pulmonary emboli. In the hospitalized patient with new fever and a pulmonary infiltrate in whom the clinical presentation suggests PE, screening duplex examinations of both lower and upper extremities and central veins may be necessary to establish the diagnosis of occult venous thrombosis.

Another common pitfall is to assume that a new-onset lower lobe infiltrate invariably represents bacterial pneumonia. In some patients with tracheobronchitis and poor mobilization of secretions, airway plugging by mucous secretions can lead to segmental or lobar collapse mimicking bacterial pneumonia. In such instances, the most important therapeutic intervention is the initiation of aggressive bronchopulmonary toilet through the use of incentive spirometry, and, on occasion, bronchodilator therapy, continuous or intermittent positive airway pressure, and even therapeutic bronchoscopy. The use of antimicrobial chemotherapy without attention to pulmonary toilet is the wrong therapeutic choice and does not address the true problem.

Finally, as illustrated in our patient, hospitalized adults with fever and a new pulmonary infiltrate may have more than one cause for the problem. This is especially common in the post-operative patient with several underlying medical problems, such as chronic lung disease and CHF. Successful evaluation and management of such patients requires ongoing vigilance by the respiratory clinician, and attention to the possibility that more than one process may be ongoing in such patients.

▼ BIBLIOGRAPHY

Goldhaber SZ: Pulmonary embolism, *N Engl J Med* 339:93-104, 1998.

Mayhall GC: Nosocomial pneumonia: diagnosis and prevention, *Infect Dis Clin N Am* 11:427-458, 1997.

McEachern R, Campbell GD: Hospital-acquired pneumonia: epidemiology, etiology, and treatment, *Infect Dis Clin N Am* 12:761-780, 1998.

CHAPTER 23

ACUTE HYPOXEMIA

Lucy Kester
Douglas Orens
Edward Hoisington
James K. Stoller

Key Terms

- ▼ Post-operative hypoxemia
- ▼ Pulmonary embolism (PE)
- ▼ Atelectasis
- ▼ Pleural effusion
- ▼ Pleuritic pain

▼ THE CLINICAL PROBLEM

A 47-year-old obese woman is status-post removal of a large ovarian tumor. She is 5-foot 6-inches tall and weighs 186 lbs. She smoked 1 pack/day for 25 years and led an inactive lifestyle. She is currently employed as a data processor. She stopped smoking 2 weeks before surgery. Her surgery was uneventful, and she left the recovery room on oxygen at 2 L/min by nasal cannula with an oxygen saturation of 97% as measured by pulse oximetry. In her hospital room, in addition to the oxygen, she was using a patient-controlled anesthesia (PCA) pump and an incentive spirometer. Her vital capacity was 1.19 L (normal predicted, 3.5 L), and laboratory values were WBC 8900/mm^3, hemoglobin 10.9 g/dL, and platelets 252,000. At the beginning of her second post-operative day, her vital capacity had increased to

1.92 L, she was able to come off the oxygen (SpO₂ 94% on room air), and she was able to ambulate to the bathroom unassisted.

In the evening of the second post-operative day, she developed a cough, became acutely short of breath and diaphoretic, and complained of right-sided pleuritic chest pain. A room air arterial blood gas (ABG) level was drawn, and oxygen by nasal cannula was started at 4 L/min. An electrocardiogram (ECG) demonstrated a sinus tachycardia. Her vital signs were heart rate 118, respiratory rate 26, blood pressure 146/86, and temperature 99.3° F. Crackles could be heard in the right lung base on auscultation. A chest x-ray was done.

The ABG results showed pH 7.48, PaCO₂ 34 mm Hg, PaO₂ 59 mm Hg, and oxygen saturation 92% on room air. After the administration of oxygen at 4 L/min, her SpO₂ increased to 95%. On examination, she did not exhibit tenderness, warmth, or redness in her calves. The chest x-ray showed an elevation of the right hemidiaphragm with possible associated atelectasis but was otherwise clear and free of infiltrates.

What is the differential diagnosis for this patient?

Differential Diagnosis of Acute Hypoxemia

Hypoxemia in the post-operative patient can be classified in general as early or late. The early phase, attributed to a decrease in functional residual capacity (FRC) caused by anesthetic drugs, absorption atelectasis, and/or surgical technique, lasts approximately 2 hours. The late phase, occurring over the next 48 hours, may be caused by hypoventilation for narcotic analgesics and atelectasis resulting from splinting due to pain and retained secretions. During and immediately after upper abdominal surgery, the patient's FRC is reduced by 70% to 80%, and the vital capacity, essential for effective coughing, is decreased by 40% to 50%. The reduction in lung volumes may persist for 7 to 14 days. As shown in Box 23-1, the impact of surgery on lung function increases as the incision approaches the diaphragm.

Non-laparoscopic abdominal surgeries also pose a significant risk for post-operative pulmonary complications. Morbidity after abdominal surgery remains

Box 23-1
Surgeries Listed by Degree of Effect on Lung Function (from Greatest to Least Effect)

Thoracic with lung resection
Thoracic without lung resection
Upper abdominal
Lower abdominal
Non-thoracic, non-abdominal

Modified from Lawrence VA, Duncan CA: Respiratory complication of surgery and anesthesia: overview. In Lubin MF, Walker K, Smith RB, (editors): *Medical management of the surgical patient*, ed 3, Philadelphia, 1995, Lippincott, pp 111-116.

20% to 25% with a mortality rate of 3% to 5% for those with significant post-operative pulmonary complications.

In addition to atelectasis, other post-operative pulmonary complications that may cause hypoxemia that may occur following abdominal surgery include pneumonia, pleural effusions, and pulmonary embolism (Box 23-2).

Several factors that increase the risk for developing these complications are listed in Box 23-3.

Table 23-1 lists specific common causes for post-operative hypoxemia, along with the mechanism of hypoxemia and the clinical features for each cause.

Clinical Features that Suggest a Specific Cause of Hypoxemia

The current patient has several clinical features that predispose her to post-operative hypoxemia. She had upper abdominal surgery, is somewhat obese, and has a smoking history greater than 20 pack years. Her inactive lifestyle and post-operative state put her at risk for deep vein thrombosis (DVT) and possible pulmonary embolism (PE). Currently, she presents with shortness of breath, right-sided pleuritic chest pain, and hypoxemia demonstrated by ABG levels. This presentation invites consideration of several causes, including atelectasis and PE.

Box 23-2
Differential Diagnosis
of Post-Operative Hypoxemia

Common Causes	Less Common Causes
Atelectasis	Pulmonary hypertension
Pneumonia	Pneumothorax
PE	
Pulmonary edema	

PE, Pulmonary embolism.

Box 23-3
Risk Factors for Developing
Post-Operative Pulmonary
Complications

Age >60
Obesity
Smoking more than 1 pack/day
Duration of anesthesia greater than 3½ hrs
Poor general physical condition

TABLE 23-1
Interpreting Signs and Symptoms in the Patient with Post-Operative Hypoxemia

Possible Causes	Mechanisms	Suggestive Clinical Features
Atelectasis	Decreased FRC, collapsed alveoli, airways blocked by retained secretions	Elevated diaphragm on chest x-ray, decreased lung volumes, weak cough, upper abdominal surgery
Pneumonia	Inflammation of the parenchyma and consolidation	Cough, fever, low SpO_2, dyspnea, chest pain, parenchymal infiltrate with air bronchograms on x-ray
Pleural effusion	Associated atelectasis, decreased lung volumes	Chest pain, low SpO_2, dyspnea, upper abdominal surgery, obscured costophrenic angle on x-ray
PE	Decreased perfusion to alveoli	Pleuritic chest pain, cough, low SpO_2, tachycardia, tachypnea, dyspnea, inactivity, elevated diaphragm on x-ray, acute hypoxemia with a relatively clear chest x-ray

FRC, Functional residual capacity; *PE,* pulmonary embolism.

Differential Aspects of Atelectasis

Atelectasis can be defined as partial or complete collapse of previously expanded lung tissue and is a common post-operative event. Atelectasis may lead to impaired gas exchange, causing an increased work of breathing, and can predispose the patient to pulmonary infection. As in the current patient, those who have recently undergone upper abdominal surgery are especially at risk. The closer the surgical incision is to the diaphragm, the greater the risk for developing atelectasis.

Knowledge of the patient's medical history is foremost in forecasting the potential for developing atelectasis. Risk factors include chronic lung disease, restrictive disorders, obesity, and a smoking history.

A significant reduction in lung volumes may occur in any post-operative patient who has been anesthetized and immobilized, has neurologic impairment, or is experiencing pain. Failure to take a deep breath periodically or to cough effectively to re-expand the lungs after surgery may cause a progressive decrease in the patient's FRC and secretion retention, resulting in atelectasis. This is especially true during the first 48 hours after surgery.

Clinical signs and symptoms of severe atelectasis include tachypnea, weak cough, and decreased breath sounds. Fine, late inspiratory crackles may be heard over the atelectatic lobe. With an increase in consolidation, bronchial breath sounds may be heard over the affected area. Atelectasis that causes severe hypoxemia frequently leads to tachycardia. Patients with underlying lung disease exhibit an increased respiratory rate and tachycardia with even moderate atelectasis.

TABLE 23-2
Differential Diagnosis for Pneumonia

Type of Surgery	Incidence of Pneumonia (%)
Thoracic	34
Craniotomy	25
Head and neck	25
Coronary artery bypass	21
Cardiac	21
Vascular	20
Cholecystectomy (open)	19
Exploratory laparotomy	18
Colonic	15
Appendectomy	8
Cesarean section	3
Cholecystectomy (laparoscopic)	<1

Adapted from Horan TC, Culver DH, Gaynes RP, et al: *Infect Control Hosp Epidemiol* 14:73, 1993.

The physical examination and the chest x-ray can confirm the diagnosis of atelectasis. Chest x-ray findings suggesting atelectasis are as follows:

1. Increased opacity in the atelectatic region of the lung
2. Displacement of the interlobar fissures
3. Crowding of the pulmonary vessels
4. Presence of air bronchograms, indicating consolidation and loss of volume.

With severe atelectasis, an elevation of the diaphragm and a shift of the trachea toward the affected side of the atelectasis may also be seen.

Treatment of atelectasis is based on re-expanding the collapsed lung segments. A number of therapeutic interventions are used to treat atelectasis, including cough and deep-breathing exercises, incentive spirometry, positive end-expiratory pressure devices, and intermittent or continuous positive airway pressure therapy. Recently, preoperative instruction techniques with incentive spirometry have become more common for high-risk patients who are then aggressively monitored post-operatively. Chest physiotherapy (PT) is indicated when trapped secretions are present. If chest PT is ineffective in removing the secretions, therapeutic bronchoscopy may be indicated. Hypoxemia must be ameliorated with appropriate supplemental oxygen.

Clinical Aspects of Pneumonia

Pneumonia is commonly defined as an inflammatory process of the lung parenchyma, which is usually infectious in origin. Pneumonias are generally classified as either community-acquired or hospital-acquired (nosocomial) pneumonia. This classification is helpful in determining the specific type of pneumonia and appropriate therapeutic management. The prevalence and severity of post-operative pneumonia may reflect the type of surgical procedure performed. The prevalence of post-operative pneumonia ranges from 3% to 34%, depending on the type of surgical procedure (Table 23-2).

Box 23-4
Risk Factors Associated
with Post-Operative Pneumonia

Surgical site
Duration of surgery
Medical history
Surgical history
Pulmonary status
Nutritional status
Duration of intubation/mechanical ventilation

The mortality rate associated with post-operative pneumonia has been reported to be 38% with mortality rates as high as 50% to 70% in patients with gram-negative pneumonia. The risk factors associated with development of post-operative pneumonia are listed in Box 23-4.

The longer the surgery, especially if thoracic or upper abdominal, the greater the risk of developing pneumonia. Mechanically ventilated patients have the highest nosocomial pneumonia rates. As the duration of intubation time increases, the frequency of pneumonia rises. Patients who have been intubated for 2 days or less are reported to have a pneumonia rate of 8% compared with 45% for those intubated longer than 14 days.

Most nosocomial pneumonias occur from aspiration of bacteria colonizing the patients' oropharynx or upper gastrointestinal tract. The placement of an artificial airway, such as occurs with intubation for surgical anesthesia, impairs the coughing mechanism and mucociliary transport that provide the first line of defense in fighting infections. Anesthetics may also impair mucociliary function by decreasing the effectiveness of the cough mechanism and allowing secretions to obstruct the smaller airways. Secretions generally need to be mechanically aspirated from patients with artificial airways, thus increasing the risk of introducing infectious pathogens into the lungs. Alveolar macrophages and humoral defense mechanisms in post-operative patients who are hypoxemic, anemic, malnourished, or who have pulmonary edema may be impaired, facilitating the spread of infection.

Handwashing is another important consideration in the pathogen transmission in the hospital. Meticulous handwashing by all health care providers has been shown to significantly decrease the incidence of nosocomial pneumonia.

Pneumonia can be difficult to diagnose, especially in mechanically ventilated patients. The clinical signs and symptoms suggesting pneumonia are listed in Box 23-5.

Diagnostic Testing for Pneumonia

When pneumonia is suspected, the patient should have a lower airway sample evaluated with a Gram's stain and culture. Samples may be in the form of expectorated secretions, tracheal aspirates, protected brush bronchoscopy specimens, or bronchoalveolar lavage (BAL) fluid, either obtained by bronchoscopy or by a catheter (mini-BAL). Complete blood cultures should be obtained along with a current chest x-ray, and, when hypoxemia is suspected, arterial blood analysis. Spu-

> **Box 23-5**
> **Clinical Signs and Symptoms**
> **Associated with Pneumonia**
>
> Evidence of a new or progressive pulmonary infiltrate
> Temperature >104° F
> Leukocytosis
> Rales/rhonchi
> Purulent tracheobronchial secretions
> Hypoxemia

tum cultures correctly identify the pathogen in approximately 50% of the patients tested for pneumonia, with contamination of expectorated samples by oropharyngeal secretions believed to compound the results.

Treatment for Pneumonia

Selecting the appropriate antibiotic therapy is crucial in treating pneumonia. The antibiotic should be effective against the most likely organism based on the Gram's stain findings and the clinical evidence. Patients are usually started on empiric antibiotic coverage until culture findings are reported. Appropriate antibiotic therapy can lessen the mortality rate from pneumonia, which can approach 70%.

As with the treatment of atelectasis, several respiratory therapy modalities can aid in clearing secretions for those pneumonias that cause excessive mucus production, which are generally bacterial pneumonia. Viral pneumonia seldom produces excessive secretions. When hypoxemia is present, the patient must be treated with sufficient oxygen to increase the PaO_2 to 65 mm Hg, and/or the SpO_2 to 92%. Incentive spirometry may be helpful in increasing lung volumes that may in turn increase the effectiveness of the patient's cough and improve oxygenation.

Clinical Aspects of Pulmonary Embolism

PE may be defined as an occlusion of the pulmonary artery, or one of its branches, by matter carried in the bloodstream, most commonly blood clots. Most patients (90%) develop PE as the result of fragmentation of a DVT of the lower extremities that migrates to the pulmonary circulation. The deep veins of the pelvis are also a frequent source of emboli. Approximately 650,000 patients develop PE each year, and PE is a common pathologic finding at autopsy. The mortality rate for PE is less than 10% when the condition is diagnosed promptly and correctly treated, but the mortality rate rises substantially in patients whose PE is undiagnosed. Importantly, most patients who die from a PE do so within the first hours of the event.

Pulmonary emboli can form at any time, but the three most common factors facilitating clot formation are blood stagnation, increased coagulability, and abnormal vessel wall. Increased coagulability of the blood is associated with prolonged bed rest, and immobility due to pain following trauma and major surgery. Other risk factors include obesity, pregnancy, childbirth, malignant conditions, and the use of birth-control pills.

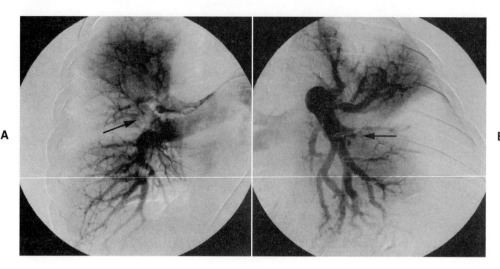

▼ **Figure 23-1** Pulmonary angiogram showing evidence of pulmonary emboli in both lungs. The arrows indicate cutoffs of the pulmonary vessels in the right **(A)** and left **(B)** pulmonary arteries, indicating the presence of acute pulmonary embolism.

PE is difficult to diagnose because the symptoms are non-specific and hard to distinguish from other diseases. Small emboli produce few or no symptoms, whereas large emboli can cause sudden death. Additionally, the primary problem bringing the patient into the hospital (e.g., pneumonia) may obscure the symptoms of PE. The classic signs of a PE are dyspnea, pleuritic chest pain, and hemoptysis. Tachypnea (respirations exceeding 16/min) is almost universally present in patients with PE, but is, of course, non-specific, as it may also accompany many other conditions being entertained in the patient with PE. Hemoptysis, although an important differentiating symptom in the diagnosis of PE, occurs infrequently. Other notable signs are the presence of rales on auscultation, and tenderness, warmth, or redness in the calves, suggesting DVT.

Diagnostic tests such as the chest x-ray, arterial blood gases, and the electrocardiogram are much more useful in ruling out other diseases than in establishing the diagnosis of PE. Test results for all three may be normal even in the presence of a pulmonary embolism. Arterial blood gas (ABG) analysis may be suggestive of pulmonary embolism, but cannot be used to rule it out. Specifically, the alveolar-arterial oxygen gradient is frequently but not universally abnormal in the presence of a pulmonary embolism. Both hypoxemia and hypocarbia may occur.

A six-view ventilation and perfusion ($\dot{V}/\dot{Q}$) lung scan (Figure 23-1) is conventionally the first step in pursuing the diagnosis of PE. If the scan shows normal perfusion, the diagnosis of PE is ruled out. A "high-probability" scan carries an 87% chance for a positive PE. However, as demonstrated by the Prospective Investigation of Pulmonary Embolism Diagnosis (PIOPED) study conducted in 1990, only 42% of patients with a pulmonary embolus had a high-probability scan. Conversely, 14% of patients with "low-probability" scans are expected to have a PE. Data from the PIOPED study also show that the results of the $\dot{V}/\dot{Q}$ scan should be interpreted in the context of the clinician's assessment of the probability of PE. As

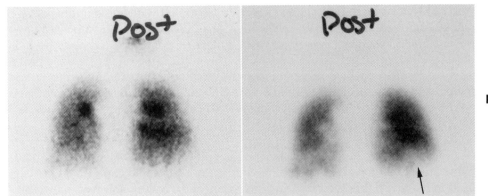

▼ **Figure 23-2** Ventilation/perfusion V̇/Q̇ scan of the lung. Comparison of the posterior views of the ventilation pattern **(A)** and perfusion pattern **(B)** show a high-probability scan. Specifically, there are several segmental perfusion deficits that show preserved ventilation. An example is shown in the right base (arrow) where the perfusion deficit is accompanied by relatively normal ventilation. Such a high-probability V̇/Q̇ scan suggests pulmonary embolism with high likelihood.

TABLE 23-3
Probability of PE Based on the Combination of Prior Clinical Probability and V̇/Q̇ Scan Patterns*

V̇/Q̇ Scan Pattern	Prior Clinical Probability (%)			All Probabilities (%)
	80-100	20-79	0-19	
High probability	96	88	56	87
Intermediate probability	66	28	16	30
Low probability	40	16	4	14
Near normal/normal	0	6	2	4
TOTAL	68	30	9	28

Adapted from Olin J: Deep venous thrombosis and pulmonary emboli. In Stoller JK, Ahmad M, Longworth DL (editors): *The Cleveland Clinic intensive review of internal medicine,* Philadelphia, 2000, Lippincott Williams & Wilkins, pp 413-427.
*PE status in 887 patients from the Prospective Investigation of Pulmonary Embolism Diagnosis (PIOPED) study is based on angiogram interpretation for 713 patients, on angiogram interpretation and outcome classification committee reassignment for 4 patients, and on clinical information alone (without definitive angiography) for 170 patients.

shown in Table 23-3, the probability of PE with a low probability V̇/Q̇ scan falls to 4% when the prior clinical probability of PE is also considered low.

In contrast, when the clinical suspicion of a PE is moderate or high, even a low-probability V̇/Q̇ scan does not reliably exclude the diagnosis, and further testing is needed. In such circumstances, if no other indication for anticoagulation is identified (e.g., DVT is found on leg studies, etc), the diagnosis of PE is often confirmed or refuted using a "gold standard" test, the pulmonary angiogram (Figure 23-2). As with any invasive procedure, there are risks associated with angiography, but the overall complication rate is about 1%. More recently, transthoracic echocardiography, magnetic resonance imaging (MRI), and spiral computed tomography (CT) have been shown to be useful tools in diagnosing PE. Spiral CT is especially promising, as results appear to compare favorably with pulmonary angiography, and the procedure is associated with less risk. However, most clinicians currently regard the spiral CT as having lower sensitivity for emboli that are present in small or peripheral branches of the pulmonary arteries.

The severity of the patient's symptoms will determine the course of therapy for treating a PE. When a reasonable likelihood of pulmonary embolism exists, a bolus of heparin should be given (assuming there are not contraindications for anticoagulation therapy), followed by an intravenous heparin infusion using a weight-based nomogram. Newer regimens of low molecular weight heparin are being evaluated. Thrombolytic therapy is indicated for patients with a PE who are experiencing hemodynamic instability causing right ventricular dysfunction or massive pulmonary embolus. Successful lysis of a thrombus with thrombolytic therapy will help correct acute hemodynamic instability, reverse right ventricular dysfunction, prevent chronic thromboembolic pulmonary hypertension, and lower mortality. Patients who are unable to be treated with anticoagulation therapy generally have a filter placed in the inferior vena cava to prevent the migration of thrombi in the legs or pelvic veins to the pulmonary circulation.

Clinical Aspects of Pleural Effusion

Pleural effusion is defined as an abnormal collection of fluid in the pleural space. As discussed in Chapters 10 and 11, the many causes of pleural effusions are classified according to their etiology and the characteristics as either transudative or exudative fluid (Box 23-6).

A transudative pleural effusion is formed as a result of abnormal hydrostatic and oncotic pressures, without loss of or damage to the integrity of the pleural

---

Box 23-6
Types of Effusions

Transudates	Exudates
Congestive heart failure	Pneumonia
Hypervolemia	PE (usually)
Hypoproteinemia	Subphrenic abscess
Ascites	Infectious disease
PE (rarely)	Gastrointestinal disease
Cirrhosis	Collagen vascular disease
Lymphatic obstruction	Pericardial disease
Atelectasis	Drug-induced pleural disease
Peritoneal dialysis	
Central venous catheter in the pleural space	

PE, Pulmonary embolism.

space. When the total protein concentration of the pleural fluid is less than 50% of the total serum protein level and the lactate dehydrogenase (LDH) values in the pleural fluid are less than 60% of the total serum value, the pleural effusion is said to be a transudate. An exudative pleural effusion occurs as the result of inflammation in the pleura or lung. In exudates, there is more protein and a greater number of inflammatory cells present than in a transudate. Protein-rich exudates are caused by the breakdown of normal reabsorption mechanisms, due to damage to the pleural surface or blockage of the lymphatics. Exudates account for approximately 70% of all pleural effusions.

A variety of surgeries involving the chest or upper abdomen may produce pleural fluid. Pleural effusions caused by cardiac surgeries occur primarily on the left side and tend to be bloody. Lung surgery that leaves the lung too small to fill the thoracic cavity may create a space under negative pressure that fills with an exudative pleural fluid. Pneumonia is among the most frequent causes of post-operative exudates. Most parapneumonic effusions resolve with antibiotic treatment for the pneumonia, although true infection of the pleural fluid (empyema) may occur and generally requires surgical drainage. Upper abdominal surgeries may cause inflammation of the diaphragm and cause an effusion. Light and George reported that 49% of patients receiving abdominal surgery developed pleural effusions.

Atelectasis may cause small transudative pleural effusions. On the other hand, patients with pleural effusions can develop atelectasis due to lung compression by the accumulating fluid.

Most patients with a pleural effusion will have a wide alveolar-arterial (A-a) gradient due to the lung process causing the effusion. Spirometry results will reveal a restrictive pattern that shows immediate improvement once the effusion resolves.

A chest x-ray is the most common method used to detect a pleural effusion. The chest film should be taken with the patient in an upright position to show the pleural fluid meniscus at the costophrenic angle. A lateral decubitus chest x-ray also helps determine the presence or absence of a pleural effusion and can help distinguish pleural thickening from an effusion and free-flowing fluid that is trapped (or loculated). Pleural effusions can also be detected by ultrasound and CT. In fact, CT is the most sensitive test for pleural effusion.

Diagnostic sampling of pleural fluid for cultures, cytology, and chemistries can be accomplished by thoracentesis, which should be performed if there is evidence of pleural effusion on chest x-ray and the fluid layer is greater than 10 mm on a decubitus view. Most parapneumonic effusions resolve with appropriate antibiotic treatment, but if bacteria invade the pleural space, a complicated parapneumonic effusion or empyema may develop. Empyemas require drainage for proper resolution in conjunction with appropriate antibiotic therapy.

Clinical Features and Diagnostic Tests that Suggest a Specific Cause of Hypoxemia

Although several diagnostic entities must be considered as potential causes of this patient's post-operative hypoxemia, the weight of clinical evidence favors a pulmonary embolism. Critical diagnostic reasoning about this patient must take into account the various candidate conditions, including PE, atelectasis, pneumonia, and pleural effusion, and distinguish among them based on information from the patient's history, physical examination, and selected diagnostic testing. Among the features suggesting PE as the cause are the many risk factors that are present (e.g., post-operative state, immobility, etc). Second, the acuity of onset with pleuritic pain and dyspnea is suggestive. Third, the hypoxemia that is unexplained by any parenchymal or pleural abnormalities on chest x-ray simultaneously greatly increases suspicion of pulmonary embolism while it lessens the likelihood of pneumonia or pleural effusion as causes of this patient's hypoxemia.

Atelectasis cannot be excluded and can, in fact, occur as a result of the splinting that accompanies pulmonary embolism. However, given the potential life-threatening nature of pulmonary embolism, especially if undiagnosed and untreated, the astute clinician will pursue the diagnosis of PE to exclusion before comfortably ascribing this patient's signs and symptoms to atelectasis.

Confirmation of the diagnosis in this patient may have been available with bilateral lower extremity duplex studies and a ventilation/perfusion lung scan. If the duplex studies are negative and the $\dot{V}/\dot{Q}$ scan is low or intermediate probability, further pursuit with an alternative procedure will be needed. Ultimately, in this patient, a pulmonary angiogram should be performed if the diagnosis of pulmonary embolism cannot otherwise be excluded or confirmed (e.g., unless the $\dot{V}/\dot{Q}$ scan has a high probability pattern or is normal, or the duplex studies show an acute above-the-knee deep venous phlebitis).

▼ BIBLIOGRAPHY

Campbell RS, Branson RD, Hurst JM: Respiratory care of the surgical patient. In Burton GG, Hodgkin JE, Ward JJ (editors): *Respiratory care: a guide to clinical practice,* ed 4, Philadelphia, 1997, Lippincott, pp 1141-1154.

Davis K, Johnson DJ: Effects of anesthesia and surgery on the respiratory system. In Pierson DJ, Kacmarek RM (editors): *Foundations of respiratory care,* New York, 1992, Churchill Livingstone, pp 389-393.

Demling RH, Wolfort S: Early postoperative pneumonia. In Wilmore DW, Brennan MF, Hasrken AH, et al (editors): *Care of the surgical patient: elective care,* vol 2, New York, 1989, Scientific American.

Farzan A: Pulmonary atelectasis. In Farzan A (editor): *A concise handbook of respiratory diseases,* ed 3, Norwalk, Conn, 1992, Appleton & Lange, pp 243-250.

Horan TC, Culver DH, Gaynes RP, et al: Nosocomial infections in surgical patients in the United States, January 1986-June 1992, *Infect Control Hosp Epidemiol* 14:73-80, 1993.

Joshi GP: Complications related to abdominal surgery with an emphasis on laparoscopy. In Benumof JL, Saidman LJ (editors): *Anesthesia and perioperative complications,* ed 2, St. Louis, 1999, Mosby, pp 665-684.

Lawrence VA, Duncan CA: Respiratory complication of surgery and anesthesia: Overview. In Lubin MF, Walker K, Smith RB (editors): *Medical management of the surgical patient,* ed 3, Philadelphia, 1995, Lippincott, pp 111-116.

Light RW, George RB: Incidence and significance of pleural effusion after abdominal surgery, *Chest* 69:621-625, 1976.

Marini JJ, Pierson DJ, Hudson LD: Acute lobar atelectasis: a prospective comparison of fiberoptic bronchoscopy and respiratory therapy, *Am Rev Respir Dis* 119:971-977, 1979.

Martin LF, Asher EF, Casey JM, et al: Postoperative pneumonia: determinants of mortality, *Arch Surg* 119:379-383, 1984.

Olin J: Deep venous thrombosis and pulmonary emboli. In Stoller JK, Ahmad M, Longworth DL (editors): *The Cleveland Clinic intensive review of internal medicine,* Philadelphia, 2000, Lippincott Williams & Wilkins, pp 413-427.

Patel VM, Honig EG: Post-operative respiratory complications. In Lubin MF, Walker K, Smith RB (editors): *Medical management of the surgical patient,* ed 3, Philadelphia, 1995, Lippincott, pp 145-154.

PIPOED Investigators: Value of the ventilation/perfusion scan in acute pulmonary embolism, *JAMA* 263(20):2753-2759, 1990

Strange C: Pleural diseases. In Scanlan CL, Wilkins RL, Stoller JK (editors): *Egan's fundamentals of respiratory care,* ed 7, St. Louis, 1999, Mosby, pp 475-490.

Wilkins RL, Pierson DJ: Assessment and management of acute atelectasis. In Pierson DJ, Kacmarek RM (editors): *Foundations of respiratory care,* New York, 1992, Churchill Livingstone, pp 851-857.

Wilkins RL, Scanlan CL: Lung expansion therapy. In Scanlan CL, Wilkins RL, Stoller JK (editors): *Egan's fundamentals of respiratory care,* ed 7, St. Louis, 1999, Mosby, pp 771-778.

CHAPTER 24

HYPERCAPNIC RESPIRATORY FAILURE

Lawrence Goldstein

Key Terms

▼ Hypercapnia
▼ Wheezing
▼ Chronic obstructive pulmonary disease (COPD)

▼ Respiratory muscle weakness
▼ Muscle fatigue
▼ Respiratory acidosis

▼ Mechanical ventilation
▼ Bi-level positive airway pressure

▼ THE CLINICAL PROBLEM

A 70-year-old man with chronic obstructive pulmonary disease (COPD) presents to a local emergency department with sudden onset of shortness of breath. He has had several previous admissions for exacerbations of COPD within the last few years. His family also notes that he became somewhat lethargic after this episode began. He previously smoked 1 pack/day for 50 years until quitting 2 years ago.

He has no other significant medical problems. His only medications are ipratropium bromide and albuterol metered dose inhalers.

Physical examination is notable for a somnolent but easily arousable elderly man who is tachycardic and tachypneic. He is using accessory muscles of respiration, and he has prominent chest retractions. Chest examination reveals hyperresonance to percussion with diminished breath sounds and expiratory wheezing.

A room air arterial blood gas reveals pH 7.20, PCO_2 65, PaO_2 56, and SaO_2 88%. A portable chest x-ray shows hyperinflation but no infiltrates.

What is the differential diagnosis for this patient's hypercapnia, and what is the most likely cause?

Differential Diagnosis of Acute Hypercapnia

The differential diagnosis of acute hypercapnic respiratory failure consists of disease processes that impair ventilation. These disorders are generally characterized as those in which the patient "won't breathe" (i.e., the central signals driving respiration are lacking, as in oversedation) versus those in which the patient "can't breathe" (i.e., the signals are intact but the respiratory system cannot respond). The most common causes of hypercapnia include exacerbations of COPD or asthma ("can't breathe"), drug overdoses ("won't breathe"), and neuromuscular diseases such as myasthenia gravis, Guillain-Barré syndrome, and myopathies (also "can't breathe") (Box 24-1). Less common causes include central sleep apnea, stroke, hypothyroidism, metabolic alkalosis, primary alveolar hypoventilation, obesity, pneumothorax, kyphoscoliosis, upper airway obstruction, ankylosing spondylosis, other neuromuscular diseases, and electrolyte disorders such as severe phosphate depletion. Potential causes of impaired ventilation are included in the following categories: decreased respiratory drive ("won't breathe"); respiratory muscle failure ("can't breathe"); or increased work of breathing ("can't breathe") (Table 24-1).

Box 24-1
Differential Diagnosis of Hypercapnia and Classification According to "Can't" Versus "Won't" Breathe

Common Causes	Less Common Causes
Acute exacerbation of COPD (can't breathe)	Stroke (won't breathe)
Status asthmaticus (can't breathe)	Hypothyroidism (won't breathe)
Drug overdose (won't breathe)	Kyphoscoliosis (can't breathe)
Myasthenic crisis (can't breathe)	Metabolic alkalosis (won't breathe)
Polymyositis (can't breathe)	Primary alveolar hypoventilation (won't breathe)
Guillain-Barré syndrome (can't breathe)	Pneumothorax (can't breathe)
Amyotrophic lateral sclerosis (can't breathe)	Pulmonary embolism (ventilated patients, can't breathe)
	Electrolyte abnormality (can't breathe)
	Upper airway obstruction (can't breathe)

COPD, Chronic obstructive pulmonary disease.

Decreased ventilatory drive is caused by decreased output by the respiratory centers within the medulla in the brainstem. This can be due to either exogenous or endogenous causes. The most common exogenous cause of acute hypercapnia is a drug overdose involving narcotics, benzodiazepines, or barbiturates, frequently mixed with alcohol. These medications reduce activity within respiratory centers, which leads to reduced responsiveness to elevation in CO_2 tension. This reduced responsiveness causes a cycle of worsening hypercapnia, which triggers decreased central nervous system activity, which, in turn, causes further retention of CO_2.

Endogenous causes of decreased ventilatory drive include brainstem tumors, stroke or infection, hypothyroidism, primary alveolar hypoventilation, central sleep apnea, and severe metabolic alkalosis. Brainstem tumors, stroke, and infection reduce respiratory center activity by a direct structural effect, while hypothyroidism and metabolic alkalosis have a suppressive effect on respiratory center activity. The causes of primary alveolar hypoventilation and central sleep apnea are currently unclear.

Respiratory muscle failure occurs when there is a signal generated by the central nervous system that either does not reach the muscle because of impaired neuromuscular transmission or because of impairment of the respiratory muscles. Respiratory muscle failure is frequently preceded by muscle fatigue. Muscle fatigue is a reversible loss of ability to develop force because of muscle activity under load that improves with rest. This can be due to an exertion-induced loss of respiratory drive, exertion-induced impairment of neuromuscular transmission, or loss of contraction due to muscle overload. Neuromuscular diseases, such as myasthenia gravis or amyotrophic lateral sclerosis, are the most common causes of respiratory muscle fatigue and failure. These diseases trigger fatigue by requiring expenditure

TABLE 24-1
Interpreting Signs and Symptoms in the Patient with Hypercapnia

Possible Causes	Mechanisms	Suggestive Clinical Features
Acute exacerbation of COPD or asthma	Bronchospasm leads to increased work of breathing and respiratory muscle fatigue	Presence of accessory muscle contraction, chest retraction, and wheezing
Drug overdose	Loss of central ventilatory drive	Presence of gradual decrease in level of consciousness
Stroke	Loss of central ventilatory drive	Presence of sudden decrease in level of consciousness
Myasthenic crisis	Respiratory muscle fatigue	Presence of a prior history and progressive weakness
Amyotrophic lateral sclerosis	Respiratory muscle fatigue and weakness	Presence of weakness and fasciculations

COPD, Chronic obstructive pulmonary disease.

of increasing amounts of energy to do normal physiologic activities such as electrical conduction of impulses or muscle contraction. Other diseases such as COPD can also lead to respiratory muscle fatigue and failure by increasing the work of breathing (WOB).

Increased WOB is the increased force required to bring in a given amount of air into the chest. Increased WOB can be broken down into physiologic and imposed processes. Physiologic WOB is the work required to overcome the elastic recoil of the chest and the resistance of the airways during normal breathing. Imposed work is the work required to overcome the resistance from an endotracheal tube or ventilator tubing when someone is being mechanically ventilated. Increased WOB further stresses a fatiguing muscle, leading to worsening of fatigue and culminating in hypercapnic respiratory failure.

Clinical Features that Suggest a Specific Cause of Hypercapnia

In the patient presented here, the physical examination and the past history of COPD are the most important clinical features that suggest a cause for this patient's hypercapnia. The presence of tachypnea, accessory muscle (e.g., sternocleidomastoid muscle prominence) use, hyperresonance to percussion, and diminished breath sounds with wheezing all suggest an exacerbation of obstructive lung disease. The absence of other clinical features also argues against other causes.

For example, the absence of focal neurologic signs argues against neurologic causes as well as certain types of drug overdoses. Specifically, the absence of pinpoint pupils argues against a narcotics overdose. The absence of any cranial nerve abnormalities (e.g., palsies) argues against a brainstem lesion. The absence of symptoms of weakness or muscle twitching argues against motor neuron disease (amyotrophic lateral sclerosis), muscle disease (polymyositis), nerve transmission disorders (exacerbations of myasthenia gravis, Guillain-Barré syndrome, or botulism), or peripheral nerve processes due to electrolyte deficiencies. Also, the absence of combinations of symptoms such as focal lower extremity weakness and bladder or bowel incontinence argues against spinal cord injury. The clear chest x-ray excludes other contributing factors such as pneumonia, pneumothorax, or pleural effusion.

Clinical features such as intense diuretic therapy and intractable vomiting would lead to consideration of metabolic alkalosis as a cause of acute hypercapnia. However, hypoventilation purely in response to metabolic alkalosis rarely allows the Pco_2 to exceed 55 mm Hg. Physical examination readily identifies other uncommon causes of acute hypercapnia such as obesity and kyphoscoliosis.

Diagnostic Testing in the Evaluation of the Patient with Hypercapnia

The most important "tests" in evaluating a patient with hypercapnia are the clinical history and physical examination. The prior history of any condition that leads to hypercapnia directs the clinician down the right clinical path. At the same time, the clinician must look for other causes that may have contributed to the process such as a bronchitis, pneumonia, or pneumothorax in a patient with COPD. Also, the clinician must be wary of a second unrelated disease process playing a role.

If a patient presents with an altered mental status and has a history of depression, then clearly a toxicology screen would be an appropriate starting point. Likewise, the new onset of headache, confusion, slurred speech, double vision, incoordination, dizziness, or focal weakness leads the clinician to look for a central nervous system process such as stroke or infection. Usually, a computed tomography (CT) scan of the brain followed by lumbar puncture would be the appropriate starting point in this situation.

Patients with a history of underlying neuromuscular disease need to be evaluated for exacerbations of their problem or the effects of overmedication. The classic example is a patient with myasthenia gravis who presents with weakness and hypercapnic respiratory failure. This patient should have an edrophonium (Tensilon) test to differentiate between an exacerbation of myasthenia or overmedication with drugs used to treat myasthenia (e.g., cholinesterase inhibitors). A patient with similar symptoms and no prior history of myasthenia should undergo an electromyogram (EMG) to look for findings of nerve conduction impairment.

A patient who presents with numbness and weakness after a viral prodrome who is found to be hypercapnic should be evaluated with an EMG for Guillain-Barré syndrome. Likewise, a patient who presents with gradual onset weakness, dysphagia, and muscle twitching (fasciculations) should also undergo an EMG to look for motor neuron disease. In any patient with known neurologic disease, a chest x-ray is indicated to look for contributing factors such as atelectasis or pneumonia.

A patient who presents with fatigue, weight gain, weakness, or muscle pain should be evaluated for hypothyroidism with a thyroid stimulating hormone level. It should be pointed out that this is not a common cause of acute-onset hypercapnia. Other important historical factors that suggest decreased respiratory drive include snoring or observed apneas in patients with obstructive sleep apnea. Although this is an uncommon cause of acute onset hypercapnia, minor precipitating factors may lead to significant worsening of a patient's respiratory status. In all of these conditions, the patient should be stabilized before the diagnostic evaluation is undertaken.

For patients with known chronic obstructive lung disease, the history and physical examination usually give a strong clue about the cause of the exacerbation. A history of an upper respiratory tract infection with the development of purulent sputum should suggest a chest x-ray to look for pneumonia. Similarly, patients who present with an acute onset of shortness of breath and pleuritic chest pain should undergo a chest x-ray to exclude a pneumothorax. Patients undergoing mechanical ventilation for any cause who develop hypercapnia should be evaluated for pulmonary thromboembolism.

Assessment of the Effect of Therapy

The simplest way to evaluate the effect of therapy in acute-onset hypercapnia is relief of the patient's respiratory difficulty. Improvement may be recognized in reduced accessory muscle use and the disappearance of chest retractions. Respiratory rate also decreases. Lethargic patients should arouse to their normal level of wakefulness when hypercapnia resolves.

The only way to be sure that hypercapnia has resolved is to check an arterial blood gas. Pneumothorax and atelectasis can be assessed by improved air entry on lung auscultation, and, more definitively, with a chest x-ray. Improved air entry and reduced wheezing on auscultation indicate response to bronchodilators and corticosteroids in patients with chronic obstructive pulmonary disease. Patients with Guillain-Barré syndrome or myasthenic crisis will manifest improved muscle strength after plasma exchange or immunoglobulin therapy.

Pitfalls and Common Mistakes in the Assessment and Treatment of Hypercapnia

The most common pitfall in the assessment of a patient who is acutely hypercapnic is failure to obtain an adequate history. Although it is occasionally true that clinical circumstances preclude a history, a careful history, either from the patient, a friend or family member, is usually available. As an example of the way in which subtle features can suggest an etiology, the patient with early amyotrophic lateral sclerosis may experience weakness that is ignored or rationalized as clumsiness. More commonly, as in acute exacerbations of COPD, an unexpected trigger (e.g., a small pneumothorax) will be missed if not sought. A small pneumothorax may be missed on a chest x-ray, especially if the film is done when the patient is supine. A pneumothorax would also be easy to miss if the patient presents with purulent sputum and is thought to have a tracheobronchitis. In these settings, it is important to remember that bronchitis leads to worsening bronchospasm, which can then lead to a spontaneous pneumothorax.

Another pitfall is failing to look for other complications of the underlying problem. For example, a patient who suffers hypercapnia due to a drug overdose or neuromuscular cause can develop aspiration pneumonitis, which can cause worsened hypercapnia.

Finally, a major pitfall in treating hypercapnia is not knowing when the patient is a candidate for non-invasive ventilation. Patients who are unconscious or otherwise unable to protect their airway should be immediately intubated and mechanically ventilated. Patients who are alert and cooperative may be candidates for non-invasive ventilation with bi-level positive airway pressure. This therapy is highly effective in acute exacerbations of COPD and certain neuromuscular disorders. It is, however, contraindicated if the patient is unable to protect the airway or is uncooperative. It should be remembered that any mode of ventilation that may be given via endotracheal tube or tracheostomy tube can be given non-invasively via a facemask. The most commonly used ventilator mode used non-invasively is pressure support ventilation.

▼ BIBLIOGRAPHY

Meduri GU: Noninvasive positive pressure ventilation in patients with acute respiratory failure, *Clin Chest Med* 17:513-554, 1996.

Pierson DJ: Indications for mechanical ventilation in acute respiratory failure, *Respir Care* 28:5, 1983.

Schmidt GA, Hall JB: Acute on chronic respiratory failure, *JAMA* 261(23):3444-3453, 1989.

Slutsky A: Consensus statement on mechanical ventilation, *Intensive Care Med* 20:64-79, 1994.

CHAPTER 25

ATELECTASIS

Eric D. Bakow

▼ THE CLINICAL PROBLEM

JT is a 54-year-old man who recently underwent a coronary artery bypass graft (CABG). The surgery was uneventful with grafts to three vessels. Before surgery, the patient reported frequent cough with some sputum production in association with a 20 pack-year smoking history, although he reports to have quit smoking 1 month before surgery. Pre-operative spirometry revealed mild-to-moderate airway obstruction that showed a 21% improvement in expiratory flow rates after administering a beta-agonist.

The post-operative course began with 8 hours of mechanical ventilation followed by weaning from assisted ventilation "per protocol." Two days after the surgery, the patient's post-operative forced vital capacity (FVC) is 40% predicted; he is on a nasal cannula 4 L/min with an SpO_2 of 92%. Pain medicine seems adequate, although ambulation is quite limited at this point. Physical findings include diminished breath sounds bilaterally with dullness to chest percussion, respiratory rate of 32 with some accessory muscle use and a temperature of 96.8° F. The chest x-ray shows left lower lobe (LLL) infiltrate/atelectasis.

In addition to the standard post-operative care, the patient is receiving incentive spirometry (IS) every hour while awake (IS volume is 800 cc), deep breathing and coughing by the nursing staff, and an aerosolized beta-agonist every 6 hours. His cough effort is minimal, and the respiratory therapist has noted some congestion.

What is the differential diagnosis, and what is the most likely cause?

Differential Diagnosis of Atelectasis

The term *atelectasis* means "incomplete expansion" and refers to the partial or complete collapse of lung tissue. Clinically significant atelectasis is an important cause of morbidity after thoracic surgery and CABG that can result in pneumonia and an increased hospital stay.

A variety of auscultatory findings can present with atelectasis that range from diminished or absent breath sounds to late inspiratory crackles and bronchial breath sounds. The general response to chest percussion is a dulled note and evidence of an elevated diaphragm over the affected area. With significant parenchymal involvement, the patient may evidence a tachypneic and hypopneic breathing pattern that also involves the use of accessory muscles; tracheal deviation to the affected side may also be apparent.

These findings are very general in nature and may represent several disease entities. The differential diagnosis of patients after CABG with radiologic evidence of atelectasis/infiltrate should include an evaluation for atelectasis, lung infection, pleural fluid, hemothorax/pneumothorax, and left diaphragm hemi-paralysis. The chest x-ray is the primary diagnostic tool for this evaluation. A key radiologic finding is the loss of lung volume, which, when present, should be interpreted as atelectasis. In contradistinction, an increase in thoracic volume of the affected side that is associated with central air bronchograms may favor the diagnosis of pleural effusion.

Fever is not a requisite finding in lung collapse. Engoren examined 100 consecutive patients who underwent CABG and found no association between fever and the presence atelectasis (as confirmed by daily portable chest x-rays) in those patients. Whereas lung infection may mimic the x-ray findings of atelectasis, fever and leukocytosis are important findings in patients with pneumonia.

Atelectasis can be etiologically related to a variety of pathogenic factors. Table 25-1 illustrates these possible causes of lung collapse.

What is the pathophysiologic basis by which each differential diagnostic entity gives rise to the symptom?

Clinical Features that Suggest Atelectasis

Atelectasis can have a quite insidious onset, and the development of lung collapse may be undetected until a substantial amount of lung volume is involved. As the process of alveolar collapse progresses, the stage is set for a "spiral" of clinical sequelae that may end in serious consequences unless intervention occurs (Figure 25-1). Small reductions in alveolar volume result in reductions in the radius of the acinus so that the pressure tending to collapse the air sac increases (the law of Laplace). The end result of this progression is that the compliance of the lung unit

TABLE 25-1
TABLE 25-1
Interpreting Signs and Symptons of Atelectasis

Possible Causes	Mechanisms
Resorption atelectasis	Use of high FIO_2 denitrogenizes alveolar space, reduces alveolar volume
Adhesive atelectasis	Surfactant deficiency, intra-operative manipulation leads to collapse of alveoli; once collapsed alveoli adhere to each other, they require a great inflating pressure to reexpand
Passive atelectasis	Pneumothorax, hypoventilation, diaphragm dysfunction; all interfere with the normal inflation of the alveolus
Cicatrization atelectasis	Alveolar volume loss due to reduced lung compliance associated with diffuse diseases such as pulmonary fibrosis
Gravity dependent atelectasis	Collapse of basilar alveoli due to a hypopneic ventilatory pattern; conditions that increase the weight of the lungs: pneumonia, pulmonary edema

From Massard G, Wihlm J: *Chest Surg Clin N Amer* 8(3):503-528, 1998.
FIO₂, Fraction of inspired oxygen.

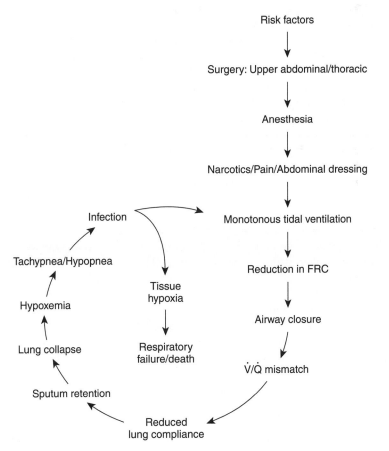

▼ **Figure 25-1** Pathogenic mechanisms and sequelae of atelectasis. *FRC,* Functional residual capacity; *V̇/Q̇,* ventilation/perfusion. From Dantzker DR, MacIntyre NR, Bakow ED: *Comprehensive respiratory care,* Philadelphia, 1995, WB Saunders.

is reduced, which further impairs alveolar ventilation. This cycle self-perpetuates to complete collapse unless a significant intervention can reinflate the alveolus, restore alveolar compliance, and simultaneously reduce the pressure tending to collapse the air space.

There is a concomitant increase in the work of breathing needed to maintain a physiologic alveolar minute volume due to the increase in lung impedance (reduced lung compliance, increased airway resistance) caused by atelectasis. This may translate into a more energy-conserving breathing pattern that is typically hypopneic (shallow tidal breathing) and tachypneic, resulting in accessory muscle use and the complaint of shortness of breath. Patients at risk with pre-existing respiratory muscle dysfunction will quickly demonstrate these signs and symptoms.

Alterations in gas transport will also be seen in clinically important lung collapse. Physiologic shunt fractions will increase in areas of collapsed lung leading to hypoxemia and possible tissue hypoxia. An arterial blood gas would typically reveal a widened A-a DO_2 gradient and a mild respiratory alkalosis. Tissue hypoxia would result in a concomitant metabolic acidosis. Monitoring of SpO_2 is now commonplace, and reductions in arterial saturation will parallel the degree of collapsed lung tissue.

Assessment of Therapy for Atelectasis

The coexistence of pain, pre-existing lung disease that tends to produce secretions, and a limited ability to deep breathe and cough are key variables that predispose to lung collapse. This constellation of findings, as demonstrated by this patient, frequently leads to clinically important atelectasis that requires supplemental oxygen. Interventions at this point must stress two immediate goals of therapy: improve airway patency and provide adequate lung inflation.

Endobronchial secretions reduce alveolar ventilation, which in turn reduces lung volume and puts into place the above mechanisms that result in atelectasis. The task of removing these secretions is made more difficult with the addition of incisional pain, narcotics, binders, and wound dressings. Inhaled beta-agonists play a role in increasing the diameter of small airways, which are then capable of ventilating more distal regions of lung parenchyma. An array of therapeutic alternatives has a proven ability to remove secretions from the airway. Percussion and postural drainage therapy, directed coughing, the Flutter valve, and airway suctioning are some of the possible options for this purpose. These therapies require an analysis of patient-specific indications, hazards, and contraindications to determine a therapeutic approach for a given patient. Standardized protocols have been used with good success in the appropriate application of respiratory care modalities. Regardless of the treatment modality, a key treatment strategy is to perform a *frequent re-assessment* of clinical outcomes (such as cough effort, sputum production, slow vital capacity, breath sounds, SpO_2, etc) to assure the reversal of this pathologic process. The physiologic response to each treatment requires some objective measure of outcome from that treatment and a comparison of that outcome to the results of previous therapies. Serial chest x-rays may also be helpful in assessing the efficacy of these therapeutic interventions.

Perhaps less well defined is therapy to re-expand collapsed lung parenchyma. The "ideal" lung inflation maneuver is one in which a large transpulmonary pressure gradient (the difference between alveolar pressure and pleural pressure) and a large inflating volume are maintained for several seconds. It is the transpulmonary pressure gradient that is responsible for "stretching" the lung and maintaining alveolar volume. It stands to reason that an inspiratory maneuver that can reliably reproduce these criteria will be useful in treating atelectasis. Current inspiratory maneuvers for this purpose now include sustained maximum inspiration (SMI), with or without an incentive spirometer; intermittent positive-pressure breathing (IPPB); face mask continuous positive airway pressure (CPAP) breathing or biphasic positive airway pressure (BiPaP); and positive expiratory pressure (PEP). Controversy persists regarding the precise role of IS in the treatment of atelectasis. However, few would dispute the routine inclusion of IS into the treatment plan of a patient with atelectasis if given attention to inspiratory volume, encouragement to use the device every hour, and careful monitoring of actual use of the spirometer.

Atelectasis can progress to collapse of a lobe or an entire lung and therapeutic fiberoptic bronchoscopy (FOB) may be an effective approach for these critical conditions. The principle mechanism of action for FOB is the ability to selectively remove secretions from the lumen of the airway, thereby restoring the channel for inflating volume and pressure to enter the collapsed lung unit. FOB also stimulates cough and may produce a localized "PEP effect" in the airway due to partial occlusion of the airway and increased airway pressure. Considerable risks accompany this technique, and at least one randomized trial involving 31 patients with acute lobar atelectasis concluded there may be no additional benefit to bronchoscopy in the treatment of these patients.

A less commonly used treatment of persistent atelectasis involves the use of "directed manual recruitment" of the lung. Scholten and colleagues described this technique in a case report involving the treatment of 4 patients with radiographic evidence of atelectasis. They used a handbag resuscitator that provided large inflating volumes and pressures over 10 to 30 seconds. A pressure manometer was placed in-line between the bag and the patient's artificial airway for precise monitoring of distending pressure. Chang-Yao et al described a similar technique using "air insufflation" in combination with a fiberoptic bronchoscope to successfully treat atelectasis in 12 patients in a medical intensive care unit (ICU). These authors reported no significant complications from the procedure, but there was significant potential for barotrauma and cardiac compromise. This treatment modality should be reserved for carefully selected and appropriately monitored patients with refractory atelectasis.

This patient's portable chest x-ray demonstrated LLL atelectasis, which was effectively managed with an increase in the frequency of the inhaled beta-agonist to every 4 hours, followed by postural drainage and percussion to the left side. Coordinating this therapy with the administration of pain medication increased the cough effort and sputum production. The patient's inspiratory capacity, measured with IS that was monitored every 2 hours, increased to 1.2 L. A repeat chest x-ray showed significant resolution of the LLL collapse over the next 48 hours, and the patient was then weaned to room air by pulse oximetry.

Pitfalls and Common Mistakes in the Assessment and Treatment of Atelectasis

Interpreting the radiographic signs of atelectasis can be a challenge. Technical variables inherent in the process of producing a portable chest x-ray are considerable: patient positioning, the degree of lung inflation, and exposure/projection variations that can greatly alter the final image.

Distinguishing lobar atelectasis from pneumonia may be problematic. Volume loss on the affected side is a key variable in this distinction. LLL collapse may also be confused with pneumomediastinum or pneumopericardium in the anteroposterior (AP) projection when the major fissure of a partially aerated lobe is lateral to and parallel with the heart border.

The radiographic appearance of atelectasis is evidence most often of lobar involvement, and there tends to be a recognizable pattern of radiographic changes as a function of the lobar anatomy that is involved. Woodring and Reed summarized the work of others to describe direct and indirect radiographic signs of atelectasis. Direct radiographic signs of atelectasis include crowded pulmonary vessels, crowded air bronchograms, and displacement of interlobular fissures. Indirect radiographic signs of atelectasis are defined with the following characteristics: pulmonary opacification, elevation of the diaphragm, mediastinal shift, displacement of the hilum, approximation of the ribs, compensatory hyperexpansion of the surrounding lung. The Woodring and Reed report is a more complete description of the radiographic signs of atelectasis.

▼ BIBLIOGRAPHY

American Association for Respiratory Care: AARC Clinical Practice Guideline: use of positive pressure adjuncts to bronchial hygiene therapy, *Resp Care* 38(5):516, 521, 1993.

Bartlett RH, Gazzaniga AB, Geraghty TR: Respiratory maneuvers to prevent postoperative pulmonary complications: a critical review, *JAMA* 224(7):1017-1021, 1973.

Chang-Yao T, Tsai Y, Lan R, et al: Treatment for collapsed lung in critically ill patients–selective intrabronchial air insufflation using the fiberoptic bronchoscope, *Chest* 97(2):435-438, 1990.

Crowe JM, Bradley CA: The effectiveness of incentive spirometry with physical therapy for high risk patients after coronary artery bypass surgery, *Physic Ther* 77(3):260-268, 1997.

Engoren M: Lack of association between atelectasis and fever, *Chest* 107(1):81-84, 1995.

Gosselink R, Schrever K, Cops P, et al: Incentive spirometry does not enhance recovery after thoracic surgery, *Crit Care Med* 28(3):679-683, 2000

Kester L, Stoller JK: Monitoring quality in a respiratory care service: methods and outcomes, *Resp Care* 44(5):512-519, 1999

Langenderfer B: Alternatives to percussion and postural drainage, *J Cardiopulmonary Rehabil* 18(4):283-289, 1998

MacMahon H: Pitfalls in portable chest radiology, *Resp Care* 44(9):1018-1032, 1999.

Marini JJ, Pierson DJ, Hudson LD: Acute lobar atelectasis: A prospective comparison of fiberoptic bronchoscopy and respiratory therapy, *Amer Rev Respir Dis* 119:971-977, 1979.

Marini JJ, Wheeler AP: Fiberoptic bronchoscopy in critical care. In Civetta JM, Taylor RN, Kirby RR (editors): *Critical care*, Philadelphia, 1988, JB Lippincott.

Massard G, Wihlm J: Postoperative atelectasis, *Chest Surg Clin N Amer* 8(3):503-528, 1998.

Miller WT: Radiographic evaluation of the chest. In Fishman AP (editor): *Pulmonary diseases and disorders*, New York, 1988, McGraw-Hill, pp 479-527.

Raoof S, Chowdhrey N, Raoof S, et al: Effect of combined kinetic therapy and percussion therapy on the resolution of atelectasis in critically ill patients, *Chest* 115(6):1658-1666, 1999.

Scholten DJ, Novak R, Snyder JV: Directive manual recruitment of collapsed lung in intubated and nonintubated patients, *American Surg* 51:330-335, 1985.

Woodring JH, Reed JC: Types and mechanisms of pulmonary atelectasis, *J Thoracic Imaging* 11:92-108, 1996.

CHAPTER 26

PRE-OPERATIVE EVALUATION

Brian M. Legere
Alejandro C. Arroliga

Key Terms

▼ Pulmonary function tests
▼ Forced expiratory volume in 1 second (FEV₁)
▼ Quantitative lung perfusion scintigraphy

▼ Predicted post-operative FEV₁
▼ Diffusing capacity
▼ Upper abdominal incision

▼ Thoracotomy
▼ Sternotomy

▼ THE CLINICAL PROBLEM

Patient 1: Peripheral Lung Mass

A 62-year-old man who is a former smoker presents for pre-operative evaluation before a planned resectional surgery for a right upper lobe (RUL) peripheral lung mass. The lesion was initially identified on a chest radiograph performed during a recent episode of bronchitis. A computed tomography (CT) scan of the chest revealed a 4-cm mass lesion in the RUL that abutted the lateral chest wall. The mass was diagnosed as adenocarcinoma by means of a transbronchial biopsy. A work-up for metastatic disease was negative. The patient has noted moderate exertional dyspnea, as well as a chronic cough productive of whitish sputum for the past 4 to 5 years.

The patient's past medical history is significant for chronic obstructive pulmonary disease (COPD) and hypertension. The patient smoked 2 packs of cigarettes per day for 35 years and quit smoking 7 years ago. Current medications include diltiazem, albuterol, and ipratropium bromide.

Physical examination revealed a blood pressure of 136/80, a heart rate of 80, and a respiratory rate of 14. Head and neck examination was normal. Lung examination revealed decreased breath sounds bilaterally with a prolonged expiratory phase and scattered wheezes. A regular rate and rhythm without murmurs, rubs, or gallops was noted on cardiac examination. The remainder of the physical examination was normal.

Pulmonary function tests (PFT) revealed a forced vital capacity (FVC) of 3.77 L (92% predicted), and a forced expiratory volume in 1 second (FEV_1) of 1.89 L (60% predicted). The FEV_1/FVC ratio was 0.50. Lung volumes utilizing body plethysmography revealed a total lung capacity (TLC) of 6.10 L (94% predicted) and a residual volume (RV) of 2.09 L (90% predicted). A diffusion capacity of lung for carbon monoxide (D_{LCO}) was 11.9 mL/min/mm Hg (56% predicted).

Diagnostic Testing in the Evaluation of Lung Resection

Evaluation of the patient with COPD who requires resectional surgery for lung cancer is a common problem in pulmonary medicine. To date, surgical resection is the only therapeutic modality that offers a significant chance of a cure for lung cancer. The primary role of the clinician is to identify patients at risk for complications from the proposed surgery and assess the magnitude of this risk. Patients who are refused surgery due to unacceptably high risk should be offered non-surgical therapy. For patients who are deemed appropriate candidates for thoracotomy and lung resection, steps (e.g., incentive spirometry, peri-operatively optimizing lung function with bronchodilators, etc.) should be taken to reduce the likelihood of peri-operative complications.

An understanding of the effects of thoracic surgery on lung and chest wall mechanics is required to adequately assess the operative candidate. Pneumonectomy and to a lesser extent lobectomy can lead to significant effects on respiratory mechanics. After thoracotomy or lung resection, chest wall compliance can be reduced by up to 75%. After pneumonectomy, the contralateral lung distends to fill the thoracic cavity. However, despite this compensatory response, the TLC and vital capacity (VC) are usually reduced. The FVC and FEV_1 can be reduced by 35% to 40% after pneumonectomy. The D_{LCO} is also expected to decrease significantly. Furthermore, the mean maximum exercise capacity can be reduced by as much as 28% after pneumonectomy. Smaller reductions in static lung volumes are encountered after lobectomy. The FEV_1 and D_{LCO} are only minimally changed after lobectomy.

Patients undergoing lung resection are at increased risk for peri-operative morbidity and mortality. It is difficult to estimate true complication rates because most studies investigating this problem are retrospective, and the definitions of peri-operative complications have differed greatly between studies. However, most studies include prolonged mechanical ventilation, pneumonia, atelectasis, and the need for reintubation as complications of lung resection.

Overall mortality rates for pneumonectomy range from 2% to 12%. The prevalence of mortality related to lobectomy is generally lower at 4% to 9%. Complications, such as pneumonia, atelectasis, prolonged air leak, and respiratory failure, occur in fewer than 6% of cases.

Many techniques have been used to identify patients at risk for complications from lung resection and to predict post-operative lung function. Commonly used modalities include spirometry, measurement of diffusion capacity for carbon monoxide, arterial blood gas analysis, lung perfusion scintigraphy, and exercise testing. It is widely held that patients with a pre-operative FEV_1 greater than 2 L or a predicted post-operative FEV_1 greater than 0.8 L or 40% of predicted, as well as a pre-operative DLCO greater than 80% of predicted can undergo a pneumonectomy. A pre-operative FEV_1 greater than 40% of predicted may be adequate if only a lobectomy is planned. Patients who do not meet these criteria should undergo further evaluation to better estimate post-operative lung function.

Cardiopulmonary exercise testing provides a readily available noninvasive means to assess candidates with borderline lung function. If the maximal measured oxygen consumption ($\dot{V}O_2$ max) is greater than 75% of predicted or 20 mL/kg/min, then a resection up to a pneumonectomy can be performed. Surgery should be reconsidered in patients with a $\dot{V}O_2$ max less than 10 mL/kg/min because of likely higher mortality. For patients whose exercise test results fall between these limits, further testing with perfusion scintigraphy is advised.

Quantitative lung perfusion scintigraphy has been used to accurately predict post-operative lung function after pneumonectomy or lobectomy. The contribution of the segments that will be resected to total lung perfusion can be assessed. The predicted post-operative FEV_1 can be calculated using the formula: post-operative FEV_1 = pre-operative FEV_1 × (1 fractional contribution of segments to be resected). It is also possible to predict post-operative lung function mathematically without relying on imaging techniques. It is estimated that each of the 19 bronchopulmonary segments contributes 5.26% to total lung function.

The American College of Physicians recommends that candidates for lung resection undergo a stepwise assessment that starts with routine spirometry and arterial blood gas analysis. Subsequently, perfusion scintigraphy or cardiopulmonary exercise testing can be performed if necessary. The algorithm outlined in Figure 26-1 provides a logical approach to evaluating candidates for lung resection.

The patient in this case has an FEV_1 of 1.89 L, which is less than 80% of predicted. His spirometry results predict that he could tolerate a lobectomy. Further testing, beginning with a cardiopulmonary stress test, would be necessary if a pneumonectomy was planned.

Patient 2: Coronary Artery Bypass Graft

A 70-year-old woman presents for pre-operative evaluation before elective coronary artery bypass graft (CABG) surgery. She was in her usual state of health until 2 months previously, when she noted left-sided substernal chest pain on exertion. Exercise echocardiography revealed anterior and lateral wall motion abnormalities with exercise. A subsequent coronary angiogram revealed three vessel coronary artery disease (CAD) amenable to surgical revascularization. Her only other complaint is that of slowly progressive moderate exertional dyspnea.

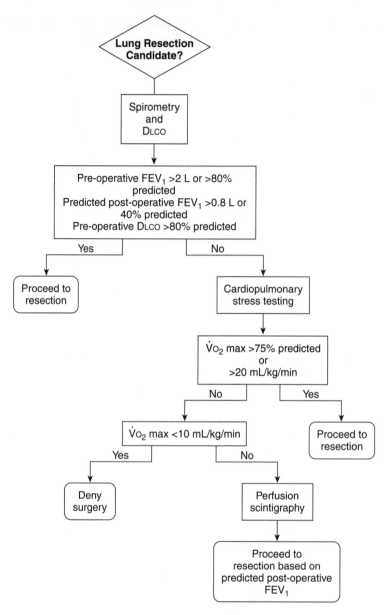

▼ **Figure 26-1** Proposed evaluation for patients undergoing lung resection.

The patient's past medical history is positive for diabetes mellitus and hypertension. She continues to smoke 1 pack of cigarettes per day and has done so for 40 years. Her current medications include glyburide, enteric-coated aspirin, isosorbide dinitrate, and enalapril.

On physical examination, her blood pressure was 128/60, heart rate was 80, and respiratory rate was 17. Head and neck examination was normal. The lungs were clear to auscultation. Cardiac examination revealed a regular rate and rhythm without murmur, rub, or gallop. The remainder of the physical examination was unremarkable.

PFT revealed an FVC of 2.38 L (91% predicted) and an FEV_1 of 1.04 L (52% predicted). The FEV_1/FVC ratio was 0.44 (57% predicted). There was a significant bronchodilator response (i.e., the FEV_1 increased by more than 200 mL and 12% after an inhaled bronchodilator). The chest radiograph revealed only mild hyperinflation and osteopenia.

Diagnostic Testing in the Evaluation of Non-Resectional Thoracic Surgery

Cardiac surgeries, specifically CABG, constitute the majority of non-resectional thoracic surgical procedures. Because of the well-known association between tobacco abuse and CAD, a significant percentage of CABG candidates have concomitant obstructive airway disease, which is the case in this patient. These patients are often referred for "clearance" before their surgeries. The utility of pre-operative pulmonary screening in this population has been hotly debated over the past few decades.

Although the majority of these procedures are performed via a median sternotomy, the alterations of the pulmonary mechanics are similar to those seen after thoracotomy. A significant decrease in pulmonary compliance is noted in the immediate postoperative period. Reduction in static lung volumes up to 33% can be observed at the time of discharge. Substantial diminution in FEV_1 and FVC by nearly 50% can also be expected after CABG. Furthermore, transient hypoxemia related to abnormalities in ventilation-perfusion matching can be seen postoperatively. Abnormalities in pulmonary function may be exacerbated by the routine harvesting of internal mammary artery (IMA) grafts, which can result in reductions in lung volumes due to phrenic nerve injury. Despite these changes in pulmonary function, the majority of patients can be extubated sooner than 24 hours after surgery. Furthermore, pulmonary function parameters can be expected to return to baseline within 3 months.

A more serious and potentially long-lasting sequela of cardiac surgery is unilateral and less commonly bilateral diaphragmatic paralysis, which can complicate up to 17% of cardiac surgeries. Such diaphragmatic dysfunction is felt to be the result of thermal injury to the phrenic nerve related to the use of ice/slush hypothermia during cardiac surgery. IMA graft harvesting, as well as the presence of diabetes mellitus, may also increase the risk of this complication. Although some patients may suffer long-term disability due to diaphragmatic dysfunction, most patients recover with time.

Several risk factors for developing peri-operative pulmonary complications have been identified in patients undergoing cardiac surgery. Low ejection fraction, clinical congestive heart failure, unstable angina, diabetes mellitus, and current to-bacco abuse have been shown to correlate with the need for prolonged mechanical ventilation post-operatively. Other risk factors for prolonged intubation include age, congestive heart failure, renal insufficiency, priority of surgery, prolonged use of intra-aortic balloon counterpulsation, recent myocardial infarction, and a history of prior cardiac surgery. Pre-operative pulmonary function abnormalities have not been shown to correlate with post-operative complications, including prolonged ventilation. Therefore surgery should not be denied to a potential candidate solely on the basis of abnormal PFTs.

It is currently recommended that PFT should be considered only in cardiac surgery candidates with a history of tobacco abuse and dyspnea. Diagnosing underlying lung disease may be helpful in planning peri-operative respiratory therapy. In this patient, with both chronic dyspnea and tobacco abuse, performing spirometry was warranted. Adding bronchodilators with or without systemic or inhaled steroids may be helpful in managing her symptoms. Furthermore, counseling the patient to stop smoking at least 2 months pre-operatively is also indicated, as this has been shown to decrease peri-operative morbidity.

Patient Number 3: Cholecystectomy

A 32-year-old man, who does not smoke, presents for evaluation before cholecystectomy. His past medical history is significant only for childhood asthma that is now quiescent. The patient has not required the use of bronchodilators for several years. He denies the presence of dyspnea or wheezing. He is on no medications and denies any known drug allergies.

Physical examination revealed a blood pressure of 110/70, a heart rate of 65, and a respiratory rate of 13. Head and neck examination was within normal limits. The lungs were clear to auscultation and percussion. The cardiac examination was normal, as was the remainder of the physical examination.

Spirometry was requested by the surgeon and is available for review. The FVC is 5.54 L (108% predicted). The FEV_1 is 4.30 L (101% predicted) and the FEV_1/FVC ratio is 0.78.

Evaluation of the Candidate for Abdominal Surgery

The likelihood of developing pulmonary morbidity after abdominal surgery depends largely on the location of the incision (upper versus lower abdomen). The major physiologic effects of abdominal surgery are exerted on the respiratory musculature, specifically the diaphragm. Therefore the closer the incision is to the diaphragm, the greater is the expected effect on pulmonary function.

After upper abdominal surgery, the clinician can expect attendant reductions in static lung volumes and the development of a rapid, shallow breathing pattern. Measurement of transdiaphragmatic pressures and diaphragmatic electromyography (EMG) confirms the presence of post-operative muscle dysfunction. To compensate for diaphragmatic weakness, intercostal and accessory muscle activity is increased. Furthermore, pain and surgical disruption of abdominal musculature can significantly reduce the contribution of abdominal muscles to respiratory effort. The result of these changes is a decreased ability to cough and an increased risk of post-operative atelectasis. Post-operative reductions in vital capacity are of a lesser magnitude and duration after lower abdominal surgery. Furthermore, impairment of diaphragmatic function is minimal after lower abdominal surgery.

The choice of surgical technique, either open or laparoscopic, can also have significant implications for post-operative pulmonary function and morbidity. Given the smaller wound size and the lesser degree of abdominal muscle disruption, one would expect laparoscopic procedures to have less impact on respiratory function. The effects of laparoscopy on pulmonary function are the direct result of the insufflation of gas (typically CO_2) into the peritoneal cavity. In addition to causing hypercarbia and acidosis, CO_2 insufflation increases the intra-abdominal pressure. This can have significant effects on respiratory mechanics. Pulmonary compliance and FRC are reduced as the diaphragm is forced upward, causing attendant reductions in both the FVC and the FEV_1. However, pulmonary function impairment is less pronounced and of shorter duration after laparoscopic procedures when compared to traditional "open" techniques.

A significant frequency of pulmonary complications is expected because of the degree of respiratory physiologic changes associated with abdominal surgery. Whereas aspiration, pneumonia, fever, and respiratory failure have been reported after both laparotomy and laparoscopy, atelectasis remains the most commonly encountered complication. Pulmonary complications can occur in over 22% of open abdominal procedures. The risk is significantly reduced with laparoscopy. Advanced age, increased body mass index, intra-peritoneal infection, prolonged pre-operative hospitalization, and upper abdominal incision site have been identified as risk factors for post-operative complications. However, neither abnormalities in pre-operative spirometry nor a history of lung disease has been shown to correlate with respiratory complications.

It is currently recommended that pre-operative spirometry be considered only for patients with a history of tobacco abuse or dyspnea before upper abdominal surgery. In the absence of overt signs or symptoms of significant respiratory disease, there is no indication for performing lung function tests before lower abdominal procedures. In this case, obtaining pre-operative spirometry was probably unwarranted.

Evaluation of the Patient Undergoing Peripheral Surgery

Few data are available regarding the pulmonary evaluation of patients undergoing surgery that does not involve the thorax or abdomen. Aside from the direct effects of anesthesia, significant peri-operative perturbations in respiratory mechanics or gas exchange are not expected. Indeed, the frequency of pulmonary complications in this setting is exceedingly low. Therefore, in the absence of signs or symptoms of significant respiratory disease, routine pulmonary evaluation is unnecessary.

▼ SUMMARY

Despite the existence of guidelines for the appropriate utilization of pre-operative PFT, it is possible that a significant proportion of these tests are performed unnecessarily. Extensive pulmonary evaluation should only be undertaken in patients who are candidates for lung resection. Patients with dyspnea or a history of significant tobacco abuse, who are about to undergo cardiac or upper abdominal surgery, are also appropriate candidates for pre-operative PFT. Before lower abdominal or peripheral surgeries, routine testing is unwarranted, unless evidence of significant occult respiratory disease exists.

▼ BIBLIOGRAPHY

Arroliga AC, Buzaid AC, Matthay RA: Which patients can safely undergo lung resection? *J Respir Dis* 12:1080-1086, 1991.

Bolton JW, Weiman DS: Physiology of lung resection, *Clin Chest Med* 14:293-303, 1993.

Brooks-Brunn JA: Predictors of postoperative pulmonary complications following abdominal surgery, *Chest* 111:564-71, 1997.

Ford GT, Rosenal TW, Clergue F, et al: Respiratory physiology in upper abdominal surgery, *Clin Chest Med* 14:237-252, 1993.

Hnatiuk OW, Dillard TA, Torrington KA: Adherence to established guidelines for preoperative pulmonary function testing, *Chest* 107:1294-1297, 1997.

Kearney DJ, Lee TH, Reilly JJ: Assessment of operative risk in patients undergoing lung resection. Importance of predicted pulmonary function, *Chest* 105:753-759, 1994.

Lawrence VA, Ohanda R, Hilsenbeck SG, et al: Risk of pulmonary complications after elective abdominal surgery, *Chest* 110:744-750, 1996.

Matsumoto M, Konishi Y, Miwa S, et al: Effect of different methods of internal thoracic artery harvest on pulmonary function, *Ann Thorac Surg* 63:653-655, 1997.

Nugent AM, Steele IC, Carragher AM: Effect of thoracotomy and lung resection on exercise capacity in patients with lung cancer, *Thorax* 54:334-338, 1999.

Schwenk W, Bohm B, Witt C, et al: Pulmonary function following laparoscopic or conventional colorectal resection: a randomized controlled evaluation, *Arch Surg* 134:6-12, 1999.

Tripp HF, Bolton JW: Phrenic nerve injury following cardiac surgery: a review, *J Card Surg* 13:218-223, 1998

Wyser C, Stulz P, Soler M: Prospective evaluation of an algorithm for the functional assessment of lung resection candidates, *Am J Respir Crit Care Med* 159:1450-1456, 1999.

Yano T, Yokoyama H, Fukuyama Y: The current status of postoperative complications and risk factors after a pulmonary resection for primary lung cancer. A multivariate analysis, *Eur J Cardiothorac Surg* 11:445-449, 1997.

Zibrak JD, O'Donnell CR, Marton K: Indications for pulmonary function testing, *Ann Intern Med* 112:763-771, 1990.

PART IV

COMMON PROBLEMS IN THE ICU ADULT

CHAPTER 27

THE DIFFICULT-TO-WEAN PATIENT

Richard D. Branson

Key Terms

▼ Weaning
▼ Polyneuropathy
▼ Intrinsic positive end-expiratory pressure (PEEP)
▼ Chronic obstructive pulmonary disease (COPD)

▼ Patient-ventilator dys-synchrony
▼ Spontaneous breathing trial
▼ Dynamic hyperinflation
▼ Respiratory muscle load
▼ Respiratory muscle capacity
▼ $P_{0.1}$

▼ Deadspace
▼ Rapid shallow breathing index
▼ Spontaneous breathing trial
▼ Auto-PEEP

▼ THE CLINICAL PROBLEM

A 63-year-old man with a history of chronic obstructive pulmonary disease (COPD) is admitted to the intensive care unit with pneumonia. The patient is well known by the pulmonary staff. He is moderately obese, has well-documented reactive airways disease, and coughs up about 1 cup of sputum per day. His arterial blood gases (ABGs) show marked hypercarbia and hypoxemia. He has significant accessory muscle use, and, over a short time, he becomes obtunded. He is intubated and placed on mechanical ventilation.

After 6 days of treatment that includes antibiotics, bronchodilators, and mechanical ventilation, his condition improves. He is awake and oriented. His current ventilator settings in the assist/control mode include a set respiratory frequency of 12 breaths/min, tidal volume of 600 mL, decelerating inspiratory flow pattern at 70 L/min, positive end-expiratory pressure (PEEP) of 4 cm H_2O, and an inspired oxygen concentration (FIO_2) of 0.40. His temperature is 99.5° F, his white blood cell (WBC) count is 10.6 per mm^3, and his hemoglobin is 10.4 g/dL. His chest x-ray shows clearing densities in the lower lobes bilaterally, flattened diaphragms, and areas of over-distension in the non-dependent (apical) segments. His breath sounds reveal diminished sounds at the bases and rhonchi throughout. He is receiving enteral nutrition (65% carbohydrate, 20% lipid, and 15% protein) at 60 mL/hr. This provides 1440 calories per day. He continues on antibiotics for his pneumonia.

Over the past 24 hours, he has been suctioned via the endotracheal tube on seven occasions. Approximately 40 mL of yellow secretions of a moderate consistency has been removed. He continues on aerosolized bronchodilators via a metered dose inhaler every 4 hours. His blood pressure is 140/73, his heart rate is 96, and his electrocardiogram shows normal sinus rhythm with occasional premature ventricular contractions. He is orally intubated with a 7.5-mm internal diameter tube that measures 29 cm at the lip. Humidification is provided with a heated humidifier set to deliver 34° C at the Y-piece. His most recent ABG values demonstrate a pH of 7.44, $PaCO_2$ of 52 mm Hg, PaO_2 of 73 mm Hg, base excess of 6 mEq/L, HCO_3^- of 27 mEq/L, and SaO_2 of 97%.

After morning rounds, the decision to attempt a spontaneous breathing trial is made. The patient remains connected to the ventilator, and the mode is switched to continuous positive airway pressure (CPAP). The CPAP control is turned to 0 cm H_2O and the FIO_2 remains 0.40. Pressure support remains off. After 10 minutes, the patient's respiratory rate is 32 and his tidal volume is 230 mL, resulting in a minute volume of 7.36 L/min. His heart rate has increased to 109 and his blood pressure is now 168/87. His frequency to tidal volume ratio (f/V_T) is 139. He is placed back on assist control at a frequency of 10 breaths/min.

Spontaneous breathing trials are attempted on four occasions over the next 3 days with similar results. After a short period of time, his f/V_T is 130-150, and he becomes noticeably uncomfortable.

This difficult-to-wean patient has a number of potential impediments to weaning. What is the differential for determining the possible causes of weaning failure, and what is the most likely cause?

Differential Diagnosis of Weaning Failure

Perhaps the most-often seen cause of weaning failure is that the patient is not ready. Before weaning attempts, the underlying cause that resulted in institution of mechanical ventilation must be alleviated. Ely and others have developed a mnemonic to describe the difficult-to-wean patient, "WHEANS NOT." This allows the clinician to evaluate the many potential causes of weaning failure.

Wheezes
Heart disease, Hypertension
Electrolyte imbalance

Anxiety, Airway abnormalities, Alkalosis (metabolic)
Neuromuscular disease, use of Neuromuscular blockers
Sepsis, Sedation
Nutrition (under- and over-feeding)
Opiates, Obesity
Thyroid disease

Weaning failure typically results as a consequence of an imbalance between respiratory neuromuscular capacity and respiratory load. This imbalance leads to respiratory muscle failure. Common causes of respiratory muscle failure include dynamic hyperinflation, respiratory acidosis, decreased oxygen delivery, malnutrition, excessive CO_2 production, increased deadspace ventilation, increased respiratory system impedance, and intrinsic PEEP (Box 27-1).

Other causes of weaning failure include a decreased output of the respiratory control center caused by oversedation, neurologic dysfunction, or use of narcotic drugs. Cardiovascular dysfunction may also impede weaning, and left heart failure has been demonstrated to be a cause of weaning failure in COPD. Myocardial ischemia may occur during weaning due to increased oxygen consumption of the respiratory muscles and stress.

Electrolyte abnormalities, acid-base disturbances, and unrecognized infection are also occasionally seen (Table 27-1). Acidosis is commonly seen as a cause of weaning failure, but metabolic alkalosis can also depress respiratory drive. After fluid resuscitation with lactated Ringers, metabolic alkalosis is a common finding. Critical illness polyneuropathy is increasingly recognized as a potential cause of weaning failure. This syndrome has been reported in up to 20% of ventilator-dependent patients. Critical illness polyneuropathy is more common in patients with sepsis, and the use of corticosteroids and neuromuscular blocking agents increases the incidence dramatically. This combination, which is common in the asthmatic patient who requires mechanical ventilation, places that population at significant risk for polyneuropathy.

Box 27-1
Differential Diagnosis of Weaning Failure

Common Causes	Less Common Causes
Respiratory muscle failure (load > capacity)	Phrenic nerve dysfunction
	Improper ventilator settings
Respiratory control center depression	Electrolyte imbalance
	Critical illness polyneuropathy, thyroid disease
Left heart failure–hemodynamic instability	Malnutrition
	Over-feeding causing excess CO_2 production
Failure to correct underlying disease/dysfunction	Pain and anxiety
Hypoxemia/reduced oxygen delivery	

TABLE 27-1
Interpreting Signs and Symptoms of Weaning Failure

Possible Causes	Mechanisms	Suggestive Clinical Features
Respiratory muscle failure (load >capacity)	Intrinsic PEEP causing ineffective triggering tachypnea and air hunger	Radiographic evidence of hyperinflation, patient respiratory efforts not recognized by the ventilator
	Increased minute volume requirements	Minute ventilation >10 L/min, fever, elevated resting energy expenditure
	Excess work of breathing, resulting in fatigue	Use of accessory muscles of respiration, airway pressure graphic demonstrating flow dys-synchrony, small artificial airway, bronchospasm, elevated $P_{0.1}$ >4.0 cm H_2O
	Respiratory muscle weakness	Reduced $P_{0.1}$, maximal inspiratory and expiratory pressures, vital capacity
Respiratory control center depression	Diminished response to increased load	Obtunded or confused patient; current use of sedatives
Left heart failure–hemodynamic instability	Impaired cardiac output and oxygen delivery	History of cardiac disease, arrhythmias consistent with ischemia, elevated wedge pressure, increased O_2 extraction
Failure to correct underlying disease/dysfunction	Organ dysfunction (lung, heart, kidney, liver) or active infection resulting in continued disease progression	Reduced pulmonary compliance, gas exchange abnormalities, fever, laboratory values consistent with organ failure
Malnutrition	Respiratory muscle weakness and impaired response to hypoxemia/hypercarbia	Reduced maximal inspiratory and expiratory pressures
Hypoxemia/reduced oxygen delivery	Impaired oxygen delivery to vital organ systems	Reduced SpO_2 and PaO_2

PEEP, Positive end-expiratory pressure; *EMG,* electromyography.

Improper ventilator settings may also interfere with weaning. Proper setting of sensitivity and matching of ventilator flow output to patient demand is necessary to eliminate patient/ventilator asynchrony. Asynchrony that leads to tachypnea in the patient with COPD can result in worsening hyperinflation and impede weaning.

Nutritional state may also affect weaning readiness. Malnourished patients may have reduced respiratory muscle strength, blunted responses to hypoxemia and hypercarbia, and electrolyte abnormalities. Adequate nutrition should be provided early with an emphasis on isocaloric feeding. Overfeeding with carbohydrate calo-

TABLE 27-1
Interpreting Signs and Symptoms of Weaning Failure—cont'd

Possible Causes	Mechanisms	Suggestive Clinical Features
Phrenic nerve dysfunction	Impaired signal conduction to the diaphragm	Post-cardiothoracic surgery, elevated diaphragm on chest x-ray, reduced maximal inspiratory and expiratory pressure, abnormal EMG
Improper ventilator settings	Patient/ventilator dys-synchrony causing respiratory muscle fatigue	Paradoxical breathing, auto-triggering, failure to trigger a breath in response to patient effort, evidence of flow dys-synchrony or neuromechanical dys-synchrony on pressure and flow graphics
Electrolyte imbalance	Respiratory muscle dysfunction/inefficiency	Use of diuretics, renal failure, liver failure, abnormal laboratory results
Critical illness poly-neuropathy, thyroid disease	Nerve dysfunction impairing respiratory muscle function	History of steroid and paralytic agent use; on examination the patient is flaccid, paretic, areflexic, or hyporeflexic; abnormal EMG
	Impaired response to increased loads	Abnormal thyroid function studies; hyporesponsivness to stimulation
Overfeeding causing excess CO_2 production	Excess CO_2 production, causing increased minute ventilation requirements	Tachypnea, respiratory quotient >1.0
Pain and anxiety	Increased O_2 consumption, patient ventilator dys-synchrony, hemodynamic instability, and stress resulting in respiratory muscle fatigue	Tachypnea, agitation, hypertension, tachycardia

EMG, Electromyography.

ries has been implicated in weaning failure. These cases generally include not only excessive carbohydrate calories but a total caloric intake in excess of patient need.

Clinical Features that Suggest a Specific Cause of Weaning Failure

In the current case, clinical features suggest that respiratory muscle failure secondary to dynamic hyperinflation and intrinsic PEEP are precipitating weaning failure. The patient's history of COPD and tachypnea during spontaneous breathing trials along with chest x-ray findings of hyperinflation should lead the clinician to suspect respiratory muscle failure. While this is the major cause of respiratory muscle failure in this case, typically the causes are multifactorial.

Respiratory muscles fail or become fatigued when the load is greater than the muscular capacity. In this patient with COPD and dynamic hyperinflation, a number of other contributing factors are evident. The "load" of the respiratory muscles is determined by the minute ventilation requirement and respiratory system impedance.

Minute ventilation requirements are increased by fever, agitation, anxiety, overfeeding, and excessive deadspace ventilation. This patient has a low grade temperature, is being fed a nominal caloric intake, and at rest is cooperative. These issues are not contributing factors in this case. However, his history of COPD and radiographic findings suggest that deadspace may be elevated. A collection of expired gases and simultaneous ABG sample would be required for measurement of deadspace.

Respiratory impedance includes both elastic and resistive forces that increase the patient's work of breathing. Resistive forces are increased by bronchospasm, presence of an artificial airway, and components of the ventilator circuitry. Elastic forces are increased by hyperinflation, pulmonary edema, abdominal distension, obesity, and chest wall edema.

This patient has a 7.5-mm internal diameter endotracheal tube, which may contribute to his hyperinflation and increased work of breathing. His history of bronchospasm and secretion production also complicates his respiratory function. He is currently receiving humidified gas via a heated humidifier, eliminating resistance issues associated with heat and moisture exchangers.

The patient has a slightly distended abdomen and is obese; both reduce the efficiency of his respiratory pump. Hyperinflation remains his main problem by increasing the work of breathing, complicating ventilator triggering and disadvantaging the respiratory muscles.

Treatment options in this patient include reducing minute ventilation requirements (control fever and agitation), secretion removal (suctioning and/or bronchoscopy), optimization of bronchodilator therapy (systemic and aerosolized therapy), and use of PEEP to counterbalance intrinsic PEEP.

Diagnostic Testing in the Evaluation of the Patient with Weaning Failure

Weaning parameters from the simple to the obtuse have been advocated to predict weaning readiness and weaning success. These parameters are listed below.

Gas Exchange
Pa_{O_2}/FI_{O_2}
Oxygenation index
Alveolar-arterial gradient
Deadspace to V_T (%)
Respiratory quotient
pH

Respiratory Muscle
Minute ventilation (L/min)
Respiratory rate (breaths/min)
V_T (mL, mL/kg)
Vital capacity (mL/kg)
Maximal voluntary ventilation
Maximal inspiratory force (cm H_2O)
Intrinsic PEEP (cm H_2O)
Dynamic and static respiratory system compliance (L/cm H_2O)
Maximal expiratory pressure (cm H_2O)

Complex Measurements
Work of breathing (j/L, j/min)
Pressure time product (cm H_2O/s/min)
Airway occlusion pressure in the first 100 ms ($P_{0.1}$)
$P_{0.1}$/ maximum inspiratory pressure
Oxygen cost of breathing
Transdiaphragmatic pressure
Tension-time index
Airway resistance

Integrative Indices
Frequency/tidal volume ratio (f/V_T), rapid shallow breathing index
Compliance, rate, oxygenation, pressure (CROP)
Weaning index

Each of these parameters has been cited as a potential predictor of weaning success. This chapter will not allow a full discussion of these variables and the context into which each fits historically. It should be mentioned, however, that none of the parameters listed above can be considered absolutely "predictive" of weaning success or failure. Each parameter must be individualized for a given patient and set of circumstances. The predictive value of a given parameter for a post-operative patient may be significantly different than the value for the COPD patient. These parameters are useful measures in elucidating the causes of weaning failure. As such, parameters that are abnormal can be used to target therapy to improve weaning success in the future. As an example, if intrinsic PEEP is found to be elevated in the current patient, measures to reduce intrinsic PEEP should be attempted.

The current literature suggests that a protocol of daily screening for weaning readiness and a spontaneous breathing trial (SBT) are the best diagnostic tests for determining weaning readiness. The daily screen consists of evaluating the overall condition of the patient through the use of the following five criteria:

1. Patient coughs when suctioned suggesting intact gag reflex
2. No continuous infusions of sedatives or vasopressors (hemodynamic stability)
3. PaO_2/FIO_2 >200 (FIO_2 <0.50)
4. PEEP ≤5 cm H_2O

5. f/V_T <105 (measured while breathing spontaneously with respiratory rate off and pressure support off for 1 minute)

If the patient passes the first 1-minute trial, then an SBT of 30-120 minutes is performed. The trial is successful if the patient tolerates 30-120 minutes of spontaneous breathing. The trial may be terminated if any of the following adverse events occur:

Respiratory rate is >35 for >5 minutes
SpO_2 <90% for >30 seconds
Heart rate increases >20% for >5 minutes
Systolic blood pressure >180 mm Hg or <90 mm Hg for >1 minute
Agitation, anxiety, or diaphoresis (compared to baseline) lasting >5 minutes

Patients who tolerate a 2-hour SBT without adverse events have a 90% chance of successfully remaining off the ventilator for 48 hours.

Determining the ability of the patient to protect the upper airway following extubation remains a subjective observation. Clearly, patients who are awake and oriented are likely to remain extubated longer than those who are obtunded. The decision to extubate a patient who has successfully completed an SBT but has an altered mental status remains with the attending physician.* The use of tracheostomy in these cases may prove useful.

Pitfalls and Common Mistakes in the Assessment and Treatment of Weaning Failure

The most common problem associated with assessing and treating weaning failure is continued weaning attempts prior to resolution of underlying pathology. The second most common pitfall is failure to recognize when a patient is ready for weaning. Both of these problems can be avoided by following the rules for daily screening and spontaneous breathing trials advocated by Ely et al.

Considerable interest in weaning modes and techniques has created controversy over the "best" method. Recent evidence from the literature appears to favor the use of pressure support compared to intermittent mandatory ventilation (IMV). However, the main finding in the literature is that the use of daily spontaneous breathing trials speeds weaning and extubation regardless of the mode of ventilation. Based on the current literature, no mode can be considered clearly superior across all patient populations. The key point is to prevent fatiguing loads in between SBTs to prevent respiratory muscle dysfunction. Within this context, the use of IMV in the COPD patient is probably unwise.

Failure to recognize overfeeding, polyneuropathy of critical illness, and malnutrition are also common problems. This results because there are no common tests to quantify these conditions. Using the WHEANS NOT mnemonic, evaluating the patient's history, and keeping a high index of suspicion can be invaluable to the clinician. When suspected, appropriate tests (indirect calorimetry, nitrogen balance, EMG) should be obtained.

---

*In patients with head injuries, a Glasgow Coma Score (GCS) of ≤8 is associated with weaning failure.

Failure to recognize patient ventilator dys-synchrony can prolong the weaning process. Observation of patient comfort and evaluation of the graphic displays of pressure and flow can aid in alleviating this problem. The clinician should stand at the bedside and evaluate patient effort and ventilator response looking for ineffective triggering and dys-synchrony. When these events are identified, more sophisticated measurements of mechanics and respiratory function may be performed. Measurement of intrinsic PEEP and $P_{0.1}$ may prove useful in determining the cause of dys-synchrony.

When possible, explaining the procedure to the patient and reassuring him or her of the events to take place can be invaluable. Too often, clinicians forget to adequately involve the patient. Patient education and cooperation are important in the weaning process.

Weaning remains as much art as science, but application of weaning protocols continues to show promise in reducing weaning times and improving weaning safety.

▼ BIBLIOGRAPHY

Brochard L, Rauss A, Benito S, et al: Comparison of three methods of gradual withdrawal of ventilatory support during weaning from mechanical ventilation, *Am J Respir Crit Care Med* 150:896-903, 1994.

Diehl JL, Lofaso F, Deleuze P, et al: Clinical relevant diaphragmatic dysfunction after cardiac operations, *J Thoracic Cardiovasc Surg* 107:487-492, 1994.

Ely EW: The utility of weaning protocols to expedite liberation from mechanical ventilation, *Respir Care Clin N Amer* 6(2):303-320, 2000.

Ely EW, Baker AM, Evans GW, et al: The prognostic significance of passing a daily screen of weaning parameters, *Intensive Care Med* 25:581-587, 1999.

Ely EW, Bennett PA, Bowton DL, et al: Large scale implementation of a respiratory therapist driven protocol for ventilator weaning, *Am J Respir Crit Care Med* 159:439-446, 1998.

Epstein SK: Endotracheal extubation, *Respir Care Clin N Amer* 6(2):321-360, 2000.

Epstein SK: Etiology of extubation failure and the predictive value of the rapid shallow breathing index, *Am J Respir Crit Care Med* 152:545-549, 1995.

Epstein SK: Weaning parameters, *Respir Care Clin N Amer* 6(2):253-301, 2000.

Esteban A, Alia I, Tobin M, et al: Effect of spontaneous breathing trial duration on outcome of attempts to discontinue mechanical ventilation, *Am J Respir Crit Care Med* 159:512-518, 1999.

Lacomis D, Petrella JT, Giuliana MJ: Causes of neuromuscular weakness in the intensive care unit: a study of ninety-two patients, *Muscle Nerve* 21:610-617, 1998.

Lemaire F, Teboul JL, Cinotti L, et al: Acute left ventricular dysfunction during unsuccessful weaning from mechanical ventilation, *Anesthesiology* 69:171-179, 1988.

Murray MJ, Marsh HM, Wochos DN, et al: Nutritional assessment of intensive care unit patients, *Mayo Clin Proc* 63:1106-1115, 1988.

Rossi A, Polese G, Brandi G: Dynamic hyperinflation. In Marini JJ, Roussos C (editors): *Update in intensive care and emergency medicine: ventilatory failure*, Berlin, 1991, Springer-Verlag, pp 199-210.

CHAPTER 28

THE WEAK PATIENT

Alison G. Morris
Fran Whalen
Michael A. DeVita

▼ Key Terms

▼ Failure to wean
▼ Weakness

▼ Critical illness poly-
neuropathy (CIP)

▼ Mechanical ventilation

▼ THE CLINICAL PROBLEM

A 55-year-old man with a history of congestive heart failure (CHF) and ischemic heart disease develops a flu-like syndrome for over a week. He comes into the hospital with chief complaints of shortness of breath and angina. He is found to have CHF and pneumonia. He is treated with a cephalosporin, an aminoglycoside, and diuretic. His fluid balance over the next 2 days is -3 L. He undergoes cardiac catheterization and then a coronary artery bypass graft (CABG). Diuretics induce 3 L of urine on the first post-operative day. The only unexpected event after surgery is failure to wean from mechanical ventilation. On his second post-operative day, he again fails to tolerate decreases in the intermittent mechanical ventilation (IMV) rate. He is afebrile, normotensive, and has a respiratory rate of 10 on IMV of 8/min and with 5 cm H_2O of pressure support. Pulmonary artery pressures are normal.

He is alert, cooperative, and pain-free but has a weak cough. His chest examination is unremarkable. Chest x-ray shows left basal atelectasis but is otherwise normal.

What is the differential diagnosis for this patient's failure to wean from the ventilator, and what are the most likely causes?

Differential Diagnosis of the Clinical Problem

The most likely causes of failure to wean from mechanical ventilation include fluid overload, chest wall restriction due to pain, cardiac insufficiency, weakness, airways obstruction, or anxiety and psychological problems. In this particular patient, many of these causes can be eliminated. The patient does not complain of pain and is awake and calm, eliminating chest wall restriction and psychological issues as causes. His chest x-ray is not compatible with fluid overload, and he has had a negative fluid balance since his hospitalization. Further, he had good cardiac function after surgery, so CHF is not a concern. Airways obstruction is a possibility; however, the patient has no previous history of obstructive lung disease and has no wheezes on physical examination. Therefore the most likely cause of this patient's failure to wean is neuromuscular insufficiency.

A difficulty that arises when evaluating the critically ill patient with prolonged failure to wean is differentiating between weakness and fatigue. The two entities are frequently confused, but the distinction is important in treating the patient. Weakness refers to a decrease in the capacity of a rested muscle to perform work. To prove weakness, one must test the strength of the rested muscle. These methods are described later in this chapter. Fatigue, on the other hand, is a reversible decrease in the ability of the muscle to contract caused by muscle activity and corrected with rest. Weak muscles may be more susceptible to fatigue, but fatigued muscles are not necessarily weak.

There are many causes of weakness in the ICU (Box 28-1), and these causes may be difficult to sort out. Common causes of weakness include critical illness polyneuropathy (CIP), electrolyte abnormalities, phrenic nerve paralysis, and

---

Box 28-1
Differential Diagnosis of Weakness

Common Causes	Less Common Causes
CIP	Myasthenia gravis
GBS	Aminoglycoside neuropathy
Phrenic nerve injury	Steroid myopathy
Fatigue	Prolonged neuromuscular blockade
Muscle atrophy	Myopathy due to neuromuscular blockers
Hypophosphatemia	Hypoadrenalism
	Refeeding syndrome
	Hypokalemia, hypomagnesemia, hypocalcemia
	Eaton-Lambert syndrome and other paraneoplastic syndromes

CIP, Critical illness polyneuropathy; *GBS,* Guillain-Barré syndrome.

Guillain-Barré syndrome (GBS). Other less common causes of weakness include myasthenia gravis and effects of drugs such as steroids, aminoglycoside antibiotics, and neuromuscular blocking agents. Each of these produces a distinctive clinical picture and occurs in a particular setting. Causes of weakness that are unlikely in this patient scenario are hypothyroidism, hypoadrenalism, post-polio syndrome, as well as Lambert-Eaton syndrome and other paraneoplastic processes.

Pathophysiology of Weakness

The causes of weakness have variable pathophysiology. The underlying problem can be classified by the location of the lesion. Problems can occur at the muscle, the nerve, or the neuromuscular junction. These abnormalities can be distinguished pathologically and by neuromuscular testing (Table 28-1).

TABLE 28-1
Interpreting Signs and Symptoms in the Patient with Weakness

Possible Causes	Mechanisms	Suggestive Clinical Features
CIP	Possibly endoneurial ischemia	Distal weakness, muscle atrophy, septic or elderly patients
GBS	Immune-mediated de-myelination of motor and sensory axons	Ascending symmetric paralysis, motor loss greater than sensory loss, loss of reflexes
Phrenic nerve injury	Hypothermic or direct injury	Recent cardiac, thoracic, mediastinal surgery; elevated left hemidiaphragm
Electrolyte abnormalities	Reduction in motor contractility, nerve conduction; decrease in ATP	Diffuse weakness; abnormal magnesium, potassium, phosphorus
Myasthenia gravis	Loss of post-synaptic acetylcholine receptors	Exercise-induced weakness, pronounced cranial nerve involvement
Aminoglycosides	Nerve end plate damage	History of aminoglycoside use
Steroid myopathy	Atrophy of type IIb muscle fibers	History of steroid use, particularly if combined with neuromuscular blockade
Prolonged neuro-muscular blockade	Accumulation of active metabolites; competitive blockade of acetyl-choline receptors	History of use of non-depolarizing agents; hepatic or renal dysfunction
Myopathy from neuro-muscular blocking agents	Thick filament degeneration and necrosis	History of use of non-depolarizing agents, especially with steroids

CIP, Critical illness polyneuropathy; *GBS,* Guillain-Barré syndrome; *ATP,* adenosine triphosphate.

CIP produces a sensorimotor axonopathy. Pathologic changes seen on biopsy include primary axonal degeneration with loss of peripheral motor and sensory fibers. There is no inflammation present. The exact cause of CIP is unclear. Endoneurial ischemia, humorally mediated cytotoxicity, or other effects of sepsis have been proposed as a possible mechanism, but a definite cause is not yet known.

GBS is characterized by demyelination of motor and sensory axons. The process is immune-mediated with the production of antibodies against myelin of peripheral and cranial nerves. The immune activation may stem from an antecedent infection. Inflammation is common and distinguishes GBS from CIP.

Hypothermic phrenic nerve injury occurs after cardiac surgery because of damage to the nerve from the cold cardioplegia solution used. The degree of exposure (e.g., whether the pericardium is shielded), the temperature of the solution, and the duration of exposure affect the incidence and severity of the phrenic neuropathy. Left phrenic nerve palsy is more common, and most injuries are reversible with time. Intra-operative stretching of the phrenic nerve occurring during thoracic or mediastinal procedures can also cause reversible nerve injury. Some patients have an idiopathic phrenic nerve palsy. Tumors or inflammatory conditions, such as pneumonia, herpes zoster, or vasculitis, can also lead to phrenic nerve paralysis.

Many of the drugs given in the intensive care unit (ICU) can lead to weakness by various mechanisms. Steroids may produce a necrotizing myopathy with loss of thick filaments seen on biopsy. They also act to increase muscle catabolism and decrease the rate of muscle synthesis. Neuromuscular blocking agents act as competitive antagonists for the acetylcholine receptor. Accumulation of the active metabolites of these drugs may lead to prolonged neurologic blockade. The drugs may also cause an acute myopathy or neuropathy, particularly when used in conjunction with corticosteroids. Pathologically, thick filament degeneration and necrosis can be seen. Aminoglycoside antibiotics produce a myasthenia gravis-like syndrome through a neuromuscular end-plate blockade. Their use may also worsen pre-existing myasthenia gravis and therefore is contraindicated in patients with the disease.

Electrolyte abnormalities can also impair both nerve and motor functioning. Disorders of calcium, potassium, magnesium, and phosphate can decrease muscle contractility and slow nerve conduction. In particular, hypophosphatemia due to depletion of intra-cellular adenosine triphosphate (ATP) can produce profound muscle weakness. An extremely low phosphate level (less than 1.5 mEq/L) by itself can lead to respiratory failure. Protein calorie malnutrition may also contribute to weakness through loss of muscle mass and diminished ATP production. Severe hypokalemia is associated with weakness and can cause paralysis. Hypomagnesemia causes mild weakness and potentiates weakness due to hypokalemia and hypophosphatemia.

Myasthenia gravis is caused by a decrease in transmission at the neuromuscular junction. Antibodies are directed against skeletal muscle acetylcholine receptors, leading to delay in production of the action potential or complete loss of conduction.

Other unusual causes of weakness include generalized motor weakness from hypothyroidism or hypoadrenalism. Eaton-Lambert syndrome, a paraneoplastic process, produces a decrease in pre-synaptic acetylcholine release. This decrease occurs because antibodies bind to calcium channels in the neuronal membrane and block synaptic release. Post-polio syndrome is another uncommon cause of weakness in patients who in the past have had polio. It results from progressive loss of motor units. Defects in neuromuscular transmission can also occur.

Clinical Features that Suggest a Specific Cause of Weakness

Each cause of weakness in patients in the ICU presents in certain patient populations and with certain clinical findings. These features can be used to generate a differential diagnosis and focus diagnostic testing. The features that suggest a specific cause in the current case are the patient's history of cardiac surgery, diuresis, his pre-admission flu-like syndrome, and the use of aminoglycosides and neuromuscular blocking agents.

CIP is the most common cause of neuromuscular weakness in ICU patients who have been mechanically ventilated for prolonged periods of time. It is more common in elderly patients, particularly those who have sepsis. The longer the patient's length of time in the ICU, the more severe the neuropathy. The weakness is usually self-limited, however, and those patients who survive their ICU stay usually have a complete recovery. The typical presentation is that of muscle atrophy in a patient who is unable to wean from mechanical ventilation. There is prominent distal motor weakness and muscle wasting. Deep tendon reflexes are usually decreased but may be normal. Sensory losses may also be present, but are often difficult to determine in the critically ill patient. Facial weakness is rare. In this particular case, the patient has not had a protracted ICU stay and does not have any of the neurologic symptoms associated with CIP, making CIP a less likely explanation of his failure to wean.

GBS is less common than CIP and typically presents with an ascending symmetric paralysis. Motor function is affected more than sensory, and deep tendon reflexes are usually absent. Some patients have autonomic instability. When cervical nerve roots 3 through 5 are arrested, diaphragmatic paralysis occurs and can lead to respiratory failure. Cranial nerve deficits are seen in some variants of the syndrome. The course may be fulminant or indolent, with symptom progression over several days or weeks. GBS is often preceded by an infection such as an upper respiratory infection, *Campylobacter jejuni,* or Epstein-Barr virus. Stressful events such as surgery can also precipitate the syndrome. The current patient had a febrile illness on hospital admission and also underwent cardiac surgery. The typical neurologic symptoms are not present in his case, however, so this diagnosis is unlikely.

Phrenic nerve paralysis often presents after cardiac bypass surgery, affecting as many as 85% of patients to some degree. Elevation of the left hemidiaphragm is the most common radiographic manifestation. Less often, the right side or both sides of the diaphragm are affected. Although many patients tolerate phrenic nerve injury, in a subset of patients, particularly those with underlying respiratory difficulties, the injury can prevent successful ventilator weaning. Regional ventilation-perfusion abnormalities occur, particularly when the patient is supine. The current patient is at risk for this problem because of his recent cardiac bypass. The abnormal findings on his chest x-ray are also consistent with a phrenic nerve injury.

Myasthenia gravis presents with weakness without sensory abnormalities. The weakness is worsened by repetitive activity and commonly affects ocular and bulbar muscles. Many patients will have ptosis, diplopia, and dysphagia. Extremity weakness is a later finding. Use of certain drugs and stressful events such as surgery can precipitate a myasthenic crisis with generalized weakness and respiratory failure. The patient presented did have recent surgery, but he had no previous history of myasthenia and none of the typical neurologic findings, making this diagnosis unlikely.

Patients in the ICU frequently require the use of drugs that have potential for producing weakness. Steroids can lead to a diffuse, flaccid quadraparesis that involves the respiratory muscles. The onset is generally gradual and initially affects proximal muscles. Muscle wasting may be noticed after several days. Sensation remains largely intact, and reflexes may be normal or decreased. Burst therapy with steroids appears to place patients at higher risk for myopathy than continuous treatment.

Neuromuscular blocking agents can also lead to weakness. Prolonged effects lasting from 6 hours to as many as 7 days after use have been reported. Patients with hepatic or renal dysfunction run a greater risk of prolonged blockade because they accumulate active metabolites of these agents. Also, concomitant acidosis, hypomagnesemia, or use of steroids or aminoglycosides significantly increase the risk of neurologic toxicity. The occurrence of acute myopathy secondary to neuromuscular blockers is less common. Patients with severe asthma who require high-dose steroids and paralysis for ventilation seem to be particularly vulnerable. These patients may have elevated creatinine kinase levels and demonstrate diffuse weakness. The current patient did have neuromuscular blockade during his cardiac surgery and has been given an aminoglycoside antibiotic. He has normal renal and hepatic function and no history of steroid use. The diagnosis of weakness secondary to prolonged neuromuscular blockade is possible but less likely than other alternatives.

Electrolyte abnormalities are another possible cause of weakness in this patient. He has been given diuretics and therefore may have low levels of potassium, phosphate, or magnesium. Also, he has not been receiving nutritional support, so he may have low levels of calcium and phosphorous. Hypophosphatemia is also a problem in patients who are fed after a prolonged period of inadequate nutrition. Electrolyte abnormalities generally present with diffuse weakness and failure to wean. Other clinical signs such as cardiac conduction abnormalities or tetany may be present but are rare.

Hypothyroidism and hypoadrenalism both result in generalized muscle weakness. Diaphragmatic weakness can occur and presents with respiratory failure and hypercapnia. Hypothyroidism also seems to decrease the ventilatory response to hypoxemia. Eaton-Lambert syndrome generally presents as limb girdle weakness in a patient with an underlying malignancy. Reflexes are decreased, and there may be mild cranial nerve involvement. The hallmark of this syndrome is improvement in strength with muscle exertion. This improvement is only temporary, and repetitive exertion eventually leads to muscle failure. Post-polio syndrome presents with progressive fatigue and weakness. Some sensory disturbances may be present. This disease should be suspected in the weak patient who has a history of polio. It is becoming increasingly uncommon with improvement in polio prevention.

Diagnostic Testing in the Evaluation of the Patient with Weakness

When a patient is thought to be weak, this observation should be verified and quantified. Neuromuscular evaluation should begin with a physical examination that specifically notes muscle strength/weakness. For respiratory muscles, this can be done by assessing the vital capacity (VC), negative inspiratory force (NIF), and the maximum minute ventilation (MMV). The first two measure strength, and the latter measures strength and, to a lesser extent, endurance. These studies should be performed on a well-rested patient to exclude fatigue as an etiology of impaired power and endurance. Generally 8 hours of rest is sufficient. If the results are normal at rest, post-exercise studies that demonstrate a diminished VC, NIF, or MMV would point toward fatigue as an etiology. Other studies may assist in determining the underlying cause and are outlined in Table 28-2. All patients who are weak should be evaluated for the etiology of the weakness, since many of the causes respond to specific treatments. The peripheral nerve stimulator should be used to assess the residual of any chemical paralysis; this also assesses the integrity of the neuromuscular junction. It is an easy bedside test to rule out pathology but is inadequate to characterize the type of neurologic injury. Nerve conduction and concomitant electromyographic (EMG) studies are essential to rule out specific neuropathies and myopathies.

TABLE 28-2
Studies Needed to Diagnose Causes of Weakness

Defect	Diagnostic Study
Electrolyte deficiency	Potassium, calcium, magnesium, phosphorus
Muscle injury	CPK; muscle biopsy
Hypothyroidism	TSH
Protein-calorie malnutrition	Albumin, prealbumin
Weakness	Careful neurologic examination, specifically noting muscle strength and weakness
Residual neuromuscular blocking agent	Review pharmacologic agents used in care of patient; peripheral nerve stimulator, using TOF
Myasthenia gravis	Peripheral nerve stimulator, using TOF; EMG; acetylcholine receptor antibodies
Steroid myopathy, steroid neuropathy	Review pharmacologic agents used in care of patient, peripheral nerve stimulator, EMG
CIP	Nerve conduction study, EMG, nerve biopsy
GBS	Nerve conduction study (delayed or absent conduction), EMG will show denervation, LP with elevated protein only

CPK, Creatine phosphokinase; TSH, thyroid-stimulating hormone; TOF, train of four (sequential muscle contraction to repeated stimuli); CIP, Critical illness polyneuropathy; EMG, electromyography; GBS, Guillain-Barré syndrome; LP, lumbar puncture.

A review of the pharmacologic agents used in the patient's management, specifically non-depolarizing muscle relaxants with steroids and aminoglycosides, can help narrow the differential diagnosis of weakness.

Patients with bilateral phrenic nerve or diaphragm injury tend to be more dyspneic in the supine versus the upright position (which may mimic CHF). VC may decrease 50% when changing the patient's position from the upright to the supine position. Simultaneous thoracic and abdominal manometry may be helpful. To perform this test, two balloon manometers are placed, one in the esophagus and another in the stomach. During inspiration, normal patients will have a fall in intra-thoracic pressure and a rise in abdominal pressure. In contrast, patients with paradoxical diaphragm motion will have a fall in abdominal pressure on inspiration and rise in pressure during expiration. Chest x-rays may show elevated diaphragms (reduced lung volumes) bilaterally. In a mechanically ventilated patient, the diaphragms are not always elevated; however, atelectasis is common on the affected side. Sonography and fluoroscopy may be misleading in bilateral paralysis because cephalad movement of the diaphragms due to negative intra-thoracic pressure generated by the still-functioning chest wall during inspiration mimics a functioning diaphragm. However, this paradoxical motion of the diaphragm (cephalad during inspiration) is rapidly distinguished from normal motion if the observer notes the phase of respiratory cycle at the time of the cephalad motion. The advantages of ultrasound over fluoroscopy are convenience and safety of the bedside evaluation in the ICU, no radiation exposure, and the ability of the sonogram to visualize the entire diaphragm from its anterior origin to its posterior insertion. In contrast, fluoroscopy visualizes the entire diaphragm well, from left to right, allowing side-to-side comparison. However, it only visualizes the top of the diaphragm well, and posterior distribution neuropathies can be missed.

Despite aggressive diuresis, this patient remained difficult to wean from the ventilator. Serum electrolytes, thyroid-stimulating hormone (TSH), and neurologic examination were normal. A sonogram of the diaphragm that was obtained while the patient was spontaneously breathing demonstrated paradoxical motion of the left hemidiaphragm and decreased excursion of the right hemidiaphragm. A phrenic nerve conduction study demonstrated absent conduction of the left phrenic nerve and normal conduction on the right. Diaphragm EMGs showed denervation potentials on the left and normal activity on the right. Therefore left phrenic nerve palsy was diagnosed.

Assessment of the Effect of Therapy on Weakness

The treatment of weakness is threefold: first, to reverse the underlying cause; second, to reduce the work of breathing; and third, to retrain the muscles to increase strength and endurance.

In this patient, there is no specific therapy to reverse the injury. However, paying careful attention to the other two components of therapy can create significant improvement. For example, weaning the patient in the upright position removes the load of the abdominal contents from the diaphragm, reduces restriction, and decreases the work of breathing. Other ways to decrease pulmonary restriction include treating pain, reducing pneumothoraces, draining effusions, and reducing lung water through diuresis. Abdominal distention is detrimental because it can decrease functional residual capacity (FRC) and increase the work of breathing. Work imposed by the ventilator and the circuit can prevent weaning from mechanical ventilation. Decreasing the trigger sensitivity to less than 1 cm H_2O in pressure-triggered ventilators or preferably changing to a flow trigger (so-called flow-by) will diminish the work required to initiate a ventilator breath. Inspiratory flow rate should exceed the patient's demand by a threefold amount to prevent adding to inspiratory work of breathing. Reducing obstruction by treating reversible airways disease and preventing and treating tracheobronchial secretions with diuresis, suction, or antibiotics as necessary is helpful as well. Other causes of increased work of breathing include narrow endotracheal tubes, organized secretions that may decrease endotracheal tube diameter, or kinking of the tube. Any such narrowing may increase resistance significantly.

There is great debate regarding the optimal way to improve muscle strength and endurance. Of course, the muscles in the distribution of impaired nerves cannot increase strength until nerve function returns. However, the other muscles of respiration can often perform the entire work of breathing once they are adequately trained. Therefore patients with even bilateral diaphragm paralysis should receive respiratory muscle training by a weaning process. Regimens that utilize tracheostomy mask trials, decrements in IMV rate, or pressure support reductions have been successful in increasing muscle strength and endurance.

This patient was rested at night in the assist-control mode, and the ventilator triggering was switched to flow-by. The patient was exercised using daily tracheostomy mask trials. Weekly measures of the VC and NIF force were followed to assess return of strength. In hypothermic phrenic nerve injury, usually there is full recovery within 1 year, although 25% of patients may have some mild persistent dysfunction or ongoing pulmonary problems. Unilateral injury usually has less frequent pulmonary sequelae and has faster recovery. This patient was weaned from the ventilator in 7 days.

Pitfalls and Common Mistakes in the Assessment and Treatment of Weakness

The most devastating pitfall in the assessment and treatment of weakness is not to consider it in a patient with respiratory insufficiency. Post-operatively in a patient with a positive fluid balance, pleural fluid, and difficulty in weaning from the ventilator, it is easy to assume that the failure is due to excess fluid or pain and not consider a broader differential. Most causes of weakness will not be found unless specifically considered and assessed. Diuresis may alter electrolyte balance and compound a previously diagnosed cause of weakness. Therefore routine laboratory evaluation is required for patients who are weak.

It is common to confuse weakness and fatigue. Careful diagnostic assessment will prevent this occurrence. Remember that weak patients fatigue more readily, so both problems may exist simultaneously. Adequate rest for weak patients can improve subsequent work performance. Failure to fully rest a patient despite being in an assist-control mode of ventilation may play a significant role in failure to wean. If the patient in the "rest" mode is uncomfortable, tachypneic, diaphoretic, tachycardic, or exhibits paradoxical breathing (abdominal retraction during inspiration and contraction with expiration), the ventilator may have too low an inspiratory flow rate, too high (too negative) a sensitivity, or auto-positive endexpiratory pressure (auto-PEEP). In fact, it is possible to have muscles fatigue or even fail during supposed rest on the ventilator.

Failure to reduce work of breathing can prevent progress. Otherwise insignificant excess workloads can be highly deleterious in a weak patient. For example, pleural effusions should be drained, and the patient should be assessed for subsequent change in performance of work. If it improves, the physician should consider continuing to minimize subsequent effusions. Auto-PEEP, which will increase the work required to trigger the ventilator, can be an occult cause of increased work of breathing.

Other complications occur in weak patients. For example, pulmonary embolism and pneumonia can complicate the course of treatment. Failure to perform work at a previously well-tolerated level should alert the physician to the possibility of this type of complication. The underlying nutritional status of the patient may be overlooked. Restitution of an anabolic state may be necessary prior to separation from the ventilator, especially after a surgical procedure with another added stress. Critically ill patients are commonly sedated and therefore move little. In that setting, weakness is easily missed and is difficult to assess even if considered.

This patient had several reasons for exhibiting difficulty in weaning from the ventilator; some of these could have been anticipated and possibly prevented. The fever and viral symptoms around the time of admission could possibly be associated with GBS or sepsis contributing to CIP; the use of aminoglycosides in addition to steroids (possibly used peri-operatively to limit the inflammatory response of surgery) and non-depolarizing muscle relaxants may combine to contribute to a critical illness myopathy. The association of phrenic nerve injury during cardiac surgery is not that uncommon, and, although there is no specific therapy for this, making the diagnosis early may give some assurance to the patient and his or her family, spare the patient multiple failed weaning trials.

▼ BIBLIOGRAPHY

Bolton C, Brown J, Sibbald W: The electrophysiological investigation of respiratory paralysis in critically ill patients, *Neurology* 33(suppl 186), 1983.

De Jonghe B, Cook D, Sharsher T, et al: Acquired neuromuscular disorders in critically ill patients: a systematic review, *Int Care Med* 24:1242-1250, 1998.

DeVita M, Robinson L, Rehder J, et al: Incidence and natural history of phrenic neuropathy occurring during open heart surgery, *Chest* 103:850, 1993.

Hund EF: Neuromuscular complications in the ICU: the spectrum of critical illness-related conditions causing muscular weakness and weaning failure, *J Neurol Sci* 136:10-16, 1996.

Sliwa, JA: Acute weakness syndromes in the critically ill patient, *Arch Phys Med Rehabil* 81:S45-S52, 2000.

Zochodne D, Bolton C, Wells G, et al: Critical illness polyneuropathy: a complication of sepsis and multiple organ failure, *Brain* 110:819, 1987.

CHAPTER 29

VENTILATOR DYS-SYNCHRONY

Neil R. MacIntyre

- ▼ Ventilator breath triggering
- ▼ Ventilator-delivered flow pattern
- ▼ Fully unloaded
- ▼ Pressure rise time adjuster
- ▼ Tracheal targeting
- ▼ Proportional assist ventilation (PAV)
- ▼ Breath cycling
- ▼ Ventilator graphics

▼ THE CLINICAL PROBLEM

A 59-year-old man with known chronic obstructive pulmonary disease (COPD) has required controlled mechanical ventilatory support for the last 2 days for hypercapnic respiratory failure thought to be secondary to a right lower lobe pneumonia. He has been treated with antibiotics, bronchodilators, and steroids and is now improving. This morning, he has adequate blood gas values on an FIO_2 of 0.3, and he is awake and following commands. A spontaneous breathing trial is attempted to assess the discontinuation potential, and he rapidly becomes tachypneic, dyspneic, and diaphoretic. He is returned to volume-targeted synchronized intermittent mandatory ventilation (SIMV) with a backup rate of 6 and 5 cm H_2O pressure support (PS). He remains quite uncomfortable, however, and appears to be "fighting" the ventilator. His airway pressure, flow, volume, and esophageal pressure graphics over time are depicted in Figure 29-1.

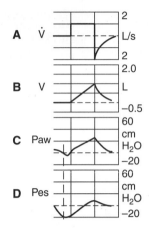

▼ **Figure 29-1** **A,** Flow; **B,** volume; **C,** airway pressure; and **D,** esophageal pressure in a patient appearing to "fight" the ventilator. The dashed line indicates the point when ventilator circuit pressure began to fall during a patient effort.

What is the differential diagnosis for this patient's discomfort after switching from controlled ventilation to an interactive form of support (SIMV + PS)?

Interactive Ventilatory Support

Mechanical ventilation modes that permit spontaneous ventilatory activity are termed *interactive* modes, since patients can affect various aspects of the mechanical ventilator's functions. These interactions can range from simple triggering of mechanical breaths to more complex processes affecting delivered flow patterns and breath timing (Table 29-1). Interactive modes require spontaneous ventilatory efforts to be present and are generally utilized when these efforts have some degree of regularity and the patient's respiratory function does not require total control by the ventilator.

There are two putative advantages to interactive modes. First, interactive modes allow for muscle "exercise," which, when done at non-fatiguing or physiologic levels, may prevent muscle atrophy and facilitate fatigue recovery. This may be particularly important during the recovering phases of respiratory failure, when total support is no longer required but the patient is still incapable of being removed from all ventilatory support. Second, permitting spontaneous patient ventilatory activity with comfortable interactive modes may reduce the need for the sedation and/or neuromuscular blockers that are often required to prevent patients from fighting machine-controlled ventilation.

Synchronizing Triggering, Flow Delivery, and Cycling

Patient ventilator interactions can either be synchronous or dys-synchronous with an interactive mode of support during any or all of the three phases of breath delivery: triggering, flow delivery, and cycling.

TABLE 29-1
Commonly Used Interactive Modes

| | Patient Can Interact with | | |
Mode	Breath Triggering	Flow Delivery	Breath Cycling
Volume assist control	Yes	No	No
Pressure assist control	Yes	Yes	No
Synchronized IMV (Volume)			
Ventilator breath	Yes	No	Yes
Spontaneous breath	Yes	Yes	Yes
Synchronized IMV (Pressure)			
Ventilator breath	Yes	Yes	No
Spontaneous breath	Yes	Yes	Yes
PS	Yes	Yes	Yes
Airway Pressure Release			
Ventilator breath	No	No	No
Spontaneous breath	Yes	Yes	Yes

IMV, Intermittent mandatory ventilation; *PS,* pressure support.

Ventilator Breath Triggering

Interactive mechanical ventilation needs to sense a spontaneous effort to trigger a mechanical response. Effort sensors are usually either pressure or flow transducers in the ventilatory circuitry and are characterized by their sensitivity (how much of a circuit pressure or flow change must be generated to initiate a ventilator response) and by their responsiveness (the delay in providing this response).

Even with modern sensors, there is unavoidable dys-synchrony in the triggering process. First, a certain level of insensitivity must be put in the sensor to avoid artifacts triggering the ventilator (i.e., "auto cycling"). Second, even when the patient effort has been sensed, demand valve systems have a certain inherent delay (up to 100 or more msec) before they physically open and achieve target flow into the airway (system responsiveness). Both of these factors can result in significant "isometric-like" pressure loads on the ventilatory muscles during the triggering process. In addition, in the setting of air trapping and intrinsic positive end-expiratory pressure (PEEP), the elevated alveolar pressure at end expiration can serve as a significant triggering threshold load on the ventilatory muscles.

Several strategies can be used to minimize the magnitude of the dys-synchrony induced during breath triggering. First, ventilators with microprocessor flow controls often have significantly better valve characteristics than those on older-generation ventilators. Second, continuous flow systems superimposed on the demand systems can improve demand system responsiveness in patients with high ventilatory drives (although such flows can reduce sensitivity in patients with very weak ventilatory drives). Third, flow-based triggers have been shown to produce a more sensitive and responsive breath-triggering process. Fourth, a small amount of applied inspiratory PS will usually increase the ventilator's initial flow delivery and can thereby improve response characteristics of the demand valve system. Fifth, in obstructive disease, patients with an inspiratory threshold load induced by intrinsic PEEP, setting applied PEEP below the intrinsic PEEP level can help equilibrate the end-expiratory alveolar and circuit pressures and improve triggering.

Improving triggering in the future may involve moving the sensors "closer" to the patient's ventilatory control center. Specifically, phrenic nerve sensors, ventilatory muscle electromyograms, or even brainstem signals are all potential sensing sites. At the present time, however, artifacts and instability of all of these signals preclude their clinical use as triggering strategies.

Ventilator-Delivered Flow Pattern

During an interactive breath, ventilatory muscles are contracting and the ventilator flow delivery should be adequate to meet one of two goals: (1) fully unload the contracting ventilatory muscles in patients with severely overloaded and fatigued muscles or (2) partially unload the contracting ventilatory muscles in patients recovering from muscle fatigue. Synchronous flow interactions can be defined by the following:

1. *Breaths designed to fully unload ventilatory muscles:* For an interactive breath to fully unload ventilator muscles, the patient should be required to only trigger the ventilator and then have the ventilator supply all of the work of the breath. Thus the goal of synchrony during a fully unloaded breath is to deliver adequate flow over the entire inspiratory effort to totally unload the contracting muscles. Achieving this goal can be assessed by comparing the pressure pattern of the patient-triggered breath with a machine-triggered breath (i.e., a breath occurring without patient activity). Synchronous flow delivery should produce nearly identical airway pressure waveforms and the only evidence of triggering in the pleural/esophageal pressure waveforms (Figure 29-2). This is usually accompanied by a near-normal spontaneous respiratory frequency.

2. *Breaths designed to partially unload ventilatory muscles:* For an interactive breath to partially unload ventilatory muscles, the patient and the ventilator need to "share" the work of the breath. Synchrony is then defined as having the ventilator provide a constant pressure "bias" on the ventilatory muscles so that their pressure-volume configuration normalizes, and "un-physiologic" high-pressure, low-volume breaths are avoided. Synchronous partially unloaded breaths will thus have a similar airway pressure waveform shape (although less magnitude) as a controlled breath, whereas the pleural/esophageal pressure waveforms will resemble a normal loading pattern. In addition, flow synchrony is usually associated with a near-normal spontaneous breathing frequency.

Over the last decade, the use of pressure-targeted breaths has been shown to improve flow synchrony as compared to flow/volume-targeted breaths, especially in patients with active ventilatory drives. This improvement is because the variable flow features of pressure targeting can adjust to patient effort while the set fixed flows of the flow/volume-targeted breaths cannot. In the last several years, the flow synchrony capabilities of the pressure-targeted breath have been further enhanced by the development of the pressure rise time adjuster (Figure 29-3). This

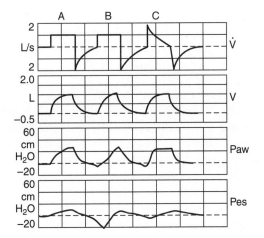

▼ **Figure 29-2** Flow *(upper panel)*, volume *(second panel)*, airway pressure *(third panel)*, and esophageal pressure *(bottom panel)* during three breaths. Breath *A* is a ventilator-controlled breath without patient effort. Breath *B* is a patient-triggered, fixed-flow breath in which flow delivery is inadequate to meet patient demand. As a consequence, significant patient muscle loading is seen in the esophageal pressure tracing, and the airway pressure graphic is literally "sucked" downward. Breath *C* is a patient-triggered breath in which a variable flow pattern with pressure targeting has resulted in better flow synchrony.

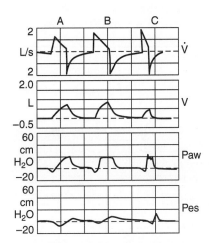

▼ **Figure 29-3** Three examples of different pressure rise times in a pressure-targeted breath of 20 cm H_2O. In breath *A*, the rise time is slow and the pressure target is achieved late in the breath. In breath *B*, the rise time is more appropriate and a smooth "square wave" of pressure is achieved. In breath *C*, the rise time is too fast, rapid oscillations ("ringing") appear in the airway pressure graphic, and the breath is terminated too early.

control allows clinicians to vary the initial flow delivery (and thus rate of rise to the pressure target) during pressure-targeted breaths. Very active ventilatory demands often require very high initial flow (and thus rate of pressure rise); less active ventilatory demands often require lower initial flow.

Two new interesting developments may enhance flow synchrony: tracheal targeting and proportional assist ventilation (PAV). Tracheal targeting is used with pressure-targeted breaths. With this approach, the ventilator interacts with a pressure sensor in the trachea (i.e., at the end of the endotracheal tube) instead of the proximal airway. The pressure damping effects of endotracheal tube resistance are thus eliminated, and flow response is enhanced. Clinical trials comparing tracheal targeting to proximal airway targeting, however, do not exist at present. PAV, in contrast to conventional interactive targeting strategies, uses "gain" settings on the patient's spontaneous flow and volume demand. Clinicians thus select a proportional "boost" to patient effort rather than setting a specific flow or pressure target during breath delivery. Selecting the proper flow and volume gain settings requires measurements of patient elastic and resistive loads for which clinicians can choose to provide a percent "unloading." Preliminary work suggests substantial flow synchrony with PAV. Concerns about overshoot from excessive gain settings exist, however, and clinical comparisons with tracheal pressure targeting strategies do not exist.

Breath Cycling

Cycling dys-synchrony can occur in one of two ways (Figure 29-4). First, if the breath lasts beyond patient effort, an inadequate expiratory time may develop (along with air trapping) and patient expiratory efforts may be required to terminate the breath. Second, if the breath terminates before the patient effort is finished, the patient may be left demanding additional flow without any being delivered. Significant imposed loading or double breath triggering may result.

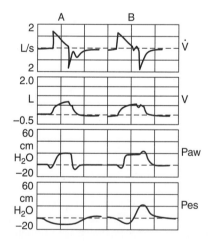

▼ **Figure 29-4** Two examples of cycle dys-synchrony. In breath *A*, gas delivery terminates early and the patient is left demanding additional flow. In breath *B*, flow continues to the point that the patient's expiratory muscles must contract to terminate gas delivery.

With volume-cycled breaths, cycling dys-synchrony requires adjustment in the set tidal volume. With time-cycled breaths, cycling dys-synchrony requires adjustment in the set inspiratory time. With flow-cycled breaths, cycling dys-synchrony can be addressed in one of two ways. First, the cycling criteria (percent of peak flow or set cycling flow) can be adjusted on some ventilators. Second, when cycling is a fraction of peak flow, the rate of rise adjustor noted above can be changed to alter the peak flow.

Changing cycling criteria may also help dys-synchrony. For example, an arbitrarily set tidal volume may be harder to synchronize than a set inspiratory time (pressure assist) or a patient-determined flow cycle (PS). Another example might be a patient who has cycling dys-synchrony with PS but who may have improvement by using a time-cycled, pressure-targeted breath (i.e., pressure assist). Finally, a number of current ventilators provide pressure-targeted breaths with a volume "guarantee." The purpose of this is to supply a certain minimum tidal volume/minute ventilation in a patient with potential instability in lung mechanics or inspiratory effort during pressure-targeted breaths. Approaches to this include a set minimum flow/tidal volume with each breath (e.g., volume-assured PS (VAPS) or pressure augmentation) or an automatic inspiratory pressure adjuster that responds to the previous breath(s) volume delivery (e.g., volume support or pressure-regulated volume control).

Assessment of the Patient with Ventilator Dys-Synchrony

Physical Examination

It is important to first assess if the problem is during triggering or breath delivery. A patient who appears to have a very active inspiratory effort but who fails to trigger the ventilator suggests either an insensitive/unresponsive assist trigger or the presence of an inspiratory threshold load imposed by intrinsic PEEP. A patient who triggers breaths but then appears to not be getting enough air suggests inadequate ventilator flow delivery. A patient who exerts expiratory muscle activity to terminate the breath suggests cycle dys-synchrony.

Ventilator Graphics

Assessment of pressure/flow/volume graphics can be very helpful in determining the cause of ventilator dys-synchrony. Insensitive/unresponsive assist triggers are characterized by significant drops in airway pressure before breath triggering. In contrast, the inspiratory threshold load imposed by intrinsic PEEP is characterized by an airway pressure drop significantly after the patient effort begins. This drop is most clearly seen with an esophageal balloon tracing that demonstrates patient effort beginning several hundred milliseconds before airway pressures change. Flow dys-synchrony is best detected in the airway pressure graphic where the assisted tracing should be compared to the controlled tracing. Significant flow dys-synchrony is manifest by pronounced downward "pulling" of the pressure graphic by patient effort (see Figure 29-2). Cycle dys-synchrony is characterized by either positive pressure elevations at end inspiration (breath too long) or negative pressure in early expiration (breath too short).

▼ SUMMARY

In the current patient, the problem visually appeared to be a delay in the triggering process with frequent missed efforts. The airway pressure graphic in Figure 29-1 showed an appropriately sensitive/responsive triggering system. However, the esophageal balloon tracing in Figure 29-1 showed a 500-msec delay between patient effort initiation and airway pressure changes, indicating significant intrinsic PEEP. The airway pressure graphic during the triggered breaths was similar to the controlled breaths, signifying adequate flow and cycle synchrony. The cause of ventilator dys-synchrony in this patient was thus the imposed triggering load imposed by intrinsic PEEP. The patient-ventilator synchrony dramatically improved after the addition of circuit PEEP, which served to "balance" PEEP throughout the airway and circuitry, thereby reducing the threshold loading.

This case serves to emphasize the need to carefully assess the patient fighting the ventilator. Optimizing patient-ventilator interactions during all three phases of breath delivery is an important clinical goal. During triggering, improved effort sensors may be the next step forward. During flow delivery, pressure-targeted breaths and pressure rise time adjusters have both been significant improvements. Tracheal targeting and proportional assist ventilation both offer future promise in this area. During cycling, better clinician understanding and adjustments of the available cycling criteria are the best way to address synchrony.

▼ BIBLIOGRAPHY

Anzueto A, Peters JI, Tobin MJ, et al: Effects of prolonged controlled mechanical ventilation on diaphragmatic function in healthy adult baboons, *Crit Care Med* 25:1187-1190, 1997.

Benner MJ, Blanch PB, Kirby RR, et al: Imposed work of breathing and methods of triggering a demand-flow, continuous positive airway pressure system, *Crit Care Med* 21:1183-1190, 1993.

Flick GR, Belamy PE, Simmons DH: Diaphragmatic contraction during assisted mechanical ventilation, *Chest* 96:130-135, 1989.

Gay PC, Rodarte JR, Hubmayr RD: The effects of positive expiratory pressure on isovolume flow and dynamic hyperinflation in patients receiving mechanical ventilation, *Am Rev Respir Dis* 139:621-626, 1990.

Gurevitch MJ, Gelmont D: Importance of trigger sensitivity to ventilator delay in advanced COPD, *Crit Care Med* 17:354-359, 1989.

Hansen-Flaschen J, Brazinsky S, Bassles C, et al: Use of sedating drugs and neuromuscular blockade in patients requiring mechanical ventilation for respiratory failure, *JAMA* 266:2870-2875, 1991.

Ho L, MacIntyre NR: Effects of initial flow rate and breath termination criteria on pressure support ventilation, *Chest* 99:134-138, 1991.

Katz J, Kraemer R, Gjerde GE: Inspiratory work and airway pressure with CPAP, *Chest* 88:519-526, 1985.

MacIntyre NR: Importance of trigger sensitivity to ventilator response delay in advanced COPD, *Crit Care Med* 18:581-582, 1990 (letter).

MacIntyre NR: Patient ventilator interactions: dys-synchrony and imposed loads. In Marini J, Slutsky A: *Physiologic basis of ventilatory support,* New York, 1997, Marcel Dekker.

MacIntyre NR: Patient-ventilator interactions. In Grenvik A, editor: *Textbook of critical care medicine,* ed 4, Philadelphia, 1999, WB Saunders.

MacIntyre NR: Tracheal pressure triggering, *Respir Care* 41:524-528, 1996.

MacIntyre NR, McConnell R, Cheng KC, et al: Pressure limited breaths improve flow dys-synchrony during assisted ventilation, *Crit Care Med* 25:1671-1677, 1997.

MacIntyre NR, McConnell R, Cheng KC: Applied PEEP reduces the inspiratory load of intrinsic PEEP during pressure support, *Chest* 111:188-193, 1997.

Marini JJ, Smith TC, Lamb VJ: External work output and force generation during synchronized intermittent mechanical ventilation, *Am Rev Respir Dis* 138:1169-1179, 1988.

Marini JJ: Strategies to minimize breathing effort during mechanical ventilation, *Crit Care Clin* 6:635-661, 1990.

Petrof BJ, Legare M, Goldberg P, et al: Continuous positive airway pressure reduces work of breathing and dyspnea during weaning from mechanical ventilation in severe chronic obstructive pulmonary disease, *Am Rev Respir Dis* 141:281-289, 1990.

Sassoon CSH, Giron AE, Ely E, et al: Inspiratory work of breathing on flow-by and demand-flow continuous positive airway pressure, *Crit Care Med* 17:1108-1114, 1989.

Sassoon CSH: Mechanical ventilator design and function: the trigger variable, *Respir Care* 37:1056-1069, 1992.

Smith TC, Marini JJ: Impact of PEEP on lung mechanics and work of breathing in severe airflow obstruction, *J Appl Physiol* 65:1488-1499, 1988.

Takahashi T, Takezawa J, Kimura T, et al: Comparison of inspiratory work of breathing in T-piece breathing, PSV, and pleural pressure support ventilation (PPSV), *Chest* 100:1030-1034, 1991.

Younes M: Proportional assist ventilation: A new approach to ventilatory support, *Am Rev Respir Dis* 145:114-120, 1992.

CHAPTER 30

HYPOTENSION WITH MECHANICAL VENTILATION

Irawan Susanto

Key Terms

▼ Mechanical ventilation
▼ Hypotension

▼ Positive end-expiratory pressure (PEEP)

▼ Pneumothorax shock
▼ Auto-PEEP

▼ THE CLINICAL PROBLEM

The patient is a 64-year-old man with a history of emphysema. He was transferred to the intensive care unit (ICU) from a medical ward several hours ago with progressive respiratory failure attributed to neuromuscular weakness of Guillain-Barré syndrome (GBS). He has had difficulty swallowing and has been fed via a nasogastric tube. According to the nursing staff, his family has on occasion surreptitiously attempted to feed the patient despite the physician's order otherwise. He has been febrile for the past 24 hours and has had difficulty clearing his secretions. He was intubated 1 hour ago and received midazolam 2 mg intravenously before the intubation. He now develops progressive hypotension. The respiratory clinician is called to the bedside to evaluate the problem.

The patient's past medical history is significant for hypertension and chronic obstructive pulmonary disease (COPD). His last pulmonary function tests 1 year ago demonstrated a forced expiratory volume in 1 second (FEV_1) of 0.96 L without significant bronchodilator response, FEV_1/forced vital capacity (FVC) ratio of 38%, total lung capacity (TLC) of 138% predicted, and residual volume (RV) of 164% predicted. He has known bullous emphysema from his prior chest x-ray.

Current medications include albuterol and ipratropium bromide inhalation therapy and unfractionated heparin 5000 U subcutaneously twice daily. His antihypertensive medication was discontinued 24 hours ago. He has just been started on broad-spectrum antibiotics. He has undergone plasmapharesis twice since admission for treatment of GBS.

His social history is significant for a caring and involved family who feels that the patient's weakness is due in part to inadequate nutrition from the nasogastric tube feeding. They have been feeding the patient by mouth despite a strict order of NPO. He was still actively smoking until he was admitted to the hospital 5 days ago.

The patient is 5-foot, 7-inches tall and weighs 161 lbs. Significant findings on physical examination include the presence of fever, a blood pressure of 92/50, pulse of 112, and respiratory rate of 24. On chest auscultation, there are decreased breath sounds throughout with crackles at both lung bases. His heart sounds are regular but distant; it is difficult to appreciate any murmur or gallop. The extremities are cool, clammy, flaccid, and non-tender, without evidence of edema, clubbing, or cyanosis. He is unable to lift his limbs against gravity and has no gag reflex. He has a very weak cough.

The frontal view chest x-ray demonstrates patchy consolidation at both lung bases with a small pleural effusion on the left. There is hyperinflation of both lung fields with proper positioning of the nasogastric tube. The tip of the endotracheal tube is about 4 cm above the main carina. Other pertinent laboratory data include a leukocytosis with left shift, a hematocrit of 32%, and a normal platelet count.

The current mechanical ventilator settings are as follows: volume synchronized intermittent mandatory ventilation (SIMV) rate 12, tidal volume 750 cc, inspiratory time of 33%, positive end-expiratory pressure (PEEP) 5, pressure support 10 cm H_2O, and FIO_2 0.45. The patient's total respiratory rate is 24.

What is the differential diagnosis of this patient's hypotension?

Differential Diagnosis of Hypotension on Mechanical Ventilation

When evaluating hypotension in mechanically ventilated patients, it is important to have a systematic approach to elucidate the underlying cause(s) and reverse the process. A working knowledge of the pathophysiology of shock and the effect of mechanical ventilation on hemodynamic parameters is essential in searching for the cause of hypotension in mechanically ventilated patients. Box 30-1 lists the common causes of hypotension in this setting, and Table 30-1 lists the clinical clues that often accompany each cause.

The causes of hypotension in a patient who is undergoing mechanical ventilation can be separated into the following broad categories: (1) as a complication of the mechanical ventilation itself and (2) as a progression of the underlying pathol-

Box 30-1
Differential Diagnosis of Hypotension on Mechanical Ventilation

Directly Caused by Mechanical Ventilation	Affected by Mechanical Ventilation
Intrinsic PEEP–inadequate expiratory time	Septic shock
Mainstem bronchus intubation	Cardiogenic shock/myocardial infarction
Tension pneumothorax	Massive pulmonary embolism
Foreign body obstruction	Cardiac tamponade
	Gastrointestinal bleeding
	Medication

PEEP, Positive end-expiratory pressure.

TABLE 30-1
Evaluating Possible Causes of Hypotension on Mechanical Ventilation with Associated Clinical Features

Possible Causes	Mechanisms	Suggestive Clinical Features
Air trapping	Increased intra-thoracic pressure	History of obstructive lung disease, intrinsic PEEP, poor lung compliance
Mainstem bronchus intubation		Contralateral diminished breath sound, position of endotracheal tube too far in, poor lung compliance, chest x-ray diagnostic
Tension pneumo-thorax		Tracheal deviation to contralateral side, ipsilateral diminished breath sound, poor lung compliance, chest x-ray diagnostic
Foreign body aspiration	Intrinsic PEEP	History of aspiration, ipsilateral dimin-ished breath sound, poor lung com-pliance, lobar collapse on chest x-ray, bronchoscopy diagnostic
Gastric ulcer bleeding	Decreased intra-vascular volume	Skin cold and clammy, tachycardic, melenic stool, coffee ground emesis or nasogastric aspirate, PAC (low PAOP, low CO, high SVR)
Septic shock	Distributive shock	Tachypneic, tachycardic, febrile, leuko-cytosis, positive blood culture, PAC (high CO, low SVR)

PEEP, Positive end-expiratory pressure; PAC, pulmonary artery catheter; PAOP, pulmonary artery occlusion pressure, equivalent to left ventricular end-diastolic pressure; CO, cardiac output; SVR, systemic vascular resistance; ECG, electrocardiogram; V̇/Q̇ scan, ventilation-perfusion scan.   Continued

TABLE 30-1
Evaluating Possible Causes of Hypotension on Mechanical Ventilation with Associated Clinical Features—cont'd

Possible Causes	Mechanisms	Suggestive Clinical Features
Congestive heart failure	Cardiogenic shock	S_3 gallop, rales, echocardiogram (decreased systolic function), PAC (high PAOP, low CO, high SVR)
Acute myocardial infarction	Cardiogenic shock	Same as congestive heart failure, with addition of acute ECG changes; positive cardiac enzymes
Valvular abnormality	Cardiogenic shock	Specific murmur on examination, echocardiogram diagnostic
Pulmonary embolism	Obstructive shock	Parasternal heave, loud P_2, right-sided S_3, ECG right heart strain, V̇/Q̇ scan diagnostic, PAC (high PAP with normal PAOP)
Cardiac tamponade	Cardiogenic shock	Narrow pulse pressure, ECG low voltage and electrical alternans, echocardiogram (pericardial effusion, diastolic collapse of cardiac chamber), PAC (equalization of pressures)

PEEP, Positive end-expiratory pressure; PAC, pulmonary artery catheter; PAOP, pulmonary artery occlusion pressure, equivalent to left ventricular end-diastolic pressure; CO, cardiac output; SVR, systemic vascular resistance; ECG, electrocardiogram; V̇/Q̇ scan, ventilation-perfusion scan.

ogy that initiated the respiratory failure (e.g., pneumonia progressing to sepsis). Even if the hypotension is a result of the progression of sepsis, mechanical ventilation may affect the course and thus the management of the sepsis.

In considering hypotension as a possible complication of mechanical ventilation, the effect of positive pressure ventilation and PEEP can be summarized as follows: Positive pressure ventilation increases the intra-thoracic pressure, which diminishes venous return into the right heart by compressing the central veins and vena cavae. Increased intra-thoracic pressure, in particular with the addition of PEEP, is transmitted to the alveolar space and the heart, therefore increasing the alveolar and juxta-cardiac pressures. Elevation of the alveolar pressure contributes to an increase in pulmonary vascular resistance and right ventricular afterload. The increase in juxta-cardiac pressure results in a decrease in left ventricular wall compliance and the effective transmural distending pressure, thereby diminishing the left ventricular end-diastolic volume (preload).

Additionally, coronary perfusion during diastole may also be diminished due to the compression of epicardial vessels by an increase in juxta-cardiac pressure, resulting in a decrease in myocardial oxygen supply. Because the two ventricles are separated by a thin septum, the increased right ventricular afterload may result in a relative movement of the interventricular septum toward the left ventricular cavity, thus further reducing the left ventricular wall compliance and preload. This phenomenon is known as *ventricular interdependence.* The overall hemodynamic effect of positive pressure ventilation and PEEP on a normal heart is a decrease in the forward cardiac output and systemic blood pressure. Most patients have an adequate hemodynamic status to start with and are readily able to compensate for these effects. However, in patients who require high positive pressures and PEEP (whether intrinsic or extrinsic) and who have a borderline low intra-vascular volume to start, the hemodynamic effects of positive pressure ventilation may be quite substantial. Development of a tension pneumothorax, which raises the intra-thoracic pressure, may create similar hemodynamic derangements.

Hypotension may also occur as a consequence of anesthetic, sedative, or analgesic agents that are commonly used to reduce a patient's discomfort associated with intubation and mechanical ventilation. The use of these agents may result in vasodilation, and, in some cases, myocardial depression. When used in patients with a low intra-vascular volume to start, the combined effects of decreased venous return by positive pressure ventilation and medication-induced vasodilation can easily precipitate hypotension.

Hypotension in a mechanically ventilated patient may also be due to a progression of the underlying pathology. In general, hypotension with its attendant complication, the hypoperfusion state or shock, can be classified into the following four categories: hypovolemic, cardiogenic, distributive, and obstructive.

Hypovolemic shock is caused by the loss of significant amount of intra-vascular volume, resulting in a low filling pressure and volume of the left ventricle at end-diastole (preload). Examples include hemorrhage from trauma, gastrointestinal bleed, retroperitoneal bleed, or excessive fluid losses such as severe diarrhea, diabetes insipidus, osmotic diuresis in diabetic hyperosmolar state, and ketoacidosis. Mechanical ventilation can worsen the hypotension by decreasing the intra-thoracic venous return caused by an increased intra-thoracic pressure, thus further decreasing the left ventricular preload and blood pressure.

Cardiogenic shock is caused by damage to the myocardium or the heart valves, resulting in an inefficient cardiac pump that fails to generate an adequate cardiac output and systemic blood pressure for tissue perfusion. The most common reason for cardiogenic shock is coronary disease that results in ischemia, leading to infarction and ultimately heart failure. The ischemia may also affect the function of the heart valves, rendering them incompetent and further diminishing the forward cardiac output from the left ventricle. Blunt chest trauma can result in cardiac contusion, or bruising of the heart muscles, which can also lead to heart failure.

The effect of positive pressure ventilation on the failing heart is different from that on a normal heart. The overall effect of positive pressure ventilation on the normal or healthy heart is a decrease in cardiac output. However, in a failing heart with decreased myocardial contractility, positive pressure ventilation results in a decrease in left ventricular afterload, thus potentially improving the cardiac output.

Distributive shock results from a loss of vasoregulatory activity of the systemic circulation, producing peripheral vasodilation and relative hypotension. Anaphylaxis and sepsis are examples of distributive shock. Classically, this type of shock is associated with high cardiac output and low systemic vascular resistance. The redistribution of cardiac output to vast vascular beds results in a relative hypoperfusion to the other organs, laying the groundwork for ischemia and multiorgan failure. The addition of positive intra-thoracic pressure from mechanical ventilation and

PEEP in patients with distributive shock reduces the venous return and cardiac output similar to patients with hypovolemic shock, and may worsen the hypotension.

Obstructive shock occurs when extra-cardiac blood flow is impeded, such as in pulmonary thromboembolism, resulting in a decreased left ventricular preload. The left ventricular preload is also diminished as a result of ventricular interdependence, a consequence of elevated pulmonary vascular resistance and right ventricular end-diastolic pressure. The increase in alveolar pressure from positive pressure ventilation and PEEP may increase the right ventricular pressure even more, leading to a further decline in left ventricular preload.

In the clinical setting, the effect of positive pressure ventilation on cardiovascular hemodynamic may be variable and sometimes difficult to predict. There are a number of other factors that may influence the hemodynamic effects of positive pressure ventilation, all of which may alter the final outcome. Some of these factors include the initial underlying cardiac function and hemodynamic status, the combination of several shock states acting together, the effect of intra-thoracic pressure changes on left atrial volume, and antidiuretic hormone. While cardiac output generally decreases with positive pressure ventilation, the actual response may vary.

In this case, the possible causes of the patient's hypotension while on mechanical ventilation are as follows:

1. *Progressive development of intrinsic PEEP and air trapping* given a relatively large tidal volume with inadequate expiratory time in a patient with known severe airway obstruction.
2. *Foreign-body aspiration with lobar collapse,* causing a redistribution of the tidal volume over a small ventilated lung volume and resulting in a high intra-thoracic pressure and an intrinsic PEEP.
3. *Tension pneumothorax,* related to item 1 or 2 above. Pneumothorax may also develop if there is an unrecognized mainstem bronchus intubation with delivery of the entire tidal volume into a hemithorax, in particular in a patient with bullous emphysema. A pneumothorax may be more difficult to detect in the patient with emphysematous lung fields on chest x-ray.
4. *Medication-induced hypotension,* which may be precipitated by anesthetics, analgesics, sedatives, and neuromuscular blocking agents.
5. *Aspiration/nosocomial pneumonia progressing to sepsis.* The patient was febrile for 24 hours before intubation, which suggests an ongoing infectious process. He also has other signs of sepsis, including tachycardia, tachypnea, and leukocytosis with a left shift.
6. *Myocardial infarction* with cardiogenic shock that complicates the stress of pneumonia, respiratory failure, and intubation is a possibility, since the patient has several risk factors for coronary disease, including gender, age, active smoking history, and history of hypertension.
7. *Venous thromboembolism* that results in obstructive shock. The patient had significant ascending limb weakness that progressed to respiratory failure associated with GBS. Lack of movement in a bedridden state results in venostasis of the lower extremities, predisposing the patient to the development of lower extremity deep venous thrombosis (DVT) and the associated pulmonary embolism (PE).
8. *Gastrointestinal bleeding* that results in hypovolemia. Patients on mechanical ventilation and under stress are at risk of developing gastric stress ulcer. Early

bleeding may not manifest in a drop in the hematocrit because of insufficient time for intra-vascular volume equilibration.

These possible causes are not necessarily mutually exclusive. Multiple etiologies may be involved in the pathogenesis of hypotension in this clinical scenario.

Clinical Features that Suggest a Specific Cause of Hypotension on Mechanical Ventilation

Although the differential diagnosis of this patient's hypotension is broad, additional information may favor or mitigate against specific causes (see Table 30-1). The following addresses each differential diagnostic possibility by number as used in the previous list:

1. In this case, the patient has severe airflow obstruction with evidence of hyperinflation and air trapping based on his baseline pulmonary function studies. He was started on positive pressure ventilation with a moderate tidal volume (~10 cc/kg) and a 1:2 inspiratory-expiratory ratio (I/E). This setting may be inadequate to allow full expiration of the mechanically generated inspiratory tidal volume. Additionally, the patient is over-breathing the ventilator significantly, effectively decreasing the I/E to almost 1:1. The increased respiratory drive is likely a consequence of pneumonia and sepsis. The inadequate expiratory time results in progressive breath stacking and development intrinsic PEEP, contributing to progressive hypotension. With progressive buildup of intrinsic PEEP, the peak pressure limit alarm will be triggered and the expiratory tidal volume diminished. Thus proper selection of alarm setting can be helpful in troubleshooting the potential contribution of mechanical ventilation in the pathogenesis of hypotension.
2. Foreign-body aspiration that results in clinically evident hypoxemia and hypotension would have demonstrated a significant finding on the chest x-ray. Common findings of foreign body aspiration on the chest x-ray include atelectasis, lobar collapse, and possibly lung collapse. Although the patient is at risk of developing foreign-body aspiration and obstruction because of the continued oral feeding given by his family members in the absence of a protective gag reflex, the clinical picture is not compatible.
3. Tension pneumothorax may develop as a sequela of increased intra-thoracic pressure from positive pressure ventilation alone or from subsequent development of intrinsic PEEP. This patient has known bullous emphysema from his prior chest x-ray, increasing the risk of pneumothorax with any positive pressure ventilation. Development of a pneumothorax while the patient is on a positive pressure ventilator generally results in a tension pneumothorax, and if not relieved promptly, results in rapid cardiovascular collapse. Unfortunately, pneumothorax in an emphysema patient is sometimes difficult to appreciate on a bedside frontal chest x-ray that results from the paucity of parenchymal lung markings. In the supine chest x-ray, a pneumothorax may not necessarily manifest at the apex of the lung; instead, it may manifest as a deep sulcus line at the ipsilateral costophrenic angle. When there is uncertainty of the presence of a pneumothorax on the frontal chest x-ray, additional chest x-ray views may be obtained such as a lordotic view or a lateral decubitus view. The mechanical

ventilator parameters and alarm triggers may be indistinguishable from those of intrinsic PEEP buildup. Bedside examination sometimes yields additional clues of the presence of a tension pneumothorax such as ipsilateral decrease in breath sound with more tympanitic percussion, deviation of the trachea contralaterally, and the development of subcutaneous emphysema. Since the chest x-ray demonstrated proper positioning of the endotracheal tube and did not show any evidence of pneumothorax, this is less likely the cause of the patient's current hypotension. If intrinsic PEEP is indeed present and is not recognized or relieved promptly, the patient is still at risk of developing a life-threatening tension pneumothorax.

4. The patient received a small dose of sedative for the intubation and has not received subsequent doses of analgesic or sedative since then. The progression of the hypotension is unlikely to be related to the medication.

5. The patient is known to have a high risk for aspiration given the absence of a gag reflex. Oropharyngeal aspiration is anticipated to occur intermittently in this patient. He is also at risk of gastric reflux aspiration due to the violation of gastroesophageal sphincter by the presence of a nasogastric tube, rendering the sphincter somewhat incompetent. Surreptitious oral feeding by the patient's family members further increases his risk of aspiration. The chest x-ray demonstrates bilateral patchy consolidation at the bases with a small pleural effusion, consistent with aspiration pneumonia. The clinical findings are compatible with sepsis, as evidenced by the presence of fever, tachypnea, tachycardia, and leukocytosis with left shift. The progressive hypotension may herald the development of septic shock from aspiration pneumonia.

6. Based on the information provided in the clinical problem, cardiogenic causes of the hypotension cannot be ruled out. This patient has multiple risk factors for coronary disease, including his age, gender, active smoking history, and hypertension. Myocardial ischemia or infarction may accompany respiratory failure. Coronary artery perfusion occurs during diastole. Hypotension from other etiologies may therefore precipitate myocardial ischemia or infarction because of the decrease in coronary perfusion, in particular in patients with an underlying coronary disease. In addition, the hyperdynamic state of sepsis increases myocardial oxygen demand, while the myocardial oxygen supply from coronary perfusion is diminished from hypotension and increased intra-thoracic pressure. In later stages of septic shock, myocardial depression may also occur independent of myocardial ischemia, resulting in a downward spiral of worsening hypotension. Acute myocardial ischemia or infarction can often be detected by specific changes in the electrocardiogram (ECG). In the setting of an underlying abnormal ECG, the diagnosis may be suspected by a rise in cardiac enzymes in the serum, or specific cardiac imaging (nuclear medicine or echocardiography). Cardiac auscultation may reveal a new regurgitant murmur (valvular incompetence) or a ventricular gallop (S_3) suggestive of ventricular systolic dysfunction.

7. Although the incidence of venous thromboembolism in patients with ascending paralysis from inflammatory polyneuropathy of GBS is unknown, data from acute spinal cord injury patients are available. Small observational studies suggest a 67% to 100% incidence of DVT in acute spinal cord injury patients. A prospective study of venous thromboembolism after major trauma reported an incidence of 35% for DVT, with spinal cord injury as the strongest risk factor.

Even with the use of low-dose unfractionated heparin prophylaxis, the incidence of DVT in spinal injury patients has been reported to be 13% to 31%. There is emerging data that low molecular heparin is superior to low-dose unfractionated heparin in the prevention of venous thromboembolism in this group of patients. The incidence of PE is generally lower than the incidence of DVT, but venous thromboembolism is still a factor to consider in patients with acute paralysis of the lower extremities. The patient in this case has the risk factors for DVT because of his age, paralysis, and smoking history. Despite the prophylaxis with low-dose unfractionated heparin, there is still a risk of DVT and subsequent PE. Even a small PE may result in a catastrophic cardiopulmonary collapse in a patient with a severely compromised pulmonary and cardiac reserve. The acute pulmonary hypertension caused by PE can sometimes be detected by the presence of a parasternal heave, a prominent pulmonic component of the second heart sound (P_2), and a right-sided S_3 gallop. In this patient, PE has not been ruled out as a contributing factor to the hypotension. Studies for evaluating lower extremity DVT (duplex ultrasound, plethysmography) are easier to perform than studies for evaluating PE (ventilation-perfusion [$\dot{V}/\dot{Q}$] scans, pulmonary angiogram). Although a positive diagnosis of DVT does not necessarily confirm the presence of PE, the treatment is similar (i.e., anticoagulation). A negative study for DVT does not rule out PE. As discussed previously, the presence of intrinsic PEEP can potentially further deteriorate the hypotension in the setting of acute PE.

8. Hypovolemia from acute bleeding also is not ruled out in this patient. Acute blood loss within the body (gastrointestinal tract, soft tissue compartment, etc) may not be accompanied by a drop in the hemoglobin concentration or hematocrit, since it takes time to equilibrate the intra-vascular and extra-vascular volumes. Hypovolemia usually triggers reflex tachycardia in an attempt to restore cardiac output. As previously discussed, positive pressure ventilation may worsen the hypotension. This patient has not received any pharmacologic gastric stress ulcer prophylaxis. The use of enteral feeding is considered as somewhat protective to the gastrointestinal mucosa from erosion and bleeding. Screening for gastrointestinal bleeding includes simple tests such as nasogastric lavage and Hemoccult examination of the stool.

The clinician should remember that several processes contribute to the development of hypotension in a ventilated patient. Narrowly focusing on a single cause may sometimes lead to an inadvertent missed opportunity to intervene in other contributing pathologies in a timely fashion.

Diagnostic Testing in the Evaluation of a Ventilated Patient with Hypotension

The work-up for a ventilated patient who develops hypotension includes the following:

- Directed physical examination: Evaluate the patient for tracheal deviation, subcutaneous emphysema, symmetry of breath sounds, presence of wheezing or rales on chest auscultation; presence of an S_3 gallop, accentuated pulmonic component of second heart sound (P_2), or new regurgitant murmur on cardiac auscultation; abdominal tenderness, gross examination of the stool color and hemoccult testing; and lower extremity tenderness or swelling.

- Evaluation of the ventilator setting and alarms: the peak pressure limit, the estimated total PEEP, and, if available, the flow-time curve.
- Medications: Review time and dosage of anesthetic, sedative, or analgesic given; time and dosage of antihypertensive and cardiodepressant agents given.
- Assessment of the patient's cardiac rhythm and electrical activity: Observe the cardiac monitor for obvious cardiac arrhythmias, obtain a 12-lead ECG, and compare with the baseline ECG.
- Radiographic reassessment: Obtain another chest x-ray if a pneumothorax or inadvertent main stem bronchus intubation is suspected. Additional views of frontal lordotic, lateral decubitus, or cross table lateral may be obtained if localized or loculated pneumothorax is suspected.
- Laboratory evaluation: Complete blood count, serum electrolytes, cardiac enzymes, blood cultures, and tracheal aspirate Gram's stain and culture.
- Additional/ancillary studies: Lower extremity imaging for DVT (venogram, plethysmography, or duplex ultrasound), $\dot{V}/\dot{Q}$ scanning for PE, echocardiogram for cardiac function, and flow-directed balloon-tipped pulmonary artery catheter (PAC) for hemodynamic monitoring.
- Therapeutic trial: If the peak pressure and intrinsic PEEP are high and the patient's oxygenation is adequate, a therapeutic trial of ventilator disconnection may be useful. This maneuver is not appropriate in patients with severe respiratory failure requiring high FIO_2 approaching 1.0 and high external PEEP. Disconnecting the patient from the ventilator allows equilibration of the intra-thoracic pressure with the atmospheric pressure. If the hypotension results from or is significantly contributed by the high intrinsic PEEP, the blood pressure may improve within minutes. If the high intra-thoracic pressure is caused by a tension pneumothorax, this maneuver will not improve the blood pressure. If tension pneumothorax is suspected from the physical examination and the hypotension is accompanied by cardiac arrhythmias, a therapeutic trial of a needle placement over the ipsilateral second intra-costal space at midclavicular line may be life-saving. Once the needle is placed, however, a chest tube has to be placed expediently. This should only be undertaken by an experienced operator, because, whether a tension pneumothorax was present or not, once the needle has been placed in the pleural space, a pneumothorax is now present.

Assessment of the Effects of Therapy for a Ventilated Patient with Hypotension

Appropriate therapy to reverse hypotension in a ventilated patient should result in improvements in the blood pressure and organ perfusion. In general, the treatment strategy should focus on treatment of the underlying pathology. The following is a brief outline of strategies to reverse the hypotension in a ventilated patient based on a specific etiology.

1. For problems related to the development of intrinsic PEEP, adjustments of the mechanical ventilator settings to prolong the expiratory phase or reduce the tidal volume are essential. If this is not possible due to the septic process and

increased CO_2 production and respiratory drive, then permissive hypercapnia with the judicious use of sedation and neuromuscular blockade may be considered. This strategy is used only as an adjunctive method while appropriate therapy for sepsis or cause of the hypermetabolic state is instituted.

2. For tension pneumothorax, placement of a chest tube to reexpand the lung is paramount to the success of treatment. The chest tube should be connected to negative suction of 20 cm H_2O.

3. When the sedative or analgesic medications are suspected to contribute to the hypotension, careful assessment of the need for the agents should be undertaken. Although most sedative or analgesic agents may exacerbate or induce hypotension, some are more so than others. Selecting an agent with fewer tendencies toward hypotension is prudent, as long as the goal of the therapy is achieved. It is important to alleviate the anxiety and discomfort of patients undergoing mechanical ventilation in order to facilitate patient-ventilator synchrony. If neuromuscular blockade is deemed necessary to achieve adequate ventilation and oxygenation, selecting an agent with less cardiovascular toxicity may reduce the risk of hypotension. Proper monitoring of the degree of paralysis can minimize the dose required. In some cases, it may be worthwhile to temporarily discontinue the medications and start over by slowly titrating up the agents to a desirable end point. When other causes of the hypotension have been ruled out and the above maneuvers have not reversed the hypotension, the clinician must then decide if vasopressor therapy should be initiated.

4. For pneumonia and sepsis, the most important therapy is treatment of the source of sepsis itself. Appropriate antibiotic therapy should be given and evacuation of an infected closed space or abscess be performed expediently. Vasopressor therapy is often needed to temporarily support the blood pressure during septic shock. Appropriate adjustment of the positive pressure ventilator may minimize the vasopressor requirement.

5. When the etiology of the hypotension itself cannot be attributed solely to the effects of mechanical ventilation, hemodynamic evaluation is warranted. A noninvasive evaluation with an echocardiogram may reveal information regarding the size and contractile state of the left and right ventricles, the wall thickness and the regional motion abnormalities of ventricles, the presence of significant valvular abnormalities, the estimate of pulmonary artery systolic pressure if a tricuspid valve regurgitant jet is demonstrable, and the presence of pericardial effusion or tamponade. Invasive hemodynamic parameters can be obtained by inserting a flow-directed balloon-tipped PAC. The PAC may give information on the cardiac output, the pulmonary artery pressure, the central venous pressure, the estimated left ventricular end-diastolic filling pressure, and allows the calculation of systemic and pulmonary vascular resistance as well as an estimation of oxygen delivery and consumption. It does not measure the juxta-cardiac pressure and gives no information on the left ventricular wall compliance, both of which are needed to fully assess the left ventricular preload. The information is often useful in distinguishing the various causes of shock or the combination thereof. Therapy for cardiogenic shock generally involves a combination of afterload reduction, preload reduction, and enhancement in contractility. Treatment of acute myocardial ischemia or infarction is beyond the scope of this chapter.

6. The presence of venous thromboembolism necessitates the initiation of systemic anticoagulation. In cases of PE-induced refractory hypotension despite appropriate adjustment of the ventilator, systemic thrombolysis may be indicated. In patients with contraindications for anticoagulation, insertion of an inferior vena cava filter should be undertaken to prevent further embolization to the pulmonary vasculature.
7. Hypovolemic shock is managed by volume repletion and correction of the underlying cause of hypovolemia. If gastrointestinal bleeding is the source of hypovolemia, blood transfusion, correction of any coagulopathy, and an endoscopic evaluation are warranted. In some cases, an angiogram may be needed to localize the source of bleeding, and, when found, may be embolized to prevent further bleeding.

Pitfalls and Common Mistakes in the Assessment and Treatment of a Ventilated Patient with Hypotension

When assessing a hypotensive patient on mechanical ventilation, a common mistake of the inexperienced clinician is to maintain a narrow focus. This chapter is designed to give a broad overview of differential diagnosis in evaluating common causes of hypotension and a systematic approach to the problem based on a clinical scenario. There may be several processes acting together, simultaneously causing and maintaining the hypotension. The clinician should remember this when the appropriate management of an apparent cause of hypotension does not result in the expected reversal of the hypotension. The mechanical ventilator itself may be the cause, a contributor, or an innocent bystander in the pathogenesis of hypotension. In general, positive pressure ventilation reduces the cardiac output and may worsen hypotension. The actual clinical effect, however, is complex and unpredictable. Even in the same patient, a properly adjusted and set mechanical ventilator on one day may not be appropriate in the next hour or day, depending on the evolving overall clinical picture.

▼ BIBLIOGRAPHY

Clagett GP et al: Prevention of venous thromboembolism, *Chest* 114(5):531S-560S, 1998.
Keith RL, Pierson DJ: Complications of mechanical ventilation: a bedside approach, *Clin Chest Med* 17(3):439-451, 1996.
Pulmonary Artery Catheter Consensus Conference Participants: Pulmonary artery catheter consensus conference: consensus statement, *Crit Care Med* 25(6):910-925, 1997.
Slutsky AS: Mechanical ventilation, *Chest* 104(6):1833-1859, 1993.

CHAPTER 31

IMMEDIATE REINTUBATION

Douglas Orens
Edward Hoisington
Lucy Kester
James K. Stoller

Key Terms

▼ Laryngospasm
▼ Stridor
▼ Tracheal obstruction

▼ Weakness
▼ Upper airway obstruction

▼ Leak test
▼ Cuff

▼ THE CLINICAL PROBLEM

A 67-year-old man has just been extubated after spending the previous 10 days on mechanical ventilation. He had been electively intubated and placed on mechanical ventilation for an episode of impending hypercapnic respiratory failure due to pneumococcal pneumonia. Weaning from mechanical ventilation has been difficult, resulting in a long duration of mechanical ventilation and intubation. The patient was treated with a course of penicillin for the pneumococcal pneumonia.

His past medical history shows moderate chronic obstructive pulmonary disease (COPD, emphysema) and coronary artery disease. His family history is significant for coronary artery disease and asthma in his sister. He is currently being treated with ipratropium bromide and a short-acting beta-agonist for COPD. He also receives a calcium channel blocker for coronary artery disease. The patient was receiving 5 mg of Valium q 4 hours prn while on mechanical ventilation. This dose was reduced to 2.5 mg every 4 hours prn, 24 hours before extubation. Immediately after extubation, the patient complained of a sore throat and was hoarse.

Physical examination at this time showed a blood pressure of 140/86 taken in the supine position. The heart rate was 94 and regular. His respiratory rate was 22 and non-labored. Examination of the head, eyes, ears, nose, and throat showed a small amount of white secretions in the oropharynx and a functional gag reflex. Breath sounds showed scattered rhonchi in the right lower lobe (RLL) but were otherwise unremarkable.

The latest chest x-ray showed an enlarged heart and resolution of the RLL infiltrate. Initial post-extubation arterial blood gas (ABG) values were pH 7.36, $PaCO_2$ 47 mm Hg, PaO_2 72 mm Hg, HCO_3^- 27, SaO_2 94% (SpO_2 93%) on an FIO_2 of 0.40 via unheated bland aerosol. Hemoximetry was performed and revealed an oxyhemoglobin of 94% and a carboxyhemoglobin of 4%. The level of methemoglobin was low. The most recent values of vital capacity (VC) and negative inspiratory force (NIF), performed before extubation, were VC 1.30 L and NIF −45 cm H_2O.

Twelve hours post-extubation, physical examination revealed a blood pressure of 165/94 in the supine position. Heart rate was 136 and regular. Respiratory rate was 35 and labored. Examination of the head, eyes, ears, nose, and throat showed stridorous sounds in the upper airway that localized to the trachea. Breath sounds were diminished bilaterally. At this time, ABG values were pH 7.30, $PaCO_2$ 60 mm Hg, PaO_2 63 mm Hg, HCO_3^- 27, SaO_2 91% on FIO_2 of 0.40. The patient was immediately reintubated.

What is the differential diagnosis of causes for this patient's reintubation, and what is the most likely cause?

Differential Diagnosis of Causes for Reintubation

Post-extubation stridor may represent several causes and requires immediate attention. Three common problems that may necessitate reintubation are airway obstruction, risk of aspiration, and difficulty with secretion clearance. Other less common causes that may require reintubation are neurologic or neuromuscular impairment, excessive secretions, tracheal stenosis, tracheomalacia, and lesions that may compress the airway such as a mass, abscess, or hematoma (Box 31-1).

Obstruction at the level of the larynx may develop as a result of laryngospasm or laryngeal edema (Table 31-1). Laryngospasm usually occurs quickly after extubation. Removal of an artificial airway can cause stimulation of the superior laryngeal nerve, which causes sustained activation of the glottic closure reflex and laryngospasm. Notably, hypoxemia and hypercarbia can depress the adductor motor response, causing relaxation of the glottic closure reflex and reducing the risk of laryngospasm. Glottic edema and vocal cord inflammation, commonly referred to as laryngeal edema, is generally less acute than laryngospasm unless it is allowed to progress and become severe, necessitating reintubation. Edema may complicate traumatic intubation, causing edema of the airway. Laryngeal edema can occur up to 24 hours post-extubation.

Box 31-1
Differential Diagnosis for Immediate Reintubation

Common Causes	Less Common Causes
Airway obstruction	Neurologic disorder
Laryngospasm	Neuromuscular disorder
Laryngeal edema	Excess secretions
Aspiration	Compression of airway
Impaired swallowing mechanism	Abscess
Gag reflex	Hematoma
Difficulty with secretion clearance	Tracheal stenosis

TABLE 31-1
Interpreting Signs and Symptoms in the Patient Who Requires Reintubation

Possible Causes	Mechanisms	Suggestive Clinical Features
Laryngeal edema	Edema or inflammation of the glottic area or vocal cords as a result of pressure from the artificial airway or traumatic intubation	Primary symptoms are hoarseness and stridor
Laryngospasm	Involuntary contraction of the laryngeal muscles that causes complete or partial closure of the glottis	Acute onset of distress soon after extubation
Aspiration	Inhalation of foreign material into the respiratory tract	Acute onset of difficulty, new appearance of copious secretions
Secretion clearance	Trouble clearing airways of excessive secretions as a result of impaired level of consciousness or cough	Can cause hypoxemia or hypercarbia
Diminished respiratory muscle strength and ability to expel secretions	Respiratory muscle fatigue may result in respiratory failure; in combination with excessive secretions, may require the need for reintubation	Abdominal paradox can occur, rapid shallow breathing

Aspiration after extubation can occur as a result of the disruption of the normal swallowing (deglutition) mechanism. Abnormal deglutition can be caused by placement of an artificial airway, trauma, lack of a functional gag reflex, or neurologic dysfunction of the normal swallowing maneuver. Swallowing occurs in four discrete phases: oral preparation, pre-oral phase, pharyngeal phase, and the esophageal phase. Each phase is necessary for normal swallowing, and the inability to perform any of these phases may predispose to aspiration. Also, peri-glottic sensation can be reduced for 4 to 8 hours after tube removal in patients who have been intubated longer than 8 hours. It has been reported that glottic function may be impaired in up to 28% of patients who have had an artificial airway in place for longer than 6 days.

For extubation to be successful, the patient must have a sufficient level of consciousness and muscular strength to produce an effective cough. Cough is one of the most important defense mechanisms for clearing the lower airways of secretions. The cough reflex is vagally mediated when irritant receptors are triggered in the airway. This reaction can be stimulated by introducing any inflammatory, thermal, chemical, or mechanical irritant into the airways. On stimulation, the cricopharyngeal muscles constrict, causing glottic closure. The intercostal muscles then contract, raising intrathoracic pressure and causing the glottis to open and air to be expelled from the thorax at a very high velocity. This maneuver causes mucus to be propelled from the lower and upper airways into the oropharynx, where it can be swallowed or expectorated. A sufficient cough reflex has been shown to be just as effective in removing secretions from the lower airways as using any of the components of bronchopulmonary hygiene (percussion, vibration, postural drainage).

Respiratory muscle weakness and excessive secretions are a worrisome combination for the post-intubation patient because they can threaten adequate oxygenation and ventilation. Inspiration is achieved at rest by contraction of the diaphragm, scalene muscles, and the intercostal muscles. Effective ventilation requires that the respiratory muscles are capable of sustaining the workload placed on them. Thus fatigue of any muscle, which can be defined as the inability to maintain the required capacity of force due to continued or repeated contractions or due to lack of sufficient nutrients, can threaten extubation success. Generally, muscle fatigue is classified as central or peripheral. Central fatigue is an exertion-induced, reversible decrease in the central respiratory drive. There are two types of peripheral fatigue: transmission and contractile. Both are reversible.

Tracheal stenosis and tracheomalacia are conditions that generally occur as a result of artificial airway placement. Tracheomalacia is caused by softening of the cartilaginous rings of the trachea, which can cause collapse during inspiration, causing airway obstruction. Tracheal stenosis is a narrowing of the lumen of the trachea, which also can cause airway obstruction. The stenosis can be due to scarring from pressure exerted on the trachea from the cuff of the endotracheal tube or as the aftermath of a traumatic intubation.

Other less common conditions, such as masses, abscesses, or hematomas, can also cause airway obstruction due to compression of the airway. Before extubation, the clinician should be aware of the potential for obstruction that may require the need for immediate reintubation.

Clinical Features that Suggest a Specific Cause for the Need for Immediate Reintubation

In the present case, several features suggest that the patient is experiencing respiratory distress due to airway obstruction from laryngeal edema. The patient's initial post-extubation physical examination showed no signs of respiratory distress. Rather, respiratory distress began only 12 hours later as laryngeal edema developed. As in this case, laryngeal edema can worsen over time and may not fully present for up to 24 hours after removal of an artificial airway. Traumatic intubation may cause edema and swelling at the time of extubation, or the presence of an endotracheal tube over a period of days may cause pressure that inflames the upper airway. Main symptoms are hoarseness and stridor, which is a high-pitched inspiratory breath sound heard over the upper airway. Hoarseness often occurs shortly after tube removal and usually resolves within a short time. Stridor should be viewed as a more serious condition and indicates that the diameter of the airway may be significantly reduced due to edema and swelling.

Laryngospasm should be the primary concern when stridor develops soon after extubation. This condition can be life-threatening and should be treated urgently. Laryngospasm presents with marked stridor and significant respiratory distress and can cause complete airway obstruction and cardiopulmonary arrest. The current patient did initially complain of some hoarseness, but did not display any signs of stridorous breath sounds or respiratory distress immediately after extubation that would have suggested laryngospasm or the presence of an airway mass, abscess, or hematoma.

Although unlikely in the current case, patients can be at risk for aspiration from trauma, inadequate gag reflex, swallowing inactivity due to artificial airway placement, or neurological dysfunction. This patient was alert post-extubation and showed evidence of an adequate gag and cough. Also, he had no history of neurologic dysfunction, which was reinforced by relatively preserved bedside measurements of VC and NIF before extubation.

Diagnostic Testing before Extubation

Before extubation, it is necessary to evaluate the patient's candidacy to start a weaning trial and then his or her likelihood to successfully be liberated from the ventilator and the endotracheal tube. Specifically, candidacy to start a weaning trial generally requires resolution of the disease state that caused the need for ventilation, hemodynamic stability, adequacy of oxygenation (FIO_2 requirement ≤ 0.50 with PEEP ≤ 5 cm H_2O), and adequacy of ventilation. Once the patient is deemed a candidate for successful weaning, assessment of various "weaning parameters" can help establish the likelihood of successful weaning.

Weaning parameters may include the patient's spontaneous minute volume, vital capacity, maximum inspiratory measurements, and a measurement of the rapid shallow breathing index (i.e., the spontaneous respiratory rate divided by the patient's measured tidal volume in liters). These parameters can collectively help determine the likelihood of successful weaning, although no single set of values perfectly predicts the patient's readiness. Favorable predictors of weaning success include a vital capacity of 10 to 20 mL/kg, maximum inspiratory force of −30 cm

H_2O or less (i.e., more negative), a tidal volume of at least 5 to 8 mL/kg, and a rapid shallow breathing index of less than 105. In addition, assurance that the patient is alert, has good neuromuscular function, minimal, thin secretions, and an effective cough are important conditions to be met before proceeding toward successful weaning and extubation.

Importantly, the patient's ability to adequately maintain spontaneous breathing while on a "T-Piece" or continuous positive airway pressure (CPAP) trial does not always predict successful extubation. Similarly, failing to maintain adequate spontaneous volumes may not disqualify a patient from successful extubation, as in the case of breathing through a small-caliber endotracheal tube.

A somewhat controversial test, called the *cuff leak test*, is available to help the clinician determine readiness for extubation. The leak test is as follows:

1. Assess the patient to ensure that he or she meets weaning criteria.
2. Suction the mouth and upper airway.
3. Deflate the cuff of the endotracheal tube.
4. Briefly occlude the end of the endotracheal tube.
5. If the patient is unable to breathe around the occluded endotracheal tube with the cuff deflated, this suggests the presence of laryngeal edema.

Miller and Cole described their experience with leak testing accomplished within 24 hours of extubation. Immediately before the test was performed, the patient was placed on the assist/control mode with the cuff around the endotracheal tube inflated. The set inspiratory and displayed expiratory tidal volumes were recorded, and the balloon pressure around the cuff was recorded using a manometer. The balloon cuff was then deflated, and the expiratory tidal volume was recorded over the next six respiratory cycles, averaging the lowest three cycles. With cuff leak volume defined as the difference between the inspiratory and averaged expiratory tidal volume, the authors concluded that a volume greater than 110 mL was associated with an absence of edema and predicted successful extubation. Although others have not confirmed the value of the leak test, especially in post-surgical patients, a leak test on the current patient could have been considered as another tool for predicting successful extubation.

In summary, the decision to proceed with extubation should be based on assessment of adequate ventilatory function (as predicted by standard weaning indexes) and a trial of spontaneous breathing, as well as assurance of upper airway patency and the ability to clear secretions.

Pitfalls and Common Mistakes in the Assessment and Treatment of the Patient with Endotracheal Extubation

Possible pitfalls in assessing the patient for weaning and extubation include (1) failure to consider upper airway edema, (2) inattention to the difficult airway, and (3) inadequate suctioning before extubation. As mentioned, it is imperative that clinicians proceed with caution concerning patients who exhibit a reduced cough or gag reflex. It is also important to minimize the risks of potential aspiration. One such safeguard is the recommendation that tube feeding be halted several hours before planned extubation. Also, some have advocated use of endotracheal tubes that permit continuous suctioning of secretions that pool above the tube cuff.

At an appropriate time well after extubation, a swallowing evaluation can be performed at the bedside. This is accomplished by having the patient in the sitting position attempt to swallow several substances, beginning with ice chips. If the patient coughs and chokes while attempting to swallow, the test should be halted and repeated at a later time. Patients failing repeated trials will need formal testing by a speech therapist and/or a barium swallow examination.

Ensuring that the patient has fully recovered from the effects of anesthesia, neuromuscular blocking agents, and sedatives is important to lessen the risk of reintubation, which is associated with an increased mortality risk.

Another pitfall to avoid is extubation with an inflated endotracheal tube cuff. Although this is much more common with inadvertent extubation, care must be given to assure that the cuff is fully deflated before extubation to avoid possible edema. Also, suctioning above and below the cuff before cuff deflation and extubation is essential.

Vocal cord paralysis, especially when unilateral, may mimic some of the signs of aspiration. On the other hand, bilateral vocal cord paralysis will typically lead to signs and symptoms of upper airway obstruction, with stridor being common.

Finally, the clinician must be prepared to reintubate the patient if post-extubation difficulty occurs. The availability of clinicians with broad experience in airway management is critical, especially in patients with a difficult airway. Again, anticipating post-extubation problems is the key to averting these pitfalls.

▼ BIBLIOGRAPHY

Barnes T: Chest physical therapy and airway care. In *Textbook of respiratory care practice*, ed 2, Chicago, 1994, Year Book Medical Publishers.

Engoren M: Evaluation of the cuff-leak test in a cardiac surgery population, *Chest* 116(4):1029-1031, 1999.

Finucane B, Santora A: Complications of endotracheal intubation between reduced cuff leak volume and postextubation stridor. In *Principles of airway management*, St. Louis, 1988, Mosby.

Miller R, Cole R: Association between reduced cuff leak volume and postextubation stridor, *Chest* 110(4):1035-1040, 1996.

Pierson D, Kacmarek R: Assessment and management of airway protection, obstruction, and secretion clearance. In *Foundations of respiratory care*, New York, 1992, Churchill Livingstone.

Weigand D: Upper airway obstruction. In *Pulmonary and critical care medicine*, St. Louis, 1993, Mosby.

CHAPTER 32

SUBCUTANEOUS EMPHYSEMA

Edgar Delgado

Key Terms

- ▼ Subcutaneous emphysema
- ▼ Pneumothorax
- ▼ Pneumomediastinum
- ▼ Tension
- ▼ Bullous lung disease
- ▼ Bullae
- ▼ Bleb
- ▼ Mechanical ventilation
- ▼ Barotrauma

▼ THE CLINICAL PROBLEM

The patient is a 56-year-old man admitted to the medical intensive care unit (MICU) with respiratory insufficiency. Physical examination reveals a heart rate of 120, respiratory rate of 32, blood pressure of 150/90 mm Hg, normal temperature, diminished breath sounds throughout all lung fields but more prominent on the right side, accompanied by fine expiratory wheezes. The patient is demonstrating signs of accessory muscle use and is also pursed-lip breathing.

He has been receiving bronchodilator therapy with 0.5 cc albuterol in 2 mL normal saline solution and chest physical therapy (CPT) q 4 hr. On the second day of his therapy, he suddenly developed an increase in shortness of breath during CPT with percussion and vibration. The respiratory therapist noted neck crepitus in the lower neck area; the treatment was immediately stopped, and the house physician was notified. Arterial blood gas (ABG) values were drawn, and a chest x-ray taken. ABG values were pH 7.32, $PaCO_2$ 70, and PaO_2 56. Past medical history revealed a history of chronic obstructive pulmonary disease (COPD) with a large emphyse-matous "bleb" on the right lower lobe (RLL).

What could have caused the increased sortness of breath, and what is the significance of palpation of subcutaneous air in the lower neck area?

Differential Diagnosis of Subcutaneous Emphysema

This phenomenon, *subcutaneous (sub-Q) emphysema,* most commonly develops from the dissection of air arising from ruptured alveoli into the subcutaneous tissue planes. It is most often expressed in the head, neck, and chest and makes the patient appear somewhat bloated and grotesque. The dissemination of air distorts facial features and can extend to very distal sites such as the abdomen and all extremities. Although this can be upsetting to patients and relatives because of its unsightly characteristics, it is not dangerous or physiologically significant. Evacuation of the subcutaneous air is rarely required, since treatment of the underlying cause leads to resolution of air in these tissue planes.

Pneumothorax is an accumulation of air or gas in the pleural space, which can occur spontaneously, as a result of trauma or due to some pathological incident. Pneumothoraces can be classified as spontaneous (either primary or secondary), traumatic, iatrogenic, or as a tension pneumothorax. It is important to recognize the significance of pneumothoraces, because they are leading contributors to the development of sub-Q emphysema.

Mechanical ventilation aids in alveolar ventilation and gas exchange in patients whose basic respiratory functions are compromised due to numerous etiologies. Although its therapeutic function is critical, mechanical ventilation can also lead to potential complications. These range from pulmonary infection to hemodynamic compromise, oxygen toxicity, nutritional and psychological issues, and barotrauma.

Barotrauma describes conditions that occur due to pressure or volume damage in the lung as a result of mechanical ventilation. The incidence of pulmonary baro-trauma has been reported in numerous studies varying from 0.5% to 38%. Baro-trauma can manifest as pneumomediastinum, pneumothorax, and subcutaneous emphysema.

Thoracic trauma, which involves injury to the contents of the chest, is divided into two categories: penetrating and non-penetrating injuries. A penetrating injury involves the invasion of the chest by a foreign body, whereas a non-penetrating injury involves damage caused by blunt trauma. Penetration of the lung by a foreign object can lead to air entering the soft tissues (sub-Q emphysema). Non-penetrating trauma involves sudden compression and decompression of the internal structures within the chest by sudden impact. Often, non-penetrating injuries cause multiple fractures of the ribs and may involve barotrauma or contusion.

Tracheobronchial injuries may be the result of blunt or penetrating trauma to the thorax or base of the neck. Three basic mechanisms of injury have been described with blunt tracheobronchial disruption: (1) compression of the chest while the glottis is closed, which can lead to a tracheal "blowout" due to an increase in endo-bronchial pressure; (2) the shear force created by rapid deceleration can result in a transverse laceration of the trachea; and (3) the increase in the diameter of the airway, due to anteroposterior compression of the chest, can lead to injury of a main-

Box 32-1
Conditions Predisposing to Subcutaneous Emphysema

Conditions	Associated Conditions
Pneumothoraces	Spontaneous
	Traumatic
	Iatrogenic
	Tension
Barotrauma	MV
	CPAP
	Bi-PAP
	IPPB
Tracheobronchial injuries	Blunt trauma
	Penetrating trauma
Other	Dental extractions
	Advanced cancers
	Hydrogen peroxide exposure
	Suicide attempts (hanging)
	Pulmonary blebs and bullae

MV, Mechanical ventilation; *CPAP,* continuous positive airway pressure; *Bi-PAP,* bi-level positive airway pressure; *IPPB,* intermittent positive pressure breathing.

stem bronchus at the level of the carina. Sub-Q emphysema may be present with any of these injuries.

Other conditions, which have been described leading to presentations of subcutaneous emphysema, range from skin contact with hydrogen peroxide, dental extractions, hangings, and advanced cancers. Box 32-1 depicts a summary of conditions predisposing to sub-Q emphysema.

Clinical Features that Suggest a Specific Cause of Subcutaneous Emphysema

As the current patient is evaluated, the clinician may begin by asking the following questions:

1. Did this patient receive positive pressure therapy? A review of the history and physician's orders did not reveal any use of positive pressure therapy since admission. It is important to note that the use of mechanical ventilation (MV), intermittent positive pressure breathing (IPPB), continuous positive airway pressure (CPAP), or bi-level positive airway pressure (Bi-PAP) can lead to development of pneumothoraces or barotrauma.
2. Is there any history of thoracic trauma? The hospital admitting diagnosis was COPD exacerbation. The medical history is insignificant for any signs of thoracic or general trauma. The patient denied any recent falls or trauma to the chest. The results of a recent chest x-ray revealed a right pneumothorax.

3. Are there any signs of tracheal injury? There is no history of tracheal trauma, and the physical examination reveals a normal trachea without evidence of tracheal shift.

4. Are there any conditions that may predispose this patient to sub-Q emphysema? The history and physical were insignificant for any advanced cancer, hydrogen peroxide exposure, or suicide attempts. The patient did have molar extractions within the past 3 months. He did demonstrate a right lower lobe emphysematous bleb, which is a significant condition that may predispose the patient to sub-Q emphysema.

Diagnostic Testing in the Evaluation of Subcutaneous Emphysema

Perhaps the most important diagnostic tool is the medical history and physical examination. Sub-Q emphysema in itself is generally not dangerous, but it is imperative to recognize its etiology. In this 56-year-old man, the clinician can rule out a variety of probable causes by the history alone. He has no history of positive pressure therapy, thoracic trauma, tracheal trauma, and he has no diagnosis of any advanced cancers, and so on.

A second and also very important diagnostic tool is the chest x-ray. By using this simple tool, the presence of a pneumothorax or many other thoracic anomalies can be identified. The chest x-ray for this patient does point to a right pneumothorax. Other technologies such as computed tomography (CT) scan or magnetic resonance imaging (MRI) can be useful tools, but they generally are more expensive, complex, not portable, and require more time to be completed.

The history of a pulmonary bleb does raise a concern as to a probable cause of the sub-Q emphysema. By definition, a *bleb* is an accumulation of air within the pleura that is not confined by connective tissue septa within the lung. Due to its thin covering, a bleb is predisposed to rupture and can often be associated with spontaneous pneumothoraces.

Diagnosis and Treatment of Subcutaneous Emphysema

It becomes evident that the presence of the RLL bleb precipitated the development of a spontaneous pneumothorax in this patient. The presence of the pneumothorax led to the dissection of air into the tissue planes, which was then manifest as sub-Q emphysema. On the patient's arrival to the MICU, a chest tube was inserted that stabilized his vital signs, including improvement in his respiratory rate and dyspnea. The sub-Q emphysema resolved within 36 hours.

In certain thoracic and cardiac surgical procedures, sub-Q emphysema can be a frequent complication, and emergency tracheostomy is often advocated as treatment. A recent case report described the use of subcutaneous drains and suction instead of tracheostomy for the treatment of a patient who developed massive subcutaneous emphysema. In that case, subcutaneous drains provided effective decompression of the head and neck areas with markedly reduced airway pressure and subcutaneous air. The use of subcutaneous drains may provide for a safe and effective means for the management of sub-Q emphysema.

▼ SUMMARY

COPD with emphysematous blebs lead to spontaneous pneumothoraces and the resultant sub-Q emphysema for this patient. This pathology may be clinically manifested by sudden changes in vital signs and respiratory status. The formation of sub-Q emphysema should alert the astute clinician to inquire into its etiology, as this becomes the target for intervention that will eliminate the source of air. Sub-Q emphysema is not dangerous in itself, but resolution of its underlying cause becomes imperative.

▼ BIBLIOGRAPHY

Ali A, Cunliffe DR, Watt-Smith SR: Surgical emphysema an pneumomediastinum complicating dental extraction, *Br Dent J* 188:589-590, 2000.

Canizares MA, Arnau A, Fortea A, et al: Hyoid fracture and traumatic subcutaneous cervical emphysema from an attempted hanging, *Arch Bronconeumol* 36:52-54, 2000.

Chu S, Glare P: Subcutaneous emphysema in advanced cancer, *J Pain Symptom Manage* 19:73-77, 2000.

Cullen DJ, Caldera DL: The incidence of ventilator-induced pulmonary barotrauma in critically ill patients, *Anesthesiology* 50:185, 1979.

Izu K, Yamamoto O, Asahi M: Occupational skin injury by hydrogen peroxide, *Dermatology* 201:61-64, 2000.

Kumar A, Pontoppidan H, Falke KJ, et al: Pulmonary barotrauma during mechanical ventilation, *Crit Care Med* 1:181, 1973.

Murphy D, Fishman A: Bullous disease of the lung. In Fishman AP: *Pulmonary diseases and disorders*, ed 2, New York, 1988, McGraw-Hill.

Olsen GN: Pre- and postoperative evaluation and management of the thoracic surgical patient. In Fishman AP: *Pulmonary diseases and disorders*, ed 2, New York, 1988, McGraw-Hill.

Peterson GW, Baier H: Incidence of pulmonary barotrauma in a medical ICU, *Crit Care Med* 11:67-69, 1983.

Sherif HM, Ott DA: The use of subcutaneous drains to manage subcutaneous emphysema, *Tex Heart Inst J* 26(2):129-131, 1999.

Zwillich CW, Pierson DJ, Creagh CE, et al: Complications of assisted ventilation: A prospective study of 354 consecutive episodes, *Am J Med* 57:161, 1974.

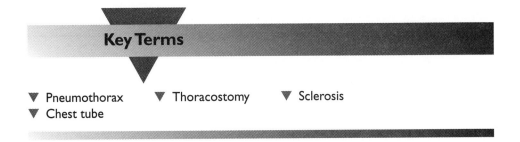

CHAPTER 33

THE PATIENT
WITH THE BUBBLING
CHEST TUBE

R. Wayne Lawson

Key Terms

▼ Pneumothorax   ▼ Thoracostomy   ▼ Sclerosis
▼ Chest tube

▼ THE CLINICAL PROBLEM

The patient is a 21-year-old man admitted through the emergency department to the surgical intensive care unit (SICU) after being thrown from an automobile and subsequently struck by another vehicle. He has multiple right-sided rib fractures with an associated flail segment and pulmonary contusions, a right pelvic fracture, a left sacral fracture, and a displaced right parietal fracture. A chest tube was inserted in the emergency room through the fifth inter-costal space at the right mid-axillary line, posteriorly, to drain a small medial effusion (Figure 33-1). Approximately 500 mL of bloody drainage was collected in the first 24 hours and an additional 200 mL of serosanguineous drainage during the second day. There is no

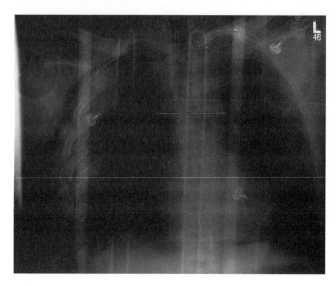

▼ **Figure 33-1**   An x-ray showing a chest tube inserted through the fifth inter-costal space at the right mid-axillary line, posteriorly, to drain a small medial effusion.

bubbling from the chest tube through the water seal. He is receiving volume-targeted mechanical ventilation to treat acute respiratory failure brought on by the flail segment.

On the morning of day 3, after the patient's bed linen was changed, the respiratory therapist noted continuous bubbling from the water seal of the patient's chest drainage system. Auscultation revealed very diminished breath sounds on the right, most notable over the right upper lobe. Peak inspiratory pressures had increased an average of 10 cm H_2O in the past 30 minutes.

What are the potential causes of bubbling from a patient's chest tube, and what is the most likely cause in this patient?

Differential Diagnosis of a Bubbling Chest Tube

Aside from a technical problem, such as a loose connection allowing ambient air into the chest drainage system, the cause of bubbling from the water seal is an air leak into the intra-pleural space, which is termed a *pneumothorax*. The potential sources of this air include (1) a disruption of the integrity of the visceral pleura, allowing air entry from the intra-pulmonary space into the intra-pleural space; (2) a disruption of the integrity of the chest wall, allowing ambient air entry into the intra-pleural space; (3) a bronchopleural fistula allowing air entry from a bronchus into the intra-pleural space; and (4) in very rare instances, gas-producing bacteria multiplying within the intra-pleural space. Box 33-1 includes common and less common causes of pulmonary air leak.

Pneumothoraces are classified in the following way. A spontaneous pneumothorax is one that occurs without trauma to the chest and is categorized as being either primary or secondary. A primary spontaneous pneumothorax occurs in the absence of any predisposing lung disease, whereas a secondary pneumothorax oc-

---

Box 33-1
Differential Diagnosis of Pulmonary Air Leak

Common Causes	Less Common Causes
Bleb rupture	Gas-producing bacteria
Bulla rupture	Catamenial
Bronchopleural fistula	Iatrogenic
Penetrating thoracic trauma	
Non-penetrating (blunt) thoracic trauma	

---

curs as the result of some underlying lung disease such as emphysema. Because the pressure in the intra-pleural space is normally less than atmospheric, except during forced expiratory maneuvers, a pressure gradient exists in the direction of the intra-pleural space, from the intra-pulmonary space. A similar gradient exists between the ambient environment and the intra-pleural space. Therefore any communication that develops between the intra-pleural space and the lung or the ambient environment results in entry of air into the intra-pleural space. The elastic recoil potential of the lung results in its partial or full collapse, with lung tissue being displaced in favor of air occupying the thoracic cavity. Positive pressure ventilation is associated with an increased incidence of pneumothorax because the positive pressure results in an increase in the pressure gradient that normally exists between the intra-pulmonary space and the intra-pleural space.

Primary spontaneous pneumothorax is believed to be caused by the rupture of an apical sub-pleural emphysematous bleb. A bleb is a small cystic air space, usually not larger than 1 cm in diameter, lying immediately under the visceral pleura. A spontaneous pneumothorax tends to occur in tall, thin individuals and is strongly associated with smoking. According to Bense et al the risk of developing a primary spontaneous pneumothorax is 7 times higher in men who smoke between 1 and 12 cigarettes per day, 21 times higher in men who smoke between 13 and 22 cigarettes per day, and 102 times higher in men who smoke more than 22 cigarettes per day. There is evidence of genetic predisposition to the development of primary spontaneous pneumothorax.

The chief symptoms of a spontaneous pneumothorax are chest pain and dyspnea, about two thirds of which begin abruptly, while the remaining third begin insidiously. Signs include diminished or absent breath sounds heard over the affected hemithorax, with hyperresonance to percussion, possible ipsilateral shift of the trachea, and a decrease in arterial oxygen saturation. The cause of the chest pain associated with a spontaneous pneumothorax is not well understood, as the lung parenchyma and visceral pleura contain no pain fibers. The parietal pleura, however, is richly innervated with pain fibers. Dyspnea occurs secondary to loss of surface area for gas exchange, resulting in hypoxemia. Dyspnea also occurs secondary to mechanical distortion of lung parenchyma, resulting in stimulation of J receptors at the alveolar level, which elicit the feeling of dyspnea along with a rapid, shallow breathing pattern. Diminished or absent breath sounds are heard over the affected lung for two reasons: (1) the affected lung is at least partially collapsed and therefore not moving as much air, thus producing less sound and (2) the presence of air in the intra-pleural space results in separation of the lung from the chest wall, thereby acoustically insulating any sound produced by air movement within the affected lung. The affected hemithorax is hyperresonant to percussion because air has replaced the lung tissue, and, the more gas a structure contains, the more resonant will be the sound produced by percussion. The reason for the ipsilateral shift of the trachea is as follows. With normal physiology, the mediastinum is held in the central position by the presence of a lung on either side. Pathologically, as air enters the intra-pleural space, thus allowing the affected lung to collapse under the force of its elastic recoil potential, the loss of tissue volume allows the mediastinal contents to shift toward the affected hemithorax. This shift pulls the trachea away from its central position, toward the affected side. Arterial oxygen saturation decreases because of lung collapse, leading to loss of ventilation, and therefore reducing gas exchange by the affected lung.

The most common cause of secondary pneumothorax is chronic obstructive pulmonary disease (COPD). The increased presence of sub-pleural blebs and bullae associated with emphysema is responsible for this phenomenon. Pneumothorax should be suspected in all patients presenting with an acute exacerbation of COPD, and careful assessment, including a chest x-ray for the possible presence of a pneumothorax, should be made.

A traumatic pneumothorax is one that occurs secondary to either penetrating or non-penetrating chest trauma. A penetrating injury to the chest can allow air into the intra-pleural space from both the ambient environment, as well as from the lung if the visceral pleura is interrupted by the penetrating object. A non-penetrating injury to the chest can result in rib fractures, which can lacerate the visceral surface of the lung, allowing air entry from the lung into the intra-pleural space.

An iatrogenic pneumothorax is one produced intentionally or unintentionally during a diagnostic or therapeutic procedure. A catamenial pneumothorax is a very rare condition that occurs in conjunction with menstruation, with the symptoms usually beginning within 24 to 48 hours of the onset of menstrual flow. The pathogenesis, while poorly understood, is thought to be related to the development of pleural and/or diaphragmatic endometriosis. Therefore a woman of child-bearing years who presents with a pneumothorax that developed within 24 to 48 hours of the beginning of menstrual flow should be suspected of having a catamenial pneumothorax.

A tension pneumothorax is one in which the air in the intra-pleural space is under positive pressure throughout the respiratory cycle. A patient with a tension pneumothorax will present with dyspnea, tachycardia, tachypnea, distended neck veins, thready pulse, and hypotension. The trachea will be contralaterally shifted because the positive pressure in the affected hemithorax pushes the mediastinal contents toward the opposite side. Treatment of a tension pneumothorax is a medical emergency. A large-bore needle should be immediately inserted into the pleural space through the second or third inter-space at the mid-clavicular line to relieve the pressure, and continuous tube thoracostomy should be implemented before removing the needle.

In addition to the signs of reduced or absent breath sounds on the affected side, hyperresonance to percussion, tracheal shift, and decreased arterial oxygen saturation (if the patient is receiving mechanical ventilatory support), peak inspiratory pressures will be elevated during volume-targeted ventilation. This elevation in inspiratory pressure occurs secondary to lung collapse. Recall that lung compliance is defined as the change in lung volume per unit of inflating pressure change. In the presence of a pneumothorax, the collapse of one lung means the tidal volume generated by the ventilator is now being delivered into a smaller space (one lung rather than two), and thus will require more pressure to deliver, which, by definition, is a reduction in compliance.

Whereas pneumothoraces that occupy less than 15% of a hemithorax are generally treated by thoracentesis and bed rest, those that occupy greater than 15% or are still actively leaking air into the intra-pleural space are generally treated with continuous thoracic drainage. This is accomplished most commonly by inserting a clear, flexible, vinyl catheter into the pleural space (via a rib inter-space) to drain the air. The term for this is closed-chest thoracostomy. The second inter-space in the mid-clavicular line or the second or third inter-space at the mid-axillary line are common insertion points for the drainage of air. The fourth, fifth, or sixth inter-spaces in the mid-axillary line are common insertion points for fluid drainage. The goal of a closed-chest drainage system is to reexpand the lung by evacuating the air and/or fluid from the intra-pleural space, while keeping the system sealed from the atmosphere, thus allowing the maintenance of normal intra-pleural pressures. Evacuation of air from the intra-pleural space is generally accomplished using a water seal system, which allows gas under positive pressure to escape from the pleural space while preventing the reentry of air into the system. It is used with one, two, and three bottle glass drainage systems. Modern preformed plastic systems perform all the functions of a multi-bottle drainage system in one compact unit and are available from a number of manufacturers. The chest tube is connected to the chest drainage system, and an extension of the tube is inserted 2 cm below the water's surface, creating an air seal that acts as a one-way valve. Gas under positive pressure from the patient's intra-pleural space bubbles out the water seal on exhalation; while on inspiration water is drawn up the tube, thus preventing the entry of air back into the space.

The most commonly used systems are pre-formed plastic systems with three chambers connected in series. Starting on the patient side, the first chamber is for the collection of any fluid that drains from the intra-pleural space (Figure 33-2). The second chamber is the water seal (Figure 33-3), in which the drainage tube is maintained at a constant depth below the water's surface of 2 cm. This allows any gas trapped in the intra-pleural space at a relative pressure difference greater than 2 cm H_2O to be vented through the water seal, while preventing ambient gas from entering the system. When functioning normally in a spontaneously breathing patient, the level of water in the water seal tube fluctuates with ventilation, rising during inspiration and falling during exhalation. This is termed *tidaling*. The third chamber in the system is the suction control chamber, which is connected to a vacuum source (Figure 33-4). This chamber is set to maintain the pressure in the entire system, including the intra-pleural space at approximately 20 cm H_2O below atmospheric pressure. The application of this sub-atmospheric pressure hastens the removal of air and fluid from the intra-pleural space. When the system is initially set up, intermittent bubbling will occur with each exhalation until all the air has been evacuated from the intra-pleural space. Continuous bubbling through the water seal is indicative of a continuing air leak. The source of the leak could be from the lung through the visceral pleura, from a bronchopleural fistula, or from a technical problem with the system itself resulting in a leak.

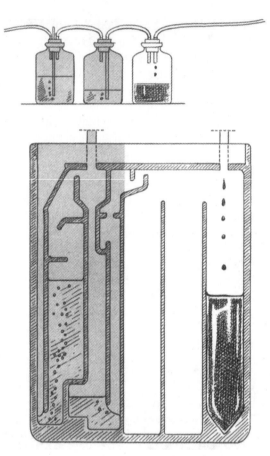

▼ **Figure 33-2** Collection chamber of a three-chambered plastic chest drainage system compared with a standard three-bottle system. The "V" at the bottom of the chamber makes it possible to measure in small increments. Fluids spill over and fill the two other channels so that increments of measurement remain small. Courtesy Pfizer Hospital Products Group, Inc, Deknatel Division, Floral Park, NY.

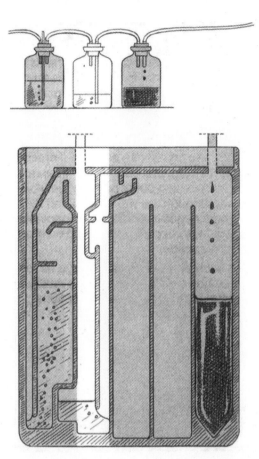

▼ **Figure 33-3**   Water seal chamber of a three-chambered plastic chest drainage system compared with a three-bottle closed chest drainage system. The narrower column on the right side of the chamber functions like the tube in the three-bottle system. Tidaling should be seen when the patient breathes. Air leaks, if present, are seen in the water to the left of the column. Courtesy Pfizer Hospital Products Group, Inc, Deknatel Division, Floral Park, NY.

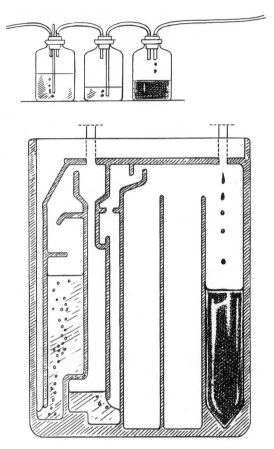

▼ **Figure 33-4** Suction-control chamber of a three-chambered plastic chest drainage system compared with a standard three-bottle system. The weight of water in the column to the left determines the amount of suction exerted on the pleural space when the system is connected to a suction source. Courtesy Pfizer Hospital Products Group, Inc, Deknatel Division, Floral

Clinical Features that Suggest a Specific Cause of a Bubbling Chest Tube

This patient's recent history of blunt trauma to the chest with multiple rib fractures, resulting in a flail segment, suggests that the cause of the continuous bubbling from the chest tube is an air leak from the lung (Table 33-1). As the patient was rotated onto his right side in the process of changing his bed linen, pressure on a broken rib segment caused laceration of the visceral pleura by the sharp edge of a broken rib. The chest tube currently in place was inserted through the fifth intercostal space in the mid-axillary line, posteriorly, for removal of a pleural effusion. The fact that it is now bubbling indicates the presence of a large amount of air in the intra-pleural space. This patient is receiving mechanical ventilation, meaning that gas under positive pressure is moving through the laceration in the visceral pleura into the intra-pleural space with every inspiratory cycle. Because the chest tube

TABLE 33-1
Interpreting Signs and Symptoms in the Patient with a Pulmonary Air Leak

Possible Causes	Mechanisms	Suggestive Clinical Features
Primary pneumothorax	Loss of visceral pleural integrity, caused by rupture of a bleb, leading to air entry into the intra-pleural space	Chest pain, dyspnea, diminished or absent breath sounds over the affected hemithorax, hyperresonance to percussion, possible ipsilateral shift of the trachea, decrease in SaO_2
Secondary pneumothorax	Loss of visceral pleural integrity, caused by rupture of a bulla, leading to air entry into the intra-pleural space	Dyspnea, chest pain, very diminished to absent breath sounds over the affected hemithorax, hyperresonance to percussion, possible ipsilateral shift of the trachea, decrease in SaO_2, cyanosis, and hypotension
Bronchopleural fistula	Loss of bronchial wall integrity leading to air entry into the intra-pleural space	Chest pain, dyspnea, diminished or absent breath sounds over the affected hemithorax, hyperresonance to percussion, possible ipsilateral shift of the trachea, decrease in SaO_2
Penetrating thoracic trauma	Loss of chest wall, and possibly visceral pleural integrity, either leading to air entry into the intra-pleural space	Recent history of penetrating trauma to the chest, movement of air into and out of the chest wall wound with ventilatory motion, pain, dyspnea, possible ipsilateral shift of the trachea, decrease in SaO_2
Non-penetrating (blunt) thoracic trauma	Loss of visceral pleural integrity, leading to air entry into the intra-pleural space	Recent history of blunt trauma to the chest, possible paradoxical motion of the chest wall with ventilatory motion, pain, dyspnea, possible ipsilateral shift of the trachea, decrease in SaO_2
Gas-producing bacteria	Bacteria multiply in the intra-pleural space, producing gas, which accumulates in the space	Recent history of pneumonia with parapneumonic effusion
Catamenial	Loss of visceral pleural integrity, leading to air entry into the intra-pleural space	Chest pain, dyspnea, diminished or absent breath sounds over the affected hemithorax, hyperresonance to percussion, possible ipsilateral shift of the trachea, decrease in SaO_2
Iatrogenic	Loss of chest wall or possibly visceral pleural integrity, either leading to air entry into the intra-pleural space	Chest pain, dyspnea, diminished or absent breath sounds over the affected hemithorax, hyperresonance to percussion, possible ipsilateral shift of the trachea, decrease in SaO_2

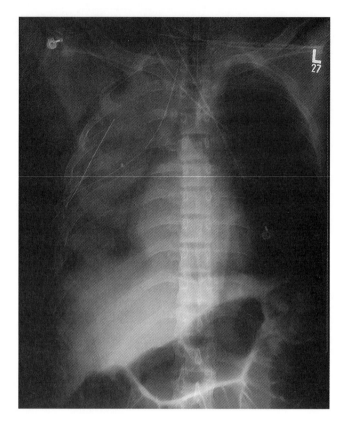

▼ **Figure 33-5** An x-ray showing a second chest tube inserted through the fourth intercostal space in the mid-axillary line, anteriorly, to drain the air.

currently in place was inserted posterior to the lung for fluid drainage, it is not in an optimal position to drain air, which will tend to collect anterior to, and around the lung. Therefore a second chest tube was then inserted through the fourth intercostal space in the mid-axillary line, anteriorly, to drain the air (Figure 33-5).

Diagnostic Testing in the Evaluation of the Patient with a Bubbling Chest Tube

The plain chest x-ray remains the most important and commonly used diagnostic tool for evaluating the presence of air within the intra-pleural space. Computed tomography (CT) and magnetic resonance imaging (MRI) scanning are valuable diagnostic tools as well but are very expensive by comparison and unnecessary in the vast majority of cases. Using the plain chest x-ray, the location and extent of the pneumothorax can be quickly and reliably ascertained. A pneumothorax that is not under tension will demonstrate a visceral pleural line separated from the chest wall with a hyperlucent hemithorax where air has replaced lung tissue. If the pneumothorax is large, it will generally show an ipsilateral shift of the mediastinum as well. A pneumothorax that is under tension will demonstrate a visible visceral pleural line as well but will also show a contralateral shift of the mediastinum and an ipsilateral depression of the hemidiaphragm, both secondary to the positive intra-pleural pressure.

Assessment and Treatment of the Patient with a Bubbling Test Tube

The astute observation by the respiratory therapist of continuous bubbling from the first chest tube where none had been observed before resulted in the therapist quickly assessing the patient for the cause of the air leak. Auscultation of the patient's chest revealed bilaterally clear breath sounds, but diminished on the right. Where peak inspiratory pressures had been averaging 24 to 26 cm H_2O before the air leak, they were now averaging 34 to 36 cm H_2O. The patient's SpO_2, which had been averaging 96% on an FIO_2 of 0.40, was now 86%. A stat chest x-ray was obtained and revealed an almost completely collapsed lung on the right with an ipsilateral shift of the mediastinum. Were it not for the presence of the first chest tube allowing some air drainage, the continuing influx of gas under positive pressure from the mechanical ventilator undoubtedly would have resulted in a tension pneumothorax. A second chest tube was inserted for drainage of the air, and the lung reexpanded (see Figure 33-5). Peak inspiratory pressures immediately returned to their prepneumothorax values, as did the SpO_2.

Over the next 2 days, the continuous bubbling gradually diminished in volume and became intermittent. By the third day, the bubbling ceased entirely. Because no further fluid or air was seen in the system, both chest tubes were removed on the fifth day.

Pitfalls and Common Mistakes in Assessment and Treatment of the Patient with a Bubbling Chest Tube

Because the diagnosis and treatment of a patient with a pneumothorax is relatively straightforward and standard in its approach, pitfalls are few. As stated in the introduction, with a properly functioning system, the cause of bubbling through the water seal of a closed chest drainage system is an air leak into the intra-pleural space, either from the intra-pulmonary space or from the ambient environment. The most likely pitfall is a leak in the closed chest drainage system itself, such as a loose connection. The integrity of the chest tube drainage system should be checked to ensure a closed, leak-free system as part of the assessment of the patient whenever initially setting up a closed drainage system on a patient, or whenever a patient with an existing closed drainage system in place develops bubbling through their underwater seal.

Also, as stated earlier, the chest x-ray is one of the most important diagnostic tools available to you in your assessment of a patient in whom you are suspicious of a pneumothorax. Therefore the quality of the film and the accuracy of the physician's interpretation of that film are critical to proper diagnosis and management. Whereas pneumothoraces that occupy a significant portion of a hemithorax are generally easy to recognize on chest x-ray, small pneumothoraces on the other hand (less than 20%) can be difficult to distinguish. Careful observation is required to distinguish separation of the visceral pleura from the parietal pleura. A poor quality film or one that is either over-penetrated or under-penetrated can make visualizing a pneumothorax much more difficult.

▼ BIBLIOGRAPHY

Bense L, Eklung G, Wiman LG: Smoking and the increased risk of contracting spontaneous pneumothorax, *Chest* 92:1009-1012, 1987.

Kircher LT Jr, Swartzel RL: Spontaneous pneumothorax and its treatment, *JAMA* 155:24-29, 1954.

Lesur O, Delorme N, Fromaget J, et al: Computed tomography in the etiologic assessment of idiopathic spontaneous pneumothorax, *Chest* 98:341-347, 1990.

Light RW: Diseases of the pleura, mediastinum, chest wall, and diaphragm. In George RB, Light RW, Matthay MA et al. (editors): *Chest medicine: essentials of pulmonary and critical care medicine*, Baltimore, 1995, Williams and Wilkins.

Light RW: Pneumothorax. In Murray JF, Nadel JA (editors): *Textbook of respiratory medicine*, vol 2, Philadelphia, 1994, WB Saunders.

Lillington GA, Mitchell SP, Wood GA: Catamenial pneumothorax, *JAMA* 219:1328-1332, 1972.

Maurer ER, Schaal JA, Mendez FL: Chronic recurrent spontaneous pneumothorax due to endometriosis of the diaphragm, *JAMA* 168:2013-2014, 1958.

Ohata M, Suzuki H: Pathogenesis of spontaneous pneumothorax, *Chest* 77:771-776, 1980.

Stern H, Toole AL, Merino M: Catamenial pneumothorax, *Chest* 78:480-482, 1980.

CHAPTER 34

REFRACTORY HYPOXEMIA

Sandra G. Adams
Jay I. Peters

Key Terms

▼ Hypoxemia　　　　　▼ Radiographic patterns　　　▼ Shunt
▼ Acute respiratory failure　▼ Pulmonary embolus (PE)

▼ THE CLINICAL PROBLEM

A 62-year-old obese woman with a long history of smoking presents with acute onset of shortness of breath and left-sided pleuritic chest pain starting approximately 36 hours ago.

Review of systems is positive for (1) generalized malaise, sore throat, rhinorrhea, increased cough with white sputum, and subjective fever causing the patient to miss work for the last 6 days; (2) chronic shortness of breath and dyspnea on exertion at one block, stable for 2 years; and (3) swelling of both legs for 3 months.

Past medical history is significant for chronic obstructive pulmonary disease (COPD), hypertension, breast cancer treated 4 years ago, and anxiety disorder. Medications include albuterol, ipratropium bromide, amlodipine (calcium channel blocker for hypertension), and alprazolam (benzodiazepine for anxiety).

On physical examination, her temperature is 100.6° F, pulse 120, respiratory rate 32, and blood pressure is 182/98. Her SpO_2 is 82% on room air (FIO_2 0.21). She is

5 foot, 6-inches tall and weighs 230 lbs. She appears somnolent and is in moderate respiratory distress. Lung examination reveals decreased breath sounds but no crackles or wheezes. Heart sounds are distant, with a positive S_4, but no audible murmurs. Her lower extremities demonstrate 2+ edema (right more than left).

Abnormal laboratory values available include a white blood cell (WBC) count of 11.4 (mildly elevated) and arterial blood gas values on room air demonstrate a pH of 7.29, a $PaCO_2$ of 54 mm Hg, a PaO_2 of 46 mm Hg, and an SaO_2 of 81%.

A chest x-ray is significant for hyperexpanded lungs with flattened diaphragms, but no specific infiltrates identified.

At this point, what is the differential diagnosis of the patient's hypoxemia? How do the radiographic results change the list of differential diagnoses in this patient?

Differential Diagnosis of Hypoxemia

Respiratory failure is defined as problems with delivering adequate oxygen to the tissues (usually with a PaO_2 <60 mm Hg) or as problems with removing adequate amounts of carbon dioxide from the tissues (usually with $PaCO_2$ of >45 to 50 mm Hg). The clinical classification of patients with severe hypoxemia is based on the appearance of the chest x-ray, which provides useful information for narrowing the differential diagnosis of common and uncommon etiologies of hypoxemia (Box 34-1). The chest x-rays of most patients with severe hypoxemia demonstrate infiltrates and thus are "white" at presentation. Others may present with a "black" (clear) chest x-ray. This classification is useful in classifying these patients and helps narrow the differential diagnosis. Patients presenting with a white x-ray (with infiltrates) usually have pneumonia, cardiogenic pulmonary edema, or non-cardiogenic pulmonary edema, also known as acute respiratory distress syndrome (ARDS). Progressive interstitial lung disease is a less common cause of hypoxemia with an abnormal chest x-ray. Patients presenting with a black x-ray (without infiltrates) usually have obstructive lung disease, pulmonary emboli, or microatelectasis. Other, less common etiologies of hypoxemia with a black chest x-ray include a right-to-left shunt, the obesity-hypoventilation syndrome, and early ARDS, associated with sepsis (Box 34-1).

Diagnostic Tests that Suggest a Specific Cause of Hypoxemia

A careful review of the history, physical examination, and laboratory data is essential in determining a specific etiology of a patient's hypoxemia. Although there can be significant overlap in these disorders, a common approach in evaluating patients with severe hypoxemia and acute respiratory failure is based on historical and clinical features and the appearance of the chest x-ray (Table 34-1). Many of these factors can help narrow the differential diagnosis in patients with hypoxemia. Some of the most important distinguishing clinical characteristics between the four main causes of severe hypoxemia with a white chest x-ray are discussed first in this section (see Table 34-1), followed by a similar but more detailed discussion of the distinguishing clinical features in the current case history of hypoxemia with a black x-ray.

Box 34-1
Differential Diagnosis of Hypoxemia

Common Causes	Less Common Causes
"White" Chest X-ray	
Pneumonia	Interstitial lung disease
Cardiogenic pulmonary edema	
Non-cardiogenic pulmonary edema (ARDS)	
"Black" Chest X-ray	
Exacerbation of underlying obstructive	Right-to-left shunt
lung disease	Obesity-hypoventilation
PE	Early ARDS (although chest CT is white)
Microatelectasis	

PE, Pulmonary embolus; ARDS, acute respiratory distress syndrome; CT, computed tomography.

As previously discussed, patients with a white x-ray usually have pneumonia, cardiogenic pulmonary edema, non-cardiogenic pulmonary edema (ARDS), or less commonly, progressive interstitial lung disease. Patients with pneumonia frequently have fever and chills, cough productive of purulent sputum, elevated WBC count, and a focal, alveolar infiltrate on chest x-ray (Figure 34-1). Many patients (approximately 50%) with pneumonia who are older than 65 do not have specific respiratory complaints and may lack fever but present with mental status changes (confusion) or hypotension.

Those with cardiogenic pulmonary edema often have a history of congestive heart failure (left ventricular dysfunction), previous myocardial infarction, severe hypertension, or valvular heart disease. Patients with cardiogenic pulmonary edema have a pulmonary artery occlusion pressure ("wedge pressure") >18 mm Hg and also frequently complain of orthopnea (shortness of breath with supine position), paroxysmal nocturnal dyspnea (awakening at night with shortness of breath due to the redistribution of peripheral edema to the chest during sleep), and lower extremity edema. The infiltrates on chest x-ray are frequently characterized by the classic central "bat wing" distribution (Figure 34-2); however, they may be patchy and indistinguishable from the other causes, due to abnormal underlying parenchymal disease such as emphysema.

ARDS is most commonly precipitated by an initial catastrophic event. Some of the common predisposing factors that have been identified include severe bilateral pneumonia, sepsis, hypotension, massive aspiration, significant trauma, multiple and rapid transfusions, pancreatitis, and toxic ingestions. The radiographic appearance in ARDS is often difficult to distinguish from that of cardiogenic pulmonary edema. However, the infiltrates in patients with ARDS are commonly more diffuse and peripheral (Figure 34-3) than those with a cardiogenic etiology. Probably the most helpful way to distinguish cardiogenic disorders from the others is by carefully observing the radiographic response to therapy. Cardiogenic pulmonary edema usually improves or clears within days of treatment, whereas the

Text continued on p. 364

TABLE 34-1
Approach to Hypoxemia

Causes	"Classic" Chest X-ray	Clinical Characteristics	Associated Co-Morbid Diseases/ Possible Precipitating Events
"White" Chest X-Ray			
Pneumonia	Focal, alveolar infiltrate	*Typical:* Fever, chills, cough, purulent sputum, elevated WBC count *Atypical:* Mental status changes (confusion), hypotension*	Post-viral upper respiratory infection, high incidence during mechanical ventilation
Cardiogenic pulmonary edema	Central vascular congestion, "bat wing" distribution, often with cardiomegaly	Orthopnea, paroxysmal nocturnal dyspnea, peripheral edema, "wedge" pressure >18 mm Hg, responds to diuretics (chest x-ray improves over days)	Myocardial infarction, severe hypertension, valvular heart disease
Non-cardiogenic pulmonary edema (ARDS)	Bilateral, diffuse infiltrates (more peripherally located)	Acute onset of symptoms, wedge pressure <18 mm Hg	Bilateral pneumonia, sepsis, hypotension, massive aspiration, trauma, pancreatitis, multiple transfusions, toxic ingestions
Interstitial lung disease	Diffuse, bilateral infiltrates fibrosis "honeycombing"	Progressive symptoms (months to years), previous chest x-ray with diffuse infiltrates	History of collagen vascular disease, malignancy

"Black" Chest X-ray			
Acute exacerbation of obstructive lung disease	Large lung volumes with flattened diaphragms or normal	Progressive symptoms over days to weeks, wheezing on examination, FEV_1/FVC <75% predicted	COPD, asthma
PE	Usually normal but occasionally abnormal†	Acute onset: Dyspnea, hemoptysis, pleuritic chest pain, history of immobility	Underlying malignancy, active smoking, hypercoagulable state, oral contraceptives, history of DVT, obesity, CHF
Microatelectasis	Normal or small lung volumes	Often associated with pain (pleuritic or abdominal), bronchial breath sounds on physical examination	Post-surgical, broken ribs
Right-to-left shunt	Normal	Usually progressive symptoms (weeks to months to years), not responsive to high levels of FIo_2	Pulmonary hypertension, pulmonary AVMs, cirrhosis (microscopic, pulmonary AVMs)

WBC, White blood cell; *ARDS*, acute respiratory distress syndrome; FEV_1/FVC, ratio of the forced expiratory volume in one second to the forced vital capacity; *PE*, pulmonary embolus; *COPD*, chronic obstructive pulmonary disease; *DVT*, deep venous thrombosis; *CHF*, congestive heart failure; *AVMs*, arteriovenous malformations.

*Approximately 50% of patients >65 years old.

†Occasionally can have oligemia (decreased blood flow to one lung), plate-like atelectasis, or an elevated diaphragm.

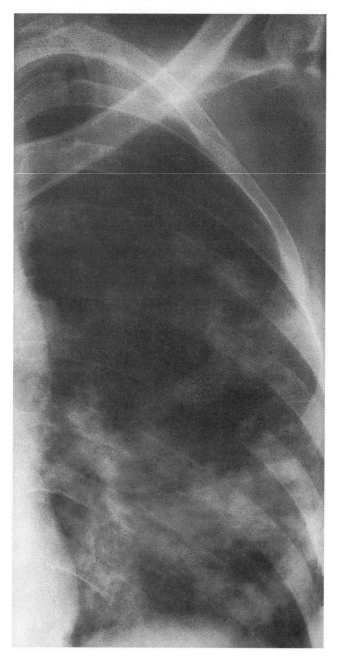

▼ **Figure 34-1**   A focal, alveolar infiltrate.

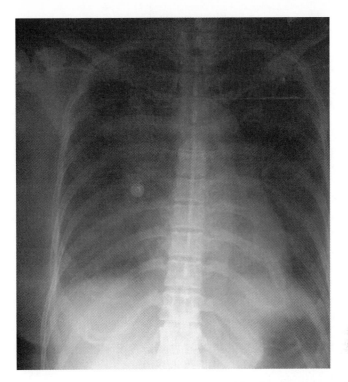

▼ **Figure 34-2**   Infiltrates are frequently characterized by the classic central "bat wing" distribution.

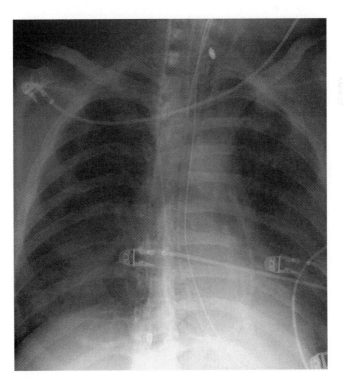

▼ **Figure 34-3**   Infiltrates in patients with acute respiratory distress syndrome (ARDS) are commonly more diffuse and peripheral than those with a cardiogenic etiology.

infiltrates from ARDS and pneumonia take weeks to months to clear. Additionally, the hypoxemia of cardiogenic pulmonary edema responds more to oxygen therapy and more often corrects with supplemental oxygen. The hypoxemia associated with ARDS often requires a higher FIO_2, mechanical ventilation, and positive end-expiratory pressure (PEEP).

One of the unusual causes of hypoxemia in a patient with infiltrates on the chest x-ray (in the white group) is chronic interstitial lung disease. Some historical features that are helpful in suggesting a diagnosis of interstitial lung disease include: (1) progressive symptoms (often over months to years); (2) a history of joint complaints, an undiagnosed rash, or other features consistent with a collagen vascular disease; (3) a previous diagnosis of malignancy that has a tendency to spread through the lymphatics to the lung (lymphangitic carcinomatosis); and (4) a prior chest x-ray with diffuse infiltrates or abnormalities.

The current patient has a black chest x-ray, which helps narrow the differential diagnosis of her hypoxemia. One of the most common causes of hypoxemia without infiltrates on radiography is an acute exacerbation of obstructive lung disease. These patients commonly have a history of asthma and/or COPD. The symptoms of shortness of breath in these patients usually occur slowly (over days to weeks), tend to progressively worsen, and are frequently associated with wheezing on physical examination. Bedside spirometry that demonstrates airflow obstruction may be helpful in confirming the diagnosis (FEV_1/FVC <75%). Although the x-ray in patients with significant COPD may demonstrate large, hyperexpanded lung volumes and flattened diaphragms, these features are generally not helpful in differentiating an acute exacerbation from chronic COPD. Often, an acute exacerbation of COPD is associated with increasing cough, shortness of breath, and sputum production over several days. The current patient has a history of COPD but does not have wheezing on her examination, and the history of the onset of symptoms is more suggestive of another diagnosis.

The diagnosis of acute pulmonary embolus (PE) is frequently elusive, and a high clinical suspicion is required to keep from missing this diagnosis. Unfortunately, many of the presenting signs and symptoms may overlap with other diagnoses. Some clues that increase the likelihood of a PE include the following: (1) acute onset of shortness of breath (especially when a patient describes the specific time the dyspnea began), (2) pleuritic chest pain, and (3) hemoptysis. In addition, risk factors for venous stasis or a hypercoagulable state also increase the chances of the patient having a PE.

The current patient has many of these risk factors, including obesity, smoking, immobility (lying in bed due to viral illness) over the last 6 days, history of breast cancer (associated with hypercoagulable state), and lower extremity edema (associated with stasis). Therefore the clinical suspicion for PE is very high.

Another cause of hypoxemia in a patient without infiltrates on chest x-ray is microatelectasis. Microatelectasis occurs in patients who take small, shallow breaths (such as post-operative patients who are in pain or those with pleuritic chest pain from a fractured rib, etc) and is diagnosed by the physical examination findings of bronchial breath sounds (loud or harsh breath sounds with expiration equal in intensity to inspiration). The chest x-ray may be normal or demonstrate slightly low lung volumes. The current patient does not have bronchial breath sounds on her examination; therefore she does not have microatelectasis.

Another etiology of severe hypoxemia is a right-to-left shunt, which should be suspected when a patient's hypoxemia fails to improve with high levels of FIo_2. The shunting of blood may occur in the heart (such as a right-to-left shunt from pulmonary hypertension) or within the vessels of the lungs (such as occurs with pulmonary arterial-venous malformations). With a careful history, the onset and time frame of worsening symptoms is commonly more insidious for shunts than for other causes of hypoxemia with a black x-ray.

Patients with obesity-hypoventilation syndrome also have a more insidious clinical course, which is similar to the slowly progressive symptoms in patients with a shunt. This syndrome is a rare cause of hypoxemia and occurs in morbidly obese individuals. It is characterized by atelectasis and chronic carbon dioxide retention; both of which are associated with hypoxemia.

Smoke inhalation is another unusual cause of hypoxemia that can be diagnosed by a careful history. The mechanism of hypoxemia involves the excessive binding of carbon monoxide to hemoglobin and the displacement of oxygen, which results in a low saturation by co-oximetry (Sao_2) but normal by pulse oximetry (Spo_2).

Although ARDS is generally classified under the white radiographic causes of hypoxemia, a few cases may present with a black x-ray, resulting in some confusion among clinicians. The patients with this confusing picture are those who present very early in the course of ARDS (during the first ~24 hours) with a black or normal-appearing chest x-ray but then uniformly progress to bilateral infiltrates (white x-ray) on follow-up studies. These infiltrates are most often seen in patients with sepsis or septic shock as the etiology of their ARDS. A computed tomography (CT) scan of the chest performed in this early stage of ARDS demonstrates significant bilateral interstitial infiltrates, which are clearly seen on CT that are not yet visible by plain radiography. Therefore, although this entity fits in the group with a white x-ray, the plain film may appear black during the early stages of the illness.

Further Diagnostic Testing in the Evaluation of Hypoxemia

After reviewing the possible causes, historical features, physical examination findings, and radiographic appearance of the current patient, the most likely etiology of her hypoxemia is PE. Although early ARDS and an acute exacerbation of COPD are still possible, the evidence available suggests that a PE is most likely. In addition, the most dangerous diagnosis to miss or overlook is an acute PE, since the mortality of an untreated embolus is about 30%. Many clinicians begin the diagnostic work-up with a ventilation-perfusion ($\dot{V}/\dot{Q}$) scan of the lungs. This study can demonstrate areas of the lung that are being ventilated but not perfused (secondary to a clot in the vessel). The problem with the $\dot{V}/\dot{Q}$ scan is that there are many disorders that can cause small defects in the perfusion portion of the scan that do not represent a PE. Therefore the results of the $\dot{V}/\dot{Q}$ scan are now standardized by defined criteria. Combining the results of the $\dot{V}/\dot{Q}$ scan with the level of clinical suspicion for a PE helps the clinician determine the likelihood of the diagnosis versus the need for further testing. A high probability scan combined with a high clinical suspicion for PE or a very low probability or normal scan with a low clinical suspicion for PE represent the optimal clinical scenarios. However, most commonly, the $\dot{V}/\dot{Q}$ scan is indeterminate (the current patient had two areas of subsegmental defects in perfusion with air trapping on the ventilation portion of the examination). Since this study does not rule out a PE and the clinical suspicion is high, the next test is a bilateral lower extremity Doppler study to evaluate for a deep venous thrombosis (DVT). This examination demonstrated a large clot in the common femoral vein of the right lower extremity. Therefore no further diagnostic work-up is indicated in this patient. The patient requires treatment with anticoagulation (warfarin) for approximately 6 months (after overlapping with heparin for about 5 days). If the lower extremity Dopplers had not demonstrated a DVT, then a further diagnostic work-up would have been indicated (with a spiral/dynamic CT of the chest or pulmonary angiography, which is still considered to be the "gold standard" for diagnosis of PE).

Pitfalls and Common Mistakes in the Management of Hypoxemia and Respiratory Failure

The initial approach in managing patients with severe hypoxemia and acute respiratory failure is supportive and includes assessing the ABCs (patency of the Airway, presence of Breathing, and adequacy of Circulatory function). The initiation of supplemental oxygen based on the arterial blood gas or on the pulse oximetry saturation is essential in the management of patients with significant hypoxemia. After the ABCs are secured, the management of acute respiratory failure involves treating the underlying disease. The most important step in the management of a patient with suspected PE is to begin empiric treatment with anticoagulation before any diagnostic studies are obtained. The standard treatment includes anticoagulation with unfractionated heparin or low-molecular-weight heparin, as long as there are no absolute contraindications (e.g., active gastrointestinal bleeding, recent hemorrhagic stroke, recent surgery, etc). An extremely unfortunate (but not uncommon) scenario is when a patient who is not empirically started on anticoagulation is in radiology undergoing diagnostic studies for PE and develops another embolus that is now fatal.

▼ SUMMARY

A careful history and review of all of the available data is critical to managing the patient with a suspected PE. A detailed history, a comprehensive physical examination, and a careful review of all of the data are necessary to successfully evaluate and manage patients with acute hypoxemia.

▼ BIBLIOGRAPHY

American Thoracic Society: Standards for the diagnosis and care of patients with chronic obstructive pulmonary disease, *Am J Respir Crit Care Med* 152:S78-120, 1995.
Brown DL, (editor): *Cardiac intensive care,* Philadelphia, 1998, WB Saunders Co.
Dalen JE, Alpert JS: Natural history of pulmonary embolism, *Prog Cardiovasc Dis* 17:259-270, 1975.
George RB et al (editors): *Chest medicine: essentials of pulmonary and critical care medicine,* ed 3, Baltimore, 1995, Williams & Wilkins.
The PIOPED Investigators: Value of the ventilation/perfusion scan in acute pulmonary embolism, *JAMA* 263:2753-2759, 1990.

CHAPTER 35

THE PATIENT WITH A HIGH PEAK AIRWAY PRESSURE

Edgar Delgado

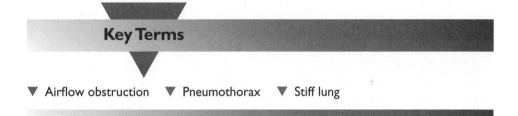

Key Terms

▼ Airflow obstruction   ▼ Pneumothorax   ▼ Stiff lung

▼ THE CLINICAL PROBLEM

As rounds begin in the medical intensive care unit (MICU), the patient in bed 2 triggers the high inspiratory pressure alarm on the ventilator. He is a 39-year-old man admitted to the unit 48 hours earlier because of bilateral pneumonia associated with respiratory distress. The patient has adequate vital signs and is being ventilated on volume-control ventilation (VCV). His settings are assist/control (A/C) mode ventilation, tidal volume (V_T) of 700 mL, set respiratory rate of 24 with a total rate of 28 breaths/minute, FIO_2 at 0.8, and positive end-expiratory pressure (PEEP) set at 10 cm H_2O. Peak inspiratory pressure (PIP) is 52 cm H_2O, and plateau pressure (P_{plat}) is 50 cm H_2O.

The patient is on a propofol drip for sedation, and he occasionally makes spontaneous breathing efforts. Assessment of breath sounds reveals mild scattered rhonchi with no wheezes. Chest x-ray from that morning depicts a ground-glass appearance with bilateral diffuse infiltrates and endotracheal tube (ETT) in good position (2 cm above the carina). The patient is suctioned via ETT with successful removal of a small amount of yellow, blood-tinged sputum. Rhonchi cleared post-suction, but peak airway pressure remains at about 52 cm H_2O.

Why is the patient's PIP still 52 cm H_2O regardless of suctioning and no audible wheezing?

Differential Diagnosis of High Peak Airway Pressure

Changes in lung volume are caused by changes in the pressure gradient created by thoracic expansion and contraction. Most commonly, these pressures are measured in centimeters of water and are influenced by several factors that include V_T, total system compliance, airway resistance, inspiratory flow ($\dot{V}$) rate, and inspiratory time (T_I).

The PIP is the maximum pressure in the airway during the inspiratory phase as measured most commonly by the ventilator at the circuit "Y" connection. Therefore any changes in the PIP generally reflect changes in ventilator parameters and/or changes in the compliance or resistance of the lungs and any ventilatory system components. For example, for a given volume, using volume-constant ventilation, the volume will not change, but the PIP will if the patient develops bronchospasm (change in resistance).

Tidal Volume

During conventional VCV and constant compliance and resistance, any changes to V_T will reflect changes to the PIP. As V_T is increased or decreased, PIP will also increase or decrease, respectively.

Compliance

The ability of the lung to expand can be evaluated by measurements of compliance. *Compliance of the lung* (C_L) is defined as the volume change (ΔV) per unit of pressure (ΔP) change and is commonly measured in liters/centimeter of water:

$$C_L = \Delta V \text{ (liter)}/\Delta P \text{ (cm } H_2O)$$

From this equation, it can be deduced that, if volume remains constant, any change in compliance will alter airway pressure. Generally, compliance and inflating pressure share an inverse relationship: when compliance increases, airway pressure decreases and as compliance decreases, peak inspiratory pressure increases.

It is imperative to understand this relationship between airway pressure and compliance when volume or pressure control modes of ventilation are applied, since the V_T delivered is the result of different flow and pressure patterns generated in the patient-ventilator system.

Resistance

As gas moves through the airways, a certain degree of impedance (most commonly termed *airway resistance*) is created. Airway resistance (Raw) has been defined as the ratio of driving pressure (ΔP) responsible for gas movement to the flow of the gas (ΔP) and is measured in centimeters of water/liter/second:

$$\text{Raw} = \Delta P \text{ (cm } H_2O)/\Delta V \text{ (L/sec)}$$

This equation illustrates that when resistance is maintained constant, flow and pressure share a direct relationship: as flow rate is increased, airway pressure also increases.

As with compliance, the clinician should understand the interactions between Raw and inspiratory flow in relation to airway pressure.

Flow and Inspiratory Time

During mechanical ventilation when compliance and resistance are unchanged, the inspiratory flow rate shares a direct relationship with the PIP. As inspiratory flow is increased or decreased, the PIP increases or decreases, respectively.

During VCV, changes in flow rate are obtained by adjusting the set flow rate parameter directly on the ventilator, by adjusting the TI or inspiratory-to-expiratory (I:E) ratio, depending on the ventilator used. As TI is increased, the ventilator decreases the delivered flow to preserve the set VT ($V_T = \dot{V} \times T_I$). The other important variable to be considered during VCV is the flow pattern, which is typically set by the clinician. The two most common patterns are decelerating (ramp) and square. The use of a square-flow pattern reaches the set flow rate quickly when the breath is initiated. This flow is maintained throughout the delivery of the VT and generally leads to increases in airway pressure.

In pressure-control ventilation (PCV), the flow waveform and rate are not predetermined (cannot be adjusted directly), thereby permitting variability of the flow characteristics as a function of patient effort. The waveform is generally decelerating (ramp) in nature and has been supported by some research as potentially responsible for improvement in gas exchange. Changes to flow are also affected by changes to TI, the ventilator's inspiratory pressure setting, and the ventilator's internal flow algorithms. During PCV, as the inspiratory pressure is increased, the ventilator increases its flow rate to target the set pressure within the prescribed TI.

The interactions between VT, compliance, resistance, flow, and inspiratory time in relation to peak inspiratory airway pressure are described in Table 35-1.

Clinical Features that Suggest a Specific Cause of High Peak Airway Pressure

The following questions should be asked in the evaluation of this 39-year-old man:

1. *Is a PIP of 52 cm H_2O harmful to the lung?* In the 1980s and early 1990s, studies in normal animals demonstrated that an acute respiratory distress syndrome (ARDS)–like injury could be provoked by ventilating with high peak airway pressures (30 to 50 cm H_2O). More recently, Amato et al demonstrated that survival could be improved in patients with ARDS when a protective ventilation strategy was utilized with PIPs below 40 cm H_2O. The literature now favors ventilation with distending pressures of $\leq$40 cm H_2O to avoid lung injury.
2. *Were there any changes in ventilator parameters to precipitate an increase in airway pressure?* As the clinician checks the ventilator history for changes in ventilator parameters over the past 48 hours, only changes to the FIO$_2$ and PEEP were implemented. The FIO$_2$ was increased from 0.4 to 0.6 to 0.8, and the PEEP was increased from 5 to 7.5 to 10 cm H_2O. Peak airway pressure has risen from 22 cm H_2O when the patient was initiated on mechanical ventilation to 52 cm H_2O, the

TABLE 35-1
Effect of Ventilator Parameters and Lung Characteristics on Peak Inspiratory Pressure

	Volume Control			Pressure Control	
	Ventilator Parameter	**PIP**		**Ventilator Parameter**	**PIP**
V_T	↑ ↓	↑ ↓	Inspiratory pressure	↑ ↓	↑ ↓
Flow	↑ ↓	↑ ↓	T_I	↑ ↓	→ →
T_I	↑ ↓	↓ ↑	Compliance	↑ ↓	→ →
Compliance	↑ ↓	↓ ↑	Resistance	↑ ↓	→ →
Resistance	↑ ↓	↑ ↓			

PIP, Peak inspiratory pressure; *VT,* tidal volume; *TI,* inspiratory time.

present pressure. Since no changes to V$_T$ and flow were made, and only an increase of 5 cm H$_2$O to the PEEP level was instituted, a change in compliance or resistance or patient-ventilator dys-synchrony must be questioned.

3. *Could the high PIP have been caused by dys-synchrony with the ventilator due to the spontaneous efforts made by the patient?* On inspection of breathing pattern, no paradoxical pattern is noted, and inspection of flow and pressure waveforms did not demonstrate any evidence of patient-ventilator dys-synchrony. When patients are on controlled modes of ventilation and with heavy sedation (propofol drip) or with paralysis, patient-ventilator dys-synchrony is highly unlikely.

4. *Is there any evidence to suggest resistance problems?* Auscultation of breath sounds revealed mild rhonchi with no wheezes. Any factors that influence the internal lumen of the airway lead to changes in resistance. Some of these elements could be secretions, bronchospasm, mucosal edema (swelling), kinks in the artificial airway or ventilator tubing, leaving the suction catheter partly into the artificial airway (ETT) and increasing inspiratory flow. From the initial evaluation, attempts to suction the airway were successful for removal of a small amount of yellow, blood-tinged sputum. Although rhonchi cleared post-suction, PIP did not improve. Follow-up inspection of ventilator tubing revealed no obvious kinks, and suctioned catheter was pulled completely out of the airway. Since no changes to ventilator flow rate were implemented, one may suspect problems in the smaller airways or deep in the lung parenchyma.

5. *Is there any evidence to suspect compliance changes?* From the clinical observation, no obvious criteria are presented indicating a probable change in compliance. Therefore diagnostic tools should be evaluated to help identify the root cause of increased PIP.

Diagnostic Testing in the Evaluation of Elevated Peak Inspiratory Pressure

Dynamic compliance calculations are used to assess changes in the non-elastic (airway) resistance to airflow, whereas static compliance is used to assess changes of the elastic (lung parenchyma) resistance to airflow:

$$C_{dyn} = \Delta V \text{ (liter)}/\Delta P \text{ (cm } H_2O)$$

where C_{dyn} is dynamic compliance in liter/cm H_2O
ΔV is corrected tidal volume (liter)
ΔP is pressure change (peak airway pressure − PEEP) in cm H_2O

$$C_{st} = \Delta V \text{ (liter)}/\Delta P \text{ (cm } H_2O)$$

where C_{st} is static compliance in liter/cm H_2O
ΔV is corrected tidal volume (liter)
ΔP is pressure change (plateau pressure − PEEP) in cm H_2O

Dynamic compliance changes with minimal or no decreases in static compliance are indicative of non-elastic airway resistance changes. When static and dynamic compliances decrease in the same proportion, it is indicative of an increase in elastic resistance. Extrapolating from these equations allows for rapid evaluation of airway resistance by simply comparing the peak versus plateau airway pressure difference. A significant peak/plateau pressure difference is due to non-elastic airway resistance, whereas a minimal peak/plateau pressure gradient indicates an elastic resistance problem.

The other diagnostic tool mentioned in the clinical problem is the chest x-ray. The findings helped determine the increase in PIP by revealing that the ETT was 2 cm above the carina (good position), which eliminated the possibility of a right mainstem intubation that would most likely cause an increase in pressure. Second, it did not mention any signs of pneumothorax or tracheal shifts, which would explain increases in pressure. Finally, it provided evidence of bilateral diffuse infiltrates and a "ground-glass" appearance, which are typical of ARDS. In ARDS, there is a decrease in compliance and therefore a gradual increase in peak inspiratory airway pressure as the disease progresses.

Another phenomenon, which should be identified in this clinical scenario, is the issue of auto-PEEP (hyperinflation), which occurs when insufficient time is dedicated to expiration. Auto-PEEP develops when alveolar units do not have enough time to completely empty inspired gas, leading to gas volume being trapped within the alveoli. When total PEEP is increased directly by adjusting the PEEP control setting on the ventilator or indirectly in the form of auto-PEEP, airway pressure will also be affected during VCV when compliance and resistance are unchanged. This can easily be explained by the compliance calculation previously discussed:

$$C_L = \Delta V \text{ (liters)}/\Delta P \text{ (cm } H_2O)$$

As a result of the direct relationship between volume and pressure in the presence of unchanged compliance, any increases in volume correspond with increases in pressure. With hyperinflation, basically more volume is introduced into the lung; therefore the result is an increase in PIP when compliance is unchanged. Since VCV targets a set VT, increasing end-expiratory pressure (same as end-expiratory lung volume) results in an increase in PIP.

In this clinical problem, evaluation of the expiratory flow waveform with the graphics monitor on the ventilator revealed that expired gas returned to baseline (zero flow) before the beginning of the next inspiration. This flow pattern is indicative of complete emptying of tidal ventilation during expiratory time and excludes the possibility of auto-PEEP as a cause of the increased PIP. Since hyperinflation was not created, then the PIP increase could not be attributed to this phenomenon.

▼ SUMMARY

A systematic approach helped identify probable causes of the elevation in PIP in this patient. The ability to measure and evaluate the peak versus plateau pressure difference indicated that the problem was within elastic resistance (lung parenchyma) and not with non-elastic (airway) variables. The addition of the chest x-ray helped diagnose the unique disease, ARDS. Also, careful analysis of the history revealed that the FIO_2 had been increased to 0.8 and the PEEP to 10 cm H_2O (common adjustments to mechanical ventilation during the progression of ARDS), which then excluded routine ventilator setting changes as a possible cause of the elevated PIP.

This clinical scenario emphasizes the importance of a systematic approach to the clinical problem of elevated peak airway pressure.

▼ BIBLIOGRAPHY

Al-Saady N, Bennett ED: Decelerating inspiratory flow waveform improves lung mechanics and gas exchange in patients on intermittent positive-pressure ventilation, *Intensive Care Med* 11:68-75, 1985.

Amato MBP, Barbas CSV, Medeiros DM, et al: Effect of a protective-ventilation strategy on mortality in the acute respiratory distress syndrome, *N Engl J Med* 338:347-354, 1988.

Dreyfuss D, Basset GT, Soler P, et al: Intermittent positive-pressure hyperventilation with high inflation pressures produces microvascular injury in rats, *Am Rev Respir Dis* 132:880-884, 1985.

Dreyfuss D, Soler P, Basset G, et al: High inflation pressure pulmonary edema: respective effects of high airway pressure, high tidal volume and positive end-expiratory pressure, *Am Rev Respir Dis* 137:1159-1164, 1988.

Kolobow T, Moretti M, Fumagalli R, et al: Severe impairment in lung function induced by high peak airway pressure during mechanical ventilation: an experimental study, *Am Rev Respir Dis* 135:312-315, 1987.

Parker J, Hernandez L, Longenecker G, et al: Lung edema caused by high inspiratory pressures in dogs: role of increased microvascular filtration pressure and permeability, *Am Rev Respir Dis* 142:321-328, 1990.

Scanlan CL, Ruppel GL: Ventilation. In Scanlan CL, Spearman CB, Sheldon RL: *Egan's fundamentals of respiratory care*, ed 6, St. Louis, 1995, Mosby.

CHAPTER 36

VENTILATOR-ASSOCIATED PNEUMONIA

David L. Longworth

Key Terms

▼ Pneumonia   ▼ Intensive care unit (ICU)   ▼ Gram-negative pneumonia
▼ Ventilator   ▼ Nosocomial

▼ THE CLINICAL PROBLEM

A 72-year-old man was admitted to hospital 10 days ago with sudden onset of chest pain radiating to the back and was found to have a dissecting thoracic aortic aneurysm. He underwent emergency surgical repair on the day of admission with placement of a Dacron tube graft to the ascending and descending thoracic aorta. His procedure was complicated by hypotension and an intraoperative stroke that involved his left middle cerebral artery. Post-operatively he has been ventilator-dependent because of pre-existing chronic obstructive lung disease and has failed to wean. Overnight, he developed a fever to 101.8° F and his FIO_2 requirement has increased from 40% to 60%. He requires 10 cm H_2O of positive end-expiratory pressure (PEEP). On suctioning through the endotracheal tube, the clinician discovers that his secretions have increased in quantity and are now brown and tinged with blood.

His past medical history is notable for hypertension, type 2 diabetes mellitus requiring insulin, and chronic obstructive pulmonary disease (COPD). He is a 60 pack-year smoker. His medications include renal dose dopamine, insulin, enalapril, and subcutaneous heparin. Post-operatively, he received 48 hours of intravenous cefuroxime and has been off antibiotics for the past 8 days. He received pneumococcal vaccine 4 years ago.

On physical examination, he is febrile to 101.5° F, intubated, and slightly agitated. The blood pressure is 140/82 mm Hg and the heart rate is 110. He is breathing over the ventilator at 16 breaths per minute. An oral endotracheal tube and nasogastric feeding tube are in place. His skin is unremarkable, and he has a right radial arterial line and left subclavian central venous line, both of which have clean exit sites. Auscultation of the chest discloses right lower lobe rales and rhonchi. A left thoracotomy incision is clean and dry, as is his former left-sided chest tube site. The cardiac examination discloses a regular rate and rhythm. There are no murmurs or gallops. The abdomen is soft, non-tender, and without organ enlargement. Bowel sounds are present. A Foley catheter is in place and the testes and epididymi are unremarkable. The lower extremities are without cords or edema. On neurologic examination, there is weakness of the right lower face, arm, and leg, consistent with his stroke.

The leukocyte count has risen from 12,000 cells/mm³ yesterday to 20,000 cell/mm³ today. His hemoglobin is 11 g/dL, and his platelet count is 325,000 cells/mm³. His serum creatinine is 1.4 mg/dL, and his random blood glucose level is elevated overnight at 280 mg%. A chest x-ray discloses a new right lower lobe infiltrate compared with the previous day's film (Figure 36-1).

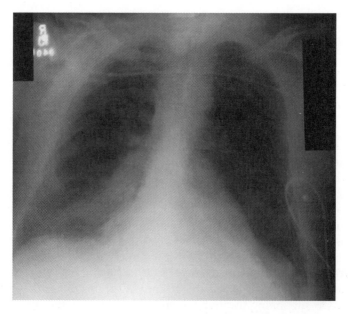

▼ **Figure 36-1** Chest x-ray with right lower lobe infiltrate.

What is the most likely diagnosis and its most common causes? What are the risk factors for this complication? What studies should be performed, and what other studies might be helpful? How should the patient be managed? What can the respiratory clinician do to minimize the likelihood of this complication recurring?

Differential Diagnosis of Ventilator-Associated Pneumonia

This patient presents with fever, leukocytosis, purulent secretions, an increasing oxygen requirement, and a new pulmonary infiltrate in the setting of mechanical ventilation for 10 days after a thoracic surgical procedure. The most likely diagnosis is ventilator-associated pneumonia (VAP), or hospital-acquired pneumonia, in which pneumonia arises in the setting of mechanical ventilation.

The differential diagnosis that should be entertained in patients with suspected VAP is similar to that of fever and a new pulmonary infiltrate in the hospitalized adult. This is summarized in Box 36-1 and discussed in detail in Chapter 22, which will not be repeated here. It includes both infectious and non-infectious causes.

VAP is a major cause of morbidity and mortality in mechanically ventilated patients in the intensive care unit (ICU). Some studies have estimated that up to 25% of such patients develop hospital-acquired pneumonia with mortality rates ranging from 30% to 70%, depending on the microorganism.

The pathogenesis of VAP differs somewhat from that of nosocomial or hospital-acquired pneumonia in the non-ventilated patient. In the latter circumstance, microorganisms may reach the lower respiratory tract through multiple mechanisms. Microaspiration of oropharyngeal secretions is the most common, but other pathogenetic mechanisms include large-volume aspiration events, inhalation of infected aerosols, hematogenous spread of infection to the lung from a remote site, contiguous spread of infection to the lung from a nearby site, or penetration of the lung by tube thoracostomy. In the subset of patients who develop

---

Box 36-1
Differential Diagnosis of Ventilator-Associated Pneumonia

Infectious Causes	Non-Infectious Causes
Common	**Common**
Pneumonia	Pulmonary embolus/infarction
	Congestive heart failure
Uncommon	ARDS
Septic pulmonary embolus	Mucous plugging with atelectasis
Intravascular device	
Right-sided endocarditis	**Uncommon**
Contiguous spread of infection	Drugs
Subdiaphragmatic abscess	Alveolar hemorrhage
Mediastinitis	Tracheoesophageal fistula
	Radiation pneumonitis

ARDS, Acute respiratory distress syndrome.

Box 36-2
Common Microorganisms Producing
Ventilator-Associated Pneumonia

Gram-Negative Bacilli
Pseudomonas aeruginosa
Acinetobacter species
Enterobacter species
Klebsiella species
Serratia marcescens
Escherichia coli
Proteus species
Legionella species

Gram-Positive Organisms
Staphylococcus aureus

nosocomial pneumonia while on the ventilator, several additional mechanisms may facilitate the development of VAP. The endotracheal tube inhibits normal host defense by its adverse effect on mucociliary clearance. In addition, secretions colonized with oropharyngeal flora may pool above the endotracheal cuff and periodically drain into the tracheobronchial tree. Deep endotracheal suctioning may even directly inoculate infected secretions into the lower airway. Finally, some organisms may adhere to the endotracheal tube through the development of a biofilm, which facilitates their persistence and migration to the lower respiratory tract.

The microorganisms responsible for VAP differ significantly from those producing community-acquired pneumonia and are summarized in Box 36-2. Community-acquired pathogens such as *Streptococcus pneumoniae* and *Haemophilus influenzae* may occasionally produce VAP in the first several days of mechanical ventilation; however, cases developing beyond 5 days of intubation are usually due to gram-negative bacilli or *Staphylococcus aureus*. The microbial differential diagnosis and antimicrobial susceptibility profiles of responsible organisms may differ significantly between institutions, and thus knowledge of local epidemiology is essential in selecting empiric and pathogen-specific therapy in patients with suspected VAP.

Clinical Features that Suggest the Diagnosis of Ventilator-Associated Pneumonia

The constellation of fever, leukocytosis, and a new pulmonary infiltrate in the mechanically ventilated patient should suggest the diagnosis of VAP. Hemodynamic instability may or may not be present and in the early stages of VAP; oxygen requirements may be stable. Purulent secretions may be absent; if present, they are not synonymous with VAP and may reflect tracheobronchitis with another cause for a new infiltrate.

Box 36-3
Risk Factors for Nosocomial Pneumonia

Patient-Related Factors
Age >70
Malnutrition
Impaired consciousness
Prolonged hospitalization
Diabetes mellitus
Renal insufficiency
Chronic obstructive lung disease

Infection Control–Related Factors
Poor hand washing
Inappropriate use of gloves
Contaminated respiratory therapy equipment
Contaminated hospital water supply
   (*Legionella* species)

Procedures and Practices
Prolonged antibiotic administration
Sedation
Immunosuppressive medications
Supine patient position
Nasogastric tubes
Gastric feeding
Prolonged surgical procedures
Fiberoptic bronchoscopy
Transportation for procedures
Prolonged mechanical ventilation

The difficulty in diagnosis of VAP and the proliferation of techniques that have been evaluated to try to improve diagnostic accuracy reflect the fact that chronically intubated patients may have pulmonary infiltrates that are unrelated to the cause of their fever, leukocytosis, or even purulent secretions. Common causes of pulmonary infiltrates that may mimic VAP include mucous plugging, atelectasis, acute respiratory distress syndrome (ARDS), or congestive heart failure (CHF). The pattern of the infiltrate is regrettably not particularly helpful in distinguishing VAP from other causes of pulmonary infiltrates. Lobar infiltrates may accompany both VAP and mucous plugging, although the sudden development over hours of dense lobar consolidation with volume loss is more suggestive of plugging with atelectasis and less characteristic of VAP. Similarly, rapidly progressive bilateral infiltrates may reflect overwhelming gram-negative pneumonia but may also be due to left-sided CHF or ARDS from another unrecognized site of infection. Hemodynamic monitoring with Swan-Ganz catheterization is frequently helpful in confirming the diagnosis of heart failure, which is characterized by the presence of an elevated pulmonary artery occlusion pressure; this is usually normal in VAP or ARDS. A major challenge to the respiratory and ICU clinician is to recognize occult sites of infection elsewhere that may produce ARDS in the mechanically ventilated patient who is often sedated. In addition, such patients may have more than one disease process evolving at any given time and thus several potential causes, both infectious and non-infectious, for a new pulmonary infiltrate, fever, and leukocytosis.

A number of risk factors have been recognized for the development of nosocomial pneumonia in general, and many are applicable to the subpopulation of patients with VAP. Risk factors for nosocomial pneumonia are summarized in Box 36-3 and include factors that are related to the patient, infection control, procedures, and practices.

Patient factors associated with an increased risk for the development of hospital-acquired pneumonia include advanced age (>70); prolonged hospital stay; malnutrition; impaired consciousness from underlying neurologic abnormalities or medications, such as sedatives or narcotics; and the presence of certain comorbid conditions such as diabetes mellitus, chronic obstructive lung disease, and renal insufficiency. Failure to strictly adhere to standard infection control practices may also contribute to the development of nosocomial pneumonia in hospitalized patients. Examples include failure to wash hands properly and to change gloves between patient contacts and faulty sterilization or decontamination techniques for respiratory therapy equipment. On rare occasion, faulty hospital water purification systems have led to contamination of the hospital water supply with *Legionella* species and outbreaks of nosocomial legionellosis.

Certain procedures and practices have also been identified as risk factors for hospital-acquired pneumonia. These include prolonged mechanical ventilation, prolonged surgical procedures (especially thoracic and abdominal), prolonged antibiotic administration (even if appropriate), the use of sedative or immunosuppressive medications, a supine position when mechanically ventilated, the presence of nasogastric tubes, enteral feeding into the stomach compared with the small bowel, recent fiberoptic bronchoscopy, and transportation out of the ICU setting for diagnostic or therapeutic procedures. In the latter circumstance, transportation is associated with supine position, disconnection of nasogastric tubes, and manipulation of ventilator tubes, all of which increase the likelihood that contaminated secretions will find their way to the lower respiratory tract. Some of these risk factors for nosocomial pneumonia represent potential targets for intervention by the respiratory care clinician, as discussed later in this chapter.

Diagnostic Testing in the Evaluation of the Patient with Suspected Ventilator-Associated Pneumonia

The accurate diagnosis of VAP is fraught with difficulty and is one of the most controversial topics in the field of pulmonary and critical care medicine. The respiratory clinician cannot rely solely on clinical manifestations, the appearance of the pulmonary infiltrate, or culture results from tracheal secretions to accurately diagnose VAP. In a minority of patients, several clinical scenarios do have a strong predictive value for the presence of VAP, as summarized in Box 36-4. In a patient with clinical signs of pneumonia and a pulmonary infiltrate, these include simultaneous isolation of the same microorganism from respiratory secretions and blood; isolation of a microorganism from empyema fluid, lung biopsy or percutaneous needle biopsy; and rapid cavitation of an infiltrate. Unfortunately, these clinical scenarios are uncommon for several reasons. First, bacteremia occurs in only a small minority of patients with VAP. Second, empyema is similarly uncommon. Third, most patients are too ill to tolerate open lung biopsy. Finally, percutaneous needle biopsy is rarely an option in mechanically ventilated patients because of the risk of pneumothorax.

A variety of diagnostic techniques have been developed and evaluated in clinical studies in an attempt to improve diagnostic accuracy in patients with suspected VAP. These are summarized in Box 36-5. Quantitative cultures of tracheal aspirates have been assessed in several studies of patients with suspected VAP. The gold

Box 36-4
Clinical Scenarios with a High Predictive Value
for the Presence of VAP in a Mechanically Ventilated Patient

Rapid cavitation of a pulmonary infiltrate
Simultaneous recovery of the same microorganism from blood and respiratory secretions
In a patient with a pulmonary infiltrate and clinical signs of pneumonia, recovery of micro-
  organisms from:
• Lung biopsy
• Empyema fluid
• Percutaneous needle aspiration of the lung

Adapted from Mayhall G: *Infect Dis Clin N Am* 11:427-457, 1997.
VAP, Ventilator-associated pneumonia.

Box 36-5
Techniques Evaluated in Diagnosis
of Ventilator-Associated Pneumonia

Quantitative Culture of Tracheal Aspirates

Bronchoscopic Techniques
Protected specimen brush
Bronchoalveolar lavage

Non-Bronchoscopically Directed Protected Techniques
Protected specimen brush
Bronchoalveolar lavage
Blind aspiration into a catheter

standard for diagnosis of VAP has differed between these studies, as has the quantitative threshold of organisms in tracheal specimens considered to be significant. In most studies, quantitative tracheal cultures have been compared with cultures obtained bronchoscopically by protected specimen brush (PSB) or bronchoalveolar lavage (BAL), which are not completely reliable for diagnosis of VAP as discussed later. When diagnostic thresholds of 10^5-10^6 colony-forming units (CFU)/cc have been employed, the sensitivity and specificity of quantitative tracheal cultures compared with PSB and BAL have ranged from 65% to 85% and 84% to 96%, respectively. In addition, in some studies, isolates obtained from tracheal cultures were not present in cultures obtained by bronchoscopy, suggesting that these upper airway organisms were not true pathogens in the lower airway. In summary, quantitative tracheal cultures have inadequate sensitivity and specificity for the accurate diagnosis of VAP.

Several bronchoscopic techniques to obtain lower airway specimens for quantitative culture have been evaluated for the diagnosis of VAP. These include the PSB and BAL. PSB was invented in 1979 and consists of two telescoping catheters, which

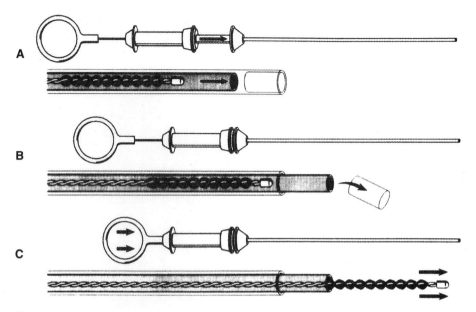

▼ **Figure 36-2** Protected specimen brush. **A,** Inner/outer catheter. **B,** Use of remote plungers for plug. **C,** Brush. From Lee FYW, Mehta AC: Basic techniques in flexible bronchoscopy. In Wang KP, Mehta AC (editors): *Flexible bronchoscopy,* Boston, 1995, Blackwell Science Publication, pp 95-118.

are passed through the bronchoscope into the lower airway (Figure 36-2). A protected brush is contained within the inner catheter; on passage into the lower airway, potentially colonized upper airway secretions are suctioned into the outer catheter to avoid contamination of the brush in the inner lumen. Once in the lower airway, the brush is advanced and specimens for quantitative culture are obtained. In most studies, the presence of greater than 10^3 CFU/cc has been considered significant.

BAL is performed by instilling a sterile physiologic solution into a segment of involved lung through the inner catheter and then suctioning back as much fluid as possible for quantitative culture. Concentrations of greater than 10^4 CFU/cc have been considered significant; some studies have also assessed the percentage of BAL cells containing intracellular organisms and have considered a threshold of greater than 5% of cells as being significant diagnostically for the presence of VAP.

Many studies have examined the sensitivity, specificity, and predictive value of quantitative cultures of specimens obtained by bronchoscopically directed BAL and PSB in the diagnosis of VAP. The best studies for diagnosis of VAP have used as a gold standard an open lung biopsy obtained immediately post-mortem, where tissue specimens have been quantitatively cultured and examined histopathologically for the presence of pneumonia. In several of these studies, bronchoscopy with PSB and BAL have also been performed immediately post-mortem and compared in their diagnostic accuracy with open lung biopsy of the same area of sampled lung. Results from these studies have been conflicting. PSB has demonstrated a sensitivity of 36% to 82%, specificity of 50% to 88%, and positive predictive value of 43% to 74% in the diagnosis of VAP when using a diagnostic threshold of greater than 10^3 CFU/cc. Bronchoscopically obtained BAL has demonstrated a sensitivity of 50% to 91%, specificity of 45% to 100%, and positive predictive value of 60% to 83% when a cutoff of $>10^4$ CFU/cc of BAL fluid is employed. In one study, the presence of greater than five cells containing microorganisms in BAL fluid had a sensitivity, specificity, and positive predictive value for the diagnosis of VAP of 89%, 91%, and 89%, respectively. Several studies have emphasized the fact that PSB and BAL are less sensitive in patients receiving antimicrobial therapy if that therapy has been changed within the preceding 72 hours. In summary, bronchoscopic techniques are more reliable than quantitative cultures of tracheal secretions in patients with suspected VAP, but are not completely sensitive or specific. Moreover, a recent change in antibiotic therapy lessens their diagnostic utility. Therefore the implication for the respiratory clinician is that such techniques, if employed, are best done before antibiotics are initiated, or before a failing regimen is modified.

Bronchoscopy requires the presence of a physician and adds expense to patient care. A number of studies therefore have examined the utility of non-bronchoscopically guided techniques to obtain lower airway samples for quantitative culture in patients with suspected VAP. In some studies, these techniques have been performed by respiratory therapists and have included aspiration of secretions through a catheter, PSB, and BAL. In a study that employed autopsy confirmation of VAP as the gold standard, the sensitivity and specificity of quantitative cultures of secretions aspirated via a Metras catheter from the lower airway were 61% and 100%, respectively. Studies examining the utility of blind PSB and BAL are more difficult to interpret, as most have used as gold standard comparators bronchoscopically obtained PSB and BAL cultures, which themselves have variable sensitivity and specificity as outlined above. Nevertheless, in most such studies, non-bronchoscopically obtained BAL and PSB cultures have similar or slightly lower sensitivities than bronchoscopically obtained samples.

In summary, the sensitivity, specificity, and indications for these various techniques remain controversial, and their use varies from center to center in the diagnosis of VAP. When such diagnostic modalities are employed, their value seems to be greatest in antibiotic-naive patients and in those on a stable failing regimen, prior to initiating a change in antimicrobial therapy. Finally, open lung biopsy appears to have a very limited role in the diagnosis of VAP and is generally only considered in the subset of immunosuppressed individuals in whom the microbial differential diagnosis also includes opportunistic pathogens, in addition to the more usual bacterial causes of VAP.

Assessment of the Effect of Therapy in the Patient with Ventilator-Associated Pneumonia

A detailed discussion of appropriate empiric and pathogen-specific therapy of VAP is beyond the scope of this chapter. However, two points merit emphasis. First, the microbial differential diagnosis and antimicrobial susceptibility profiles of the most common causes of VAP differ between institutions. Second, because of this, appropriate empiric and pathogen-specific therapy for VAP may differ from one institution to another. It is therefore essential that the respiratory clinician be aware of the local epidemiology of VAP when selecting therapy for patients with VAP.

Patients with VAP usually do not respond immediately to an appropriate antibiotic regimen. They may take several days to a week to demonstrate a clinical response, especially in the setting of overwhelming gram-negative pneumonia. Fever, leukocytosis, and hemodynamic instability are usually the first parameters to improve. Respiratory failure and radiographic improvement may lag behind these other parameters, especially in those with complicating ARDS, in which impaired oxygenation and pulmonary infiltrates may persist for many days or even weeks.

In the mechanically ventilated patient with suspected VAP, failure to improve after several days to a week of antibiotic therapy should raise several differential diagnostic concerns, including the presence of a pathogen resistant to the prescribed antimicrobial regimen, an unrecognized empyema, mucous plugging with impaired clearance of secretions, an occult and unrecognized infection elsewhere, or another non-infectious cause for sustained fever, leukocytosis, and pulmonary infiltrates such as pancreatitis. In the patient with suspected VAP who is failing therapy at 5 to 7 days, surveillance cultures and imaging studies should be performed in search of another explanation for the patient's ongoing problems, and bronchoscopy should be considered, both to obtain lower airway specimens in search of a resistant pathogen and for potential therapy if mucous plugging is present.

Pitfalls and Common Mistakes in Assessment and Treatment of Patients with Suspected Ventilator-Associated Pneumonia

As should be evident from earlier discussion, pitfalls are many and mistakes are common in the assessment and management of patients with suspected VAP. Several should be emphasized. The first relates to patient assessment. Not all mechanically ventilated patients who have fever, leukocytosis, and pulmonary infiltrates have VAP. Other causes for fever and pulmonary infiltrates must be considered, and the infiltrates are sometimes unrelated to the underlying cause of fever. In addition, patients in the ICU may have more than one cause of fever and more than one cause of pulmonary infiltrates, which makes the diagnosis of VAP especially difficult. Second, a positive culture of tracheal secretions, even if accompanied by a sputum Gram's stain that demonstrates many polymorphonuclear infiltrates and a predominant microorganism, is not synonymous with the diagnosis of VAP. Failure to recognize the limitations of these tests may lead to inappropriate management decisions with regard to antibiotic therapy. Fourth, the optimal timing of diagnostic intervention in patients with suspected VAP is sometimes overlooked. When techniques such as PSB and BAL are considered, they should be used prior to initiating therapy or when a failing regimen has been in place for at least 72 hours, as this maximizes diagnostic yield. Fifth, ignorance of local hospital epidemiology with regard to common pathogens and antimicrobial susceptibility profiles hobbles optimal decision making with regard to empiric and pathogen-specific therapy of VAP. Finally, in assessing response to therapy, a common mistake is to assume that ongoing fever and leukocytosis signifies inappropriate antimicrobial therapy. Patients with VAP may fail to respond to a regimen for several reasons, which include a missed or resistant pathogen. Such apparent failures may also have other explanations, such as mucous plugging, the presence of an occult empyema, the presence of unrecognized infection elsewhere, or other non-infectious causes of ongoing fever.

Box 36-6
Strategies for the Prevention of Ventilator-Associated
Pneumonia by the Respiratory Clinician

Wash hands between each patient contact
Change gloves between each patient contact
Discard potentially contaminated respiratory therapy equipment
Use antibiotics judiciously
Avoid supine patient position
Place enteral feeding tubes in small bowel rather than stomach
Minimize patient transport out of the ICU; when essential, avoid supine position and manipula-
   tion of ventilator tubes

ICU, Intensive care unit.

The Role of the Respiratory Clinician in the Prevention of Ventilator-Associated Pneumonia

The respiratory clinician has an important role to play in the prevention of VAP. Many of the risk factors for VAP outlined in Box 36-2 are amenable to intervention by respiratory clinicians, as summarized in Box 36-6.

Respiratory clinicians should wash hands and change gloves between each patient contact, so as to avoid spread of nosocomial pathogens between ventilated patients in the ICU. Contaminated respiratory therapy equipment should be discarded. Prolonged antibiotic use is a risk factor for the development of nosocomial pneumonia. While antibiotic use is essential in many patients, judicious use of these agents should be an important goal for the respiratory clinician. Not only will this strategy reduce the risk of VAP for a given patient, but prudent antibiotic use within the ICU setting can retard the emergence of resistant strains of organisms capable of producing VAP. Supine position is a well-recognized risk factor for aspiration and the development of hospital-acquired pneumonia; elevation of the head of the bed is a simple strategy to minimize the risk of aspiration. When enteral feeding is required, tubes should be placed in the small bowel rather than in the stomach. Finally, patient transportation out of the ICU is often necessary for diagnostic and therapeutic procedures. Nevertheless, this is a recognized risk factor for the development of VAP, and during such transport, every effort should be made to avoid supine patient position and manipulation of ventilator tubing, which can lead to aspiration of contaminated fluid in the tubing.

▼ BIBLIOGRAPHY

Mayhall CG: Nosocomial pneumonia: diagnosis and prevention, *Infect Dis Clin N Am* 11:427-457, 1997.

McEachern R, Campbell GD: Hospital-acquired pneumonia: Epidemiology, etiology, and treatment, *Infect Dis Clin N Am* 12:761-780, 1998.

Torres A, El-Ebiary M: Invasive diagnostics for pneumonia: protected specimen brush, bronchoalveolar lavage, and lung biopsy methods, *Infect Dis Clin N Am* 12:701-722, 1998.

INDEX

A

Abdomen, contiguous spread of infection from, 242t
Abdominal surgery, evaluation of patient for, 284-285
ABG; See Arterial blood gas (ABG)
Abscess, lung; See Lung abscess
Absent breath sounds, 21
Acidosis, respiratory, hypercapnic respiratory failure and, 267-272
Acute bronchitis, 52t
Acute epiglottitis, stridor and, 203t, 204
Acute exacerbation of COPD or asthma, hypercapnia and, 269t
Acute hypercapnia, differential diagnosis of, 268-270, 268b, 269t
Acute hypoxemia, 253-265
    clinical aspects of, 262-263, 262b
    diagnostic tests suggesting cause of, 255, 263-264
    differential diagnosis of, 254-255, 254b, 255b, 256-257, 256t
    pneumonia and, 257-259, 257t, 258b, 259b
    pulmonary embolism and, 259-262, 260, 261, 261t
Acute myocardial infarction, 322t
Acute pleuritic chest pain, 168
Acute respiratory distress syndrome (ARDS), 358, 359, 363
Acute respiratory failure, refractory hypoxemia and, 357-366
Adenopathy, bilateral hilar; See Bilateral hilar adenopathy
Adventitious breath sounds, 20
Air insufflation, atelectasis and, 277
Air trapping, hypotension with mechanical ventilation and, 321t, 324
Airflow obstruction
    chronic exertional dyspnea and, 65-78
    patient with high peak airway pressure and, 367-372
    wheezing and, 195-200
Airway pressure, high peak, patient with; See High peak airway pressure, patient with
Airway resistance, patient with high peak airway pressure and, 368-369, 370
Airway tumors, localized, wheezing and, 197t
Allergy, respiratory care and, 7b
Alveolar hemorrhage, fever and new pulmonary infiltrate and, 242t
Alveolar hypoventilation, chronic hypercapnia and, 145-152
Amebiasis, cavitary pulmonary infiltrate and, 218
American Academy of Sleep Medicine, 85
American College of Physicians, 281
American Gastroenterological Association, 183
American Thoracic Society (ATS), 161, 161t
Aminoglycosides, patient with weakness and, 301t
Amyotrophic lateral sclerosis, hypercapnia and, 269t
Anchoring, 36

Angina
    Ludwig's, stridor and, 203t, 204
    microvascular, non-pleuritic chest pain and, 181t
Angina pectoris, critical diagnostic thinking and, 3-38
Angioedema, stridor and, 203t, 204-205
Angiotensin-converting enzyme (ACE) inhibitor, cough and, 41-47
Ankylosing spondylitis
    inspection of chest and, 18
    upper lobe pulmonary infiltrate and, 193
Anterior chest wall syndrome, chest pain and, 172t
Anxiety, weaning failure and, 293t
Aortic dissection, chest pain and, 171
Aortic stenosis, chest pain and, 171
Apnea, obstructive, 81-82
ARDS; See Acute respiratory distress syndrome (ARDS)
Arterial blood gas (ABG) in evaluation of clinical problem, 25-29
Arterial oxygen content (CaO_2), 28
Arterial oxygen tension, 25-28
Arterial pH, 28
Arteriovenous malformation
    minor hemoptysis and, 102t
    pulmonary, digital clubbing and, 110t
    solitary pulmonary nodule and, 91t
Ascites, critical diagnostic thinking and, 3-38
Aspergilloma, solitary pulmonary nodule and, 91t
Aspergillosis
    cavitary pulmonary infiltrate and, 216
    pulmonary; See Pulmonary aspergillosis
Aspergillus
    solitary pulmonary nodule and, 91t
    upper lobe pulmonary infiltrate and, 187-193, 191
Aspiration
    cavity pulmonary infiltrate and, 211-230
    foreign body; See Foreign body aspiration
Aspiration pneumonia
    fever and new pulmonary infiltrate and, 242t
    hypotension with mechanical ventilation and, 324
    microorganisms producing, 241b
    pulmonary infiltrate and, 240-241, 244
Assessment of atelectasis, 273-278
Asthma, 42, 52t
    acute exacerbation of, hypercapnia and, 269t
    cardiac; See Cardiac asthma
    cough-variant, 42
    progressive exertional dyspnea and, 57-64
    wheezing and, 195-200, 197t
Atelectasis, 26t-27t, 29, 273-278
    acute hypoxemia and, 253-265
    assessment of therapy for, 276-277

Page numbers in italics indicate illustrations, *b* indicates boxes, and *t* indicates tables.